BIOSENSING TECHNOLOGIES FOR THE DETECTION OF PATHOGENS - A PROSPECTIVE WAY FOR RAPID ANALYSIS

Edited by **Toonika Rinken**
and **Kairi Kivirand**

Biosensing Technologies for the Detection of Pathogens - A Prospective Way for Rapid Analysis
http://dx.doi.org/10.5772/intechopen.69579
Edited by Toonika Rinken and Kairi Kivirand

Contributors

Alejandro Dinamarca, Natalia Romo, Claudia Ibacache-Quiroga, Rodrigo Díaz-Viciedo, Elizabeth Hong-Geller, Samantha Adikari, Johann F. Osma, Miguel Aroca, Juliana Noguera, Ana Lucía Campaña, Sergio Florez, Juan Carlos Cruz, Natalia Lopez-Barbosa, René Hanke, Philipp Demling, Patrick Opdensteinen, Suresh Sudarsan, Lars Blank, Michael Osthege, Florian Gohr, Nina Bailly, Wolfgang Wiechert, Ulrich Schwaneberg, Markus Joppich, Karolina Dziąbowska, Elżbieta Czaczyk, Dawid Nidzworski, Lingwen Zeng, Lihua Wang, Jiao Hu, Min-Gon Kim, Bhagwan S Batule, Seong U Kim, Hyoyoung Mun, Won-Bo Shim, Monique Lacroix, Amina Baraketi, Stéphane Salmieri, Jean-François Laurent Bodart, Corentin Spriet, Angelina Kasprowicz, Dave Trinel, Charles Adetunji, Paomipem Phazang, Bhalla Neera, Foram Madiyar, Omer Farooq, Jun Li, Toonika Rinken

Published by InTech
Janeza Trdine 9, 51000 Rijeka, Croatia

Publishing Process Manager Maja Bozicevic
Technical Editor SPi Global
Cover InTech Design team

First published March, 2018
Printed in Croatia
Legal deposit, Croatia: National and University Library in Zagreb

Additional hard copies can be obtained from orders@intechopen.com

Biosensing Technologies for the Detection of Pathogens - A Prospective Way for Rapid Analysis, Edited by Toonika Rinken and Kairi Kivirand
p. cm.
Print ISBN 978-953-51-3915-7
Online ISBN 978-953-51-3916-4

For EU product safety concerns:
IN TECH d.o.o., Prolaz Marije Krucifikse Kozulić 3, 51000 Rijeka, Croatia,
info@intechopen.com or visit our website at intechopen.com.

Meet the editors

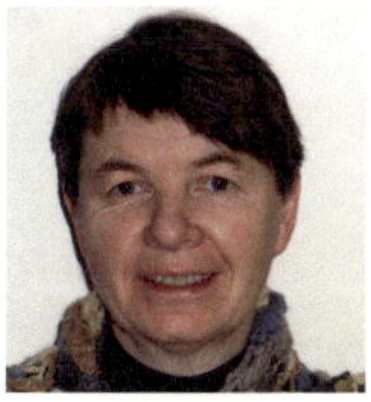

Toonika Rinken is a senior researcher of environmental chemistry and is leading a biosensor lab at the Institute of Chemistry in the University of Tartu, Estonia. She received her PhD degree in chemistry in 2000 in the same university for the modeling and calibration studies of biosensors and has passed professional self-improvement in Uppsala (Sweden) and Gröningen (the Netherlands). Dr. Rinken's research activities are focused on the design and development of biosensing systems for rapid monitoring of environment and food and the studies of signal rising, modeling and calibration of biosensor-based analytical systems.

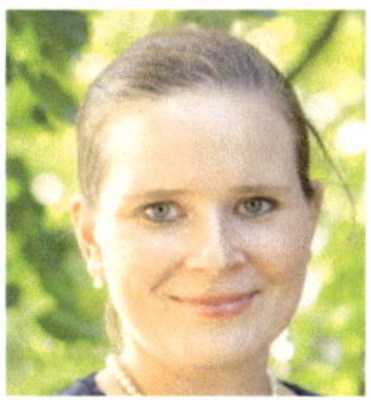

Dr. Kairi Kivirand is a researcher at the University of Tartu and at the Tallinn University of Technology. She received a PhD degree in environmental chemistry in 2011 for her studies of biosensors for biogenic amines. Her research activities are focused on the purification, identification and characterization of bioactive molecules and on the design and development of biosensing systems for a variety of applications. She is an expert in the application of liquid chromatography systems for the extraction and purification of bioactive compounds.

Contents

Preface IX

Chapter 1 **Introductory Chapter: Why Do We Need Rapid Detection of Pathogens? 1**
Kairi Kivirand and Toonika Rinken

Chapter 2 **Current and Emerging Technologies for Rapid Detection of Pathogens 5**
Lingwen Zeng, Lihua Wang and Jiao Hu

Chapter 3 **Volatile Organic Compound and Metabolite Signatures as Pathogen Identifiers and Biomarkers of Infectious Disease 21**
Elizabeth Hong-Geller and Samantha Adikari

Chapter 4 **Biosensors: A Fast-Growing Technology for Pathogen Detection in Agriculture and Food Sector 37**
Adetunji Charles Oluwaseun, Paomipem Phazang and Neera Bhalla Sarin

Chapter 5 **Foodborne Pathogens Detection: Persevering Worldwide Challenge 53**
Amina Baraketi, Stephane Salmieri and Monique Lacroix

Chapter 6 **Detection and Control of Indoor Airborne Pathogenic Bacteria by Biosensors Based on Quorum Sensing Chemical Language: Bio-Tools, Connectivity Apps and Intelligent Buildings 73**
Claudia Ibacache-Quiroga, Natalia Romo, Rodrigo Díaz-Viciedo and M. Alejandro Dinamarca

Chapter 7 **Development of a Modular Biosensor System for Rapid Pathogen Detection 89**
René Hanke, Nina Bailly, Philipp Demling, Florian N. Gohr, Patrick Opdensteinen, Michael J. Osthege, Markus Joppich, Suresh Sudarsan, Ulrich Schwaneberg, Wolfgang Wiechert and Lars M. Blank

Chapter 8 **Detection of Pathogens Using Microfluidics and Biosensors 111**
Natalia Lopez-Barbosa, Ana Lucia Campaña, Mabel Juliana Noguera, Sergio Leonardo Florez, Miguel Angel Aroca, Juan C. Cruz and Johann F. Osma

Chapter 9 **Dielectrophoresis-Assisted Pathogen Detection on Vertically Aligned Carbon Nanofibers Arrays in a Microfluidic Device 135**
Foram Ranjeet Madiyar, Omer Farooq and Jun Li

Chapter 10 **Application of Electrochemical Methods in Biosensing Technologies 151**
Karolina Dziąbowska, Elżbieta Czaczyk and Dawid Nidzworski

Chapter 11 **Development of HRPzyme-Integrated PCR Platform for Colorimetric Detection of Foodborne Pathogens 173**
Bhagwan S. Batule, Seong U. Kim, Hyoyoung Mun, Won-Bo Shim and Min-Gon Kim

Chapter 12 **FRET-Based Enzyme Activity Reporter: Practical Hints for Kinases as Indicators of Virulence 191**
Corentin Spriet, Angelina Kasprowicz, Dave Trinel and Jean-François Bodart

Preface

Biosensing technologies combining the high selectivity of biomolecular recognition and the sensitivity of modern signal detection platforms are a prospective option for automated analyses. They allow rapid detection of single molecules as well as cellular substances. Novel semisynthetic biorecognition agents along with smart materials, modern electronics and information technology are paving a way to the next generation of analytical equipment, which is miniature, robust, cheap and applicable for automatic operation.

Pathogens are infectious biological agents like viruses, fungi, or different microorganisms. We are living in a world of bacteria, which form a biomass exceeding that of all plants and animals. Although we are constantly exposed to different pathogens, a vast majority of them are eliminated by our immune system. Still, in many cases, a treatment is necessary to fight various infections.

Effective treatment of infections requires precise detection of the causative agent. However, the detection of pathogens can be time-consuming. For example, bacteria are currently identified mostly by microbiological culturing methods that take several days. Faster alternatives for microbiology are polymerase chain reaction and enzyme-linked immunoanalyses allowing to obtain results in several hours. However, they are still not suitable for on-line analysis due to relatively long detection time and complex procedures.

A prospective option for the detection of pathogens in a time frame of minutes is biosensors. Thanks to the fast development of technology, numerous novel biosensor solutions offering real-time, on-site multiplex detection of a large variety of infectious agents have been proposed. The present book, including 12 chapters from 50 authors, introduces the principles of identification of specific pathogen biomarkers along with different biosensor-based technologies applied for pathogen detection. I would like to express my appreciation to all authors for their contribution and cooperation and wish them success in their forthcoming activities. My special thanks go to InTech team, particularly the publishing process manager Maja Bozicevic for her professional commitment and dedication.

Toonika Rinken and Kairi Kivirand
University of Tartu, Estonia

Chapter 1

Introductory Chapter: Why Do We Need Rapid Detection of Pathogens?

Kairi Kivirand and Toonika Rinken

Additional information is available at the end of the chapter

http://dx.doi.org/10.5772/intechopen.74670

1. Importance of pathogens

A pathogen is defined as an infectious biological agent, which can be a virus, bacterium, fungus, or other microorganism being the first link in the chain of infections and diseases. We are all exposed to pathogens in our everyday life, but normally they cause no harm as the body's immune system eliminates them. In order to survive and multiply, pathogens must be able to colonize the host, replicate, and spread to a new host.

Pathogens can be divided into human, animal, and environmental pathogens [1, 2]. The two major subdivisions of environmental pathogens are foodborne and waterborne pathogens [3]. The key difference between environmental pathogens and human along with animal pathogens is their ability to survive and thrive outside the host [3].

Environmental pathogens are defined as microorganisms that normally spend a substantial part of their lifecycle outside hosts. They are born in the water, soil, air, food, and other elements of our surroundings, and influence individual organism [3]. Foodborne diseases are caused by the consumption of food or water contaminated with pathogens or their toxins. The common foodborne pathogens, which are responsible for most of the foodborne disease outbreaks, are *Listeria monocytogenes*, *Escherichia coli* O157:H7, *Staphylococcus aureus*, *Salmonella enterica*, *Bacillus cereus*, *Vibrio* spp., *Campylobacter jejuni*, and *Clostridium perfringens* [2].

The increasing demand for street food and for minimally processed ready-to-eat products has increased concerns about food safety [2]. We should carefully control the production processes in the food and agricultural sectors to assure high standards for food quality and safety. Most waterborne pathogens (*Salmonella typhimurium*, *Vibrio cholerae*, *Legionella*, *Escherichia coli* O157:H7, and *Campylobacter jejuni*) do not grow in water, and are introduced into drinking-water supplies with human or animal feces. These pathogens can initiate infections in the gastrointestinal tract following ingestion [1]. It has been calculated that diseases caused by waterborne pathogens have an annual economic cost around 1 billion dollars in the US and nearly 12 billon USD worldwide [1]. Based on this threat, infections caused by contaminated water have a considerable impact and testing of the safety of drinking-water should be improved.

Treating infections with broad-spectrum antibiotics in cases where timely treatment is unavoidable, but the causative agent has not yet properly identified is a common practice. This can cause major damage to the normal microbiota of host organism and pose a global threat of spreading drug-resistant bacteria [4]. Decades of research into antibiotic development has produced highly effective and safe antibiotics, giving excellent tools for prevention and focused fight with bacterial infections [4]. However, release of each new drug has been inevitably followed by a rapid propagation of resistant pathogens. This issue has become a serious threat, causing annually at least 23,000 deaths in the United States [4] and about 25,000 deaths in the European Union [5].

In US, it is suggested that around 80% of the nation's annual antimicrobial consumption is used in food animals for medical procedures, disease prevention, and growth promotion [6]. So, the misuse of antibiotics due to insufficient identification of infection-causing pathogens in veterinary has even a bigger impact on the spread of drug-resistant bacteria.

The availability of modern detection methods plays a key role in the speed and quality of monitoring, surveillance, and quantitative microbial risk assessment, and has a major influence on implementing the best practices to prevent threats [1].

2. Current methods for pathogen detection

How to detect small numbers of pathogens in large numbers of harmless microflora in a large and complex sample matrix? How to make sure that the strains recovered are indeed pathogenic?

The gold standards for pathogen detection are culture-based methods [7, 8]. The culture-based methods or count methods of culturing and colony—detecting of microorganisms—are based on the integration of the sample into a nutrient medium in which the microorganisms can multiply, thus providing visual confirmation of their growth [9]. Although these methods are simple, easily adaptable, and generally inexpensive, they are laborious, limited by low sensitivity (false negative results), and require relatively long time to perform as they depend on the ability of the microorganisms to grow in different culture media [9]. It commonly takes 2–3 days to get initial results, and up to 1 week to get final information about the specific pathogen causing the infection or disease with culture method [9].

In recent decades, many new methods have emerged for the rapid diagnostics of bacterial infections. Microbiological analysis are based on the detection of microorganisms by visual, immunological, or genetic means, either before (enumerative methods) or after enrichment of samples [9].

http://dx.doi.org/10.5772/intechopen.74670

The most widespread methods for pathogen detection are polymerase chain reaction (PCR) and enzyme-linked immunosorbent assay (ELISA). PCR method is very specific and can be used to identify microorganisms that cannot be readily cultured. However, the PCR method which requires amplification, isolation, and quantification of DNA is a complex technique to use and requires costly instruments and trained personnel [10]. In comparison with PCR analysis, ELISA is less complicated and less expensive, but real-time detection is not possible due to the need of incubation of samples for 2–3 h [10]. Therefore, neither PCR nor ELISA techniques meet the criteria of carrying out on-site rapid analysis of pathogens, therefore alternative methods are in urgent need. The main advantages of rapid detection techniques are the possibility of earlier interference and faster focused action to potential problems, but also improved throughput of analysis.

Novel technologies for the detection of pathogens are of critical importance, and extensive research and development activities are going on with the aim to reduce assay time and reduce the amount of manual labor by automating methods whenever possible [8, 9]. The sensitivity of assessment is another major parameter in cases when potential risk of infections is caused by low number or a single pathogen.

Modern biotechnologies are important in many fields: agriculture, medicine, environmental monitoring, and in food industry as they are improving the ability to detect pathogens quickly and effectively. Nevertheless, the development of new methods has many challenges. These methods should be capable of concentrating pathogens and removing matrix-associated inhibitors, should be simple, rapid, and inexpensive; they should be able to eliminate or reduce the need for culture enrichments and minimize the chance for false-positive results [8].

In recent years, there has been a constant growth in the field of pathogen biosensing due to modern developments of novel electronic devices. Biosensor-based technologies commonly rely on the specific recognition of antigen epitopes of pathogen targets by a recognition agent-like antibodies or aptamers. These immunosensing technologies offer prospective features like real-time, on-site, simultaneous multiplex detection of different pathogenic agents integrating the selectivity of biomolecules and the processing power of modern nanoelectronics [11]. One must also remember that even having established a rapid and reliable method for the detection of pathogens, we should remember that detection technology is not the only aspect to consider and we still have to follow strict sampling procedures to avoid contamination. Otherwise, the results can be meaningless or even worse—misleading.

Author details

Kairi Kivirand and Toonika Rinken*

*Address all correspondence to: toonika.rinken@ut.ee

University of Tartu, Tartu, Estonia

References

[1] Ramírez-Castillo FY, Loera-Muro A, Jacques M, Garneau P, Avelar-González FJ, Harel J, et al. Waterborne pathogens: detection methods and challenges. Pathogens (Basel, Switzerland). 2015;**4**:307-334. DOI: 10.3390/pathogens4020307

[2] Law JW-F, Ab Mutalib N-S, Chan K-G, Lee L-H. Rapid methods for the detection of foodborne bacterial pathogens: Principles, applications, advantages and limitations. Frontiers in Microbiology. 2014;**5**:1-19. DOI: 10.3389/fmicb.2014.00770

[3] Cangelosi GA, Freitag NE, Buckley MR. From Outside to Inside: Environmental Microorganisms as Human Pathogens. Washington, DC: American Academy of Microbiology. Book NLM ID: 101249346. 2004:1-16

[4] Maxson T, Mitchell DA. Targeted treatment for bacterial infections: Prospects for pathogen-specific antibiotics coupled with rapid diagnostics. Tetrahedron. 2016;**72**:3609-3624. DOI: 10.1016/j.tet.2015.09.069

[5] European Centre for Disease Prevention and Control. The Bacterial Challenge: Time to React. EMEA/576176/2009 Stockholm. 2009. DOI: 10.2900/2518

[6] Van Boeckel TP, Brower C, Gilbert M, Grenfell BT, S a L, Robinson TP, et al. Global trends in antimicrobial use in food animals. Proceedings of the National Academy of Sciences of the United States of America. 2015:1-6. DOI: 10.1073/pnas.1503141112

[7] Leonard P, Hearty S, Brennan J, Dunne L, Quinn J, Chakraborty T, et al. Advances in biosensors for detection of pathogens in food and water. Enzyme and Microbial Technology. 2003;**32**:3-13. DOI: 10.1016/S0141-0229(02)00232-6

[8] Jaykus L-A. Challenges to developing real-time methods to detect pathogens in foods. ASM News. 2003;**69**:341-347

[9] López-Campos G, Martínez-Suárez JV, Aguado-Urda M, López-Alonso V. Microarray Detection and Characterization of Bacterial Foodborne Pathogens. Boston, MA: Springer; 2012. pp. 13-32. DOI: 10.1007/978-1-4614-3250-0

[10] Zhao Y, Wang H, Zhang P, Sun C, Wang X, Wang X, et al. Rapid multiplex detection of 10 foodborne pathogens with an up-converting phosphor technology-based 10-channel lateral flow assay. Scientific Reports. 2016;**6**:1-8. DOI: 10.1038/srep21342

[11] Singh R, Das MM, Sumana G, Gupta RK, Sood S, Malhotra BD. Biosensors for pathogen detection: A smart approach towards clinical diagnosis. Sensors and Actuators, B: Chemical. 2014;**197**:385-404. DOI: 10.1016/j.snb.2014.03.005

Chapter 2

Current and Emerging Technologies for Rapid Detection of Pathogens

Lingwen Zeng, Lihua Wang and Jiao Hu

Additional information is available at the end of the chapter

http://dx.doi.org/10.5772/intechopen.73178

Abstract

Foodborne diseases, caused by pathogenic bacteria, have become an important social issue in the field of food safety. It presents a widespread and growing threat to human health in both developed and developing countries. As such, techniques for the detection of foodborne pathogens and waterborne pathogens are urgently needed to prevent the occurrence of human foodborne infections. Although traditional culture-based bacterial isolation and identification are the "gold standard" methods with high preciseness, their drawbacks in time-consuming are inadequate for rapid detection of pathogen to reduce foodborne disease occurrence. Fortunately, with the development of biotechnologies and nanotechnologies, various kinds of new technologies for rapid detection of pathogens have been developed so far, such as nucleic acid-based methods, antibody-based methods, and aptamer-based assays. In this chapter, we summarized the principles and the application of some recent rapid detection technologies for pathogenic bacteria. Moreover, the advantages and disadvantages of the established and emerging rapid detection methods are addressed here.

Keywords: pathogen, rapid detection, nucleic acid, antibody, aptamer

1. Introduction

Foodborne pathogens, which are widely responsible for many foodborne diseases, constitute a serious threat to human health. In recent years, foodborne and waterborne pathogenic microorganisms have caused numerous epidemic diseases in the world [1]. *Salmonella, Shiga bacillus, Escherichia coli* O157:H7, *Bacillus cereus, Staphylococcus aureus,* and *Listeria monocytogenes* are the primary pathogens that are responsible for most foodborne disease [2–6]. Centers for Disease Control and Prevention (CDC) reported that approximately 73,000 cases of foodborne disease occur annually. In 2013, a total of 19,056 are infected with foodborne pathogen, of which 4200 are hospitalizations, and 80 are deaths in the United States [7]. The foodborne diseases are even high prevalence in many developing countries. Worldwide, there are 600 million foodborne illnesses with 420,000 deaths in 2010, which is estimated by the World Health Organization (WHO) Foodborne Disease Burden Epidemiology Reference Group (FERG). A great proportion of these cases are due to the contamination of raw or undercooked foods and drinking water [4, 6, 8, 9]. Hence, it is urgent to detect foodborne pathogens in order to control foodborne pathogen spread and reduce foodborne disease occurrence.

Currently, culture-based bacterial isolation and identification are the "gold standard" methods for laboratory detection of foodborne pathogens [10]. However, they suffer from time consumption, which requires 2–3 days for initial culture and enrichment, and more than 1 week for confirming the target pathogenic bacteria [11, 12]. Moreover, it requires expensive instruments and professional technicians and remains problematic due to the lack of phenotypic characteristics

Method	Advantages	Disadvantages	Sensitivity	Ref.
Real-time PCR[a]	—Amplification can be monitored at real time —Confirmation of specific amplification by melting curve —Accurate quantification	—Difficulty in multiplex assay —Need skilled person and support —False-positive results	10 CFU/mL	[25]
Multiplex PCR[a]	—Highly efficient (detection of several pathogens at a time) —Systematic (suitable for detection of groups of pathogens)	—Difficulty in distinguishing live and dead cells —Requires post-PCR processing of products (electrophoresis) —Need skilled person and support —Costs more than culture-based methods and ELISA	1 CFU/mL	[26]
Antibody-based method (ELISA[b] and LFIA[c])	—More rapid than culture-based methods (1~2 h vs. 5~7 d) —Can be automated to reduce assay time and manual labor input —Able to handle large numbers of samples —Convenient and suitable for the on-site testing	—Difficulty to differentiate damaged or stressed cells —Need for pre-enrichment —High cross-reactivity with close antigens in bacteria	60 CFU/mL	[35]
Aptamer-based method (optical and electrochemical methods)	—Inexpensive, stable, and can be chemically synthesized than antibody —Time-saving (2 h vs. 5~7 d of culture-based methods) —Automated to reduce manual labor input —High throughput —Multiplex assays	—High false positive —Difficulty in detecting damaged or stressed cells —Need for pre-enrichment —Possibility of cross contamination	1.5 CFU/mL	[78]

[a] PCR, polymerase chain reaction; [b] ELISA, enzyme-linked immunosorbent assay; [c] LFIA, lateral flow immunoassays.

Table 1. Advantages and disadvantages of detection methods.

to distinguish between generic pathogens, which may largely restrict its application. It is evident that culture and colony-counting methods are inadequate for rapid detection of foodborne pathogens, especially for reduce foodborne disease occurrence. The frequent outbreak of foodborne diseases and the economic and social implications indicate that analytical methodologies that can rapidly detect and identify pathogens are urgently needed. As such, many researchers devote themselves to developing more advanced detection methods that can identify pathogens accurately and rapidly in a timely manner in the food industry [13–20].

In this chapter, we summarize the recent trends, developments, advantages, and disadvantages (listed in **Table 1**) about rapid detection of pathogens based on nucleic acid, antibodies, and aptamers and then give a perspective on the future directions of rapid analysis of pathogens.

2. Methodologies for pathogen detection

2.1. Nucleic acid-based assays

Culture- and colony-based methods are the standard methods for the detection of pathogens. They rely on the ability of microorganisms to multiply to visible colonies [21]. The major drawbacks of these microbiological methods are their labor intensiveness and time consumption as it usually takes 2–3 days for initial results and up to 7–10 days for confirmation. In comparison, nucleic acid-based assays can greatly shorten the testing time.

2.1.1. Real-time PCR

Real-time PCR technology is a reliable method in identification and quantitative detection of bacteria due to its accuracy, rapidity, specificity, and low detection limit. In addition, it is a promising alternative approach to estimating the number of bacteria [22, 23]. For example, Gyawali et al. [22] presented a specific and sensitive real-time PCR method to detect *Ancylostoma caninum* ova in wastewater matrices. This method exhibited high sensitivity with the ability to detect *Ancylostoma caninum* DNA up to dilution of 10^{-4} (equivalent to 500 fg) consistently. Moreover, the precise copy number of a specific nucleic acid sequence can be quantified with the real-time PCR technique based on a calibration curve created with known concentrations of DNA [24, 25]. Gokduman et al. [25] established a recombinant plasmid-based quantitative real-time PCR assay for *Salmonella enterica* serotypes with the detection limit of 10 CFU/mL. Obviously, the real-time quantitative PCR has already been a promising quantitative method for the quantitative detection of bacteria, due to its lower cost than that of culture-based method.

2.1.2. Multiplex PCR

Multiplex PCR, also known as multiple primer PCR, which is a PCR reaction system with two or more primers, can amplify a plurality of nucleic acid fragments in a system. Compared to other methods, multiplex PCR is very useful as it allows the simultaneous detection of several pathogenic bacteria by introducing different primers to amplify DNA regions coding for specific genes of each bacterial strain targeted [26]. Methods for multiplexing PCR have considerably improved over the last years, thereby decreasing genotyping costs and increasing throughput. Examples of multiplex PCR technique for the simultaneous detection pathogens include multiplex PCR assay for rapid and simultaneous detection of *Escherichia coli* O157:H7, *Salmonella, Staphylococcus aureus, Listeria monocytogenes,* and *Vibrio parahaemolyticus* [27]; simultaneous detection of bacteria of the genus *Listeria, Listeria monocytogenes,* and major serotypes and epidemic clones of *Listeria monocytogenes* [28]; and simultaneous detection of *Escherichia coli* O157:H7 and *Listeria monocytogenes* [29]. Multiplex real-time PCR-based assay can rapidly detect 25 clinically important pathogens directly from whole blood in <6 h [30].

2.2. Antibody-based assays

Antibodies are a unique natural family of immune system-related glycoproteins known as immunoglobulins, produced by differentiated B cells in response to the attendant of an immunogen during an immune response. Because of the specific interactions and the extremely high equilibrium association constants (10^{10}/M and greater) attainable between an antibody and its corresponding antigen, antibodies are employed as an excellent biorecognition element for the highly sensitive and selective immunoassays [31]. Their utilization in biosensors brings new tools for analysis in the biochemical, clinical, and environmental fields. Without exception, antibody-based assays such as enzyme-linked immunosorbent assay (ELISA), lateral flow immunoassay (LFIA), and so on are very popular for the detection of pathogens.

2.2.1. Enzyme-linked immunosorbent assay (ELISA)

ELISA-based approaches are the most prevalent antibody-based assay for pathogen detection [32]. Compared with the culture-based methods, this immunological approach has been used to detect pathogens in poultry production (poultry feed, feces, litter, carcass rinsing, and water samples) and has provided a better sensitivity and shorter time frame [33]. Recently, improvements by combination with other advanced nanomaterials such as novel enzyme-based signal probes have been made in the basic ELISA method for pathogen detection. For example, by using silica nanoparticles (NPs) carrying poly(acrylic acid) brushes as a "catalase (CAT) container" to increase enzyme loading, Chen et al. [34] presented an improved plasmonic ELISA (pELISA) method for detection of *Listeria monocytogenes* at ultralow concentrations with the sandwich format. The limit of detection (LOD) obtained by this method (80 CFU/mL) was two and five orders of magnitude lower than that of conventional CAT-based pELISA and horseradish peroxidase (HRP)-based conventional ELISA, respectively. To further simplify the preparation of enzyme-labeled antibody, Lin's group innovatively prepared an all-in-one organic–inorganic nanoflower, which integrated biorecognition unit (concanavalin A or antibody), signal amplification unit (glucose oxidase or HRP), and carrier unit within a one-pot reaction. And then, it was used for a portable sensitive ELISA detection of *Escherichia coli* O157:H7. Under the optimal conditions, the detection sensitivity can reach as low as 10 CFU/mL for the case of concanavalin A-glucose oxidase [17] and 60 CFU/mL for the case of antibody-HRP [35].

2.2.2. *Lateral flow immunoassay (LFIA)*

LFIA-based methods are a form of immunoassay, which emerge for the first time at the end of the 1960s and consist of a chromatographic system and immunochemical reaction [36–38]. The principle of LFIA is based on antibody–antigen specific interaction. After the sample is applied to the sample pad, it migrates along the test strip *via* capillary action, and a signal response is obtained about 5–10 min later [39, 40]. Due to its simplicity, rapidity, low cost, portability, and facile interpretation without external reagent or external instrumentation, LFIA has held great potential for foodborne pathogen detection [15, 16, 41]. In addition, the LFIA can realize visual detection and quantitative detection by employing different labels, such as colloid gold, fluorescent materials, and magnetic beads [40, 42, 43]. Descriptions on some of the labels that are applied for pathogenic bacteria detection are presented in the following sections.

2.2.2.1. *Colloid gold as label*

Colloid gold is the most widely used label of LFIA due to its intense color and direct visualization [44], and it has been widely used for the detection of foodborne pathogens [45–48]. Jung et al. [45] used a colloid gold-based LFIA to detect *Escherichia coli* O157:H7 in enriched samples, and the LOD was 1.8×10^5 CFU/mL without enrichment and 1.8 CFU/mL after enrichment. Preechakasedkit et al. [49] also developed a colloid gold immunochromatographic strip for the detection of *Salmonella typhimurium* with a minimum detection limit of 1.14×10^5 CFU/mL. Park et al. [15] presented a detection method of *Escherichia coli* O157:H7 and *Salmonella typhimurium* with a pressed paper-based dipstick by employing colloid gold as labels. The detection limit of *Escherichia coli* O157:H7 was around 10^5 CFU/mL, while that of *Salmonella typhimurium* was around 10^6 CFU/mL. In the case of the work of Song et al. [41], *Shigella boydii*, and *Escherichia coli* O157:H7 can be detected simultaneously in bread, milk, and jelly samples using colloid gold-based LFIA, and the detection limit of 10^6 CFU/mL for both *Shigella boydii* and *Escherichia coli* O157:H7 was achieved.

2.2.2.2. *Quantum dots as label*

As the low sensitivity of colloid gold, fluorescent materials have gained more and more interest due to their higher sensitivity than colloid gold in the field of lateral flow assay [50]. Furthermore, the fluorescent materials enable lateral flow assay to detect the target quantitatively. Compared with colloid gold, which can only provide qualitative or semiquantitative results, quantitative detection can offer more information [42, 51, 52]. In particular, quantum dots show unique fluorescence properties, such as high and stable fluorescence signal [53–55]. During the last decade, quantum dot-based lateral flow assays have been applied to the detection of foodborne pathogen [56–58]. Bruno [56] utilized quantum dot-conjugated antibody as the signal reporter of the lateral flow assay to detect *Escherichia coli* O157:H7. With the assay, the detection limit of *Escherichia coli* O157:H7 is calculated to be 600 cells per test, while that of colloid gold-based lateral flow assay is 6000 cells per test, indicating the higher sensitivity of quantum dots than colloid gold as labels of lateral flow assay. Chen et al. [58] also developed a competitive format lateral flow assay with quantum dots for the detection of *Staphylococcus aureus* in food. The detection limit is 3 CFU/mL.

2.2.2.3. *Magnetic beads as label*

Magnetic beads are another type of label, which can realize quantitative detection of targets by measuring the magnetic signal [40, 57, 59]. Due to the fact that they are strongly colored and can enrich and separate targets from complex matrix, magnetic beads are new attractive materials to construct a lateral flow assay, which will probably replace traditional labels. Especially, magnetic beads can simultaneously provide visual signal and magnetic signal. Several researches have recently focused on the use of magnetic bead-based lateral flow assay to detect pathogenic bacteria [60–62]. Wang et al. [60] employed antibody-coated magnetic beads with the diameter of 300 nm as signal reporter of lateral flow assay for *Bacillus anthracis* spore detection. A detection limit of 6×10^4 spores/g of milk powder, 2×10^5 spores/g of starch, and 5×10^5 spores/g of baking soda was obtained, respectively. Suaifan et al. [63] described a magnetic bead-based lateral flow assay, which can specifically and simultaneously detect *Escherichia coli* O157:H7 proteases in complex food matrices. The limits of detection were 12 CFU/mL in broth and 30–300 CFU/mL in food matrices. Xia et al. [64] developed a gold magnetic bifunctional nanobead-based lateral flow assay for the detection of *Salmonella choleraesuis*. Results indicated that the assay was specific and rapid with the detection limit of 5×10^5 CFU/mL, which was much more sensitive than that of colloid gold-based LFIA (5×10^6 CFU/mL), suggesting that magnetic beads were indeed superior to colloid gold.

2.3. Aptamer-based assays

Besides antibodies, other biomolecules have been investigated to selectively capture and enrich pathogens from cultures, among which aptamer is the most prevalent one [65]. Aptamers, as short single-stranded nucleic acids (DNA or RNA), can bind with high affinity and specificity to a wide range of target molecules, such as ions, small organic molecules, and proteins [66–68]. The affinities of aptamers for their targets are comparable to, or even higher than most monoclonal antibodies. More importantly, compared with antibodies, they also exhibit a number of advantages. First of all, aptamers can be routinely produced by chemical synthesis, avoiding the use of animals required for antibody production. Furthermore, they are generally more chemically stable, and their binding properties are easier to manipulate. To this end, a number of aptasensors based on optics and electrochemistry have been recently reported for pathogenic microorganism typing and detection.

2.3.1. *Optical strategies*

Surface-enhanced Raman scattering (SERS) possesses several attractive properties, such as ultrahigh sensitivity, high speed, comparatively low cost, and multiplexing ability and portability [69–71], which enable SERS to be widely used for sensitive detection of chemical and biological agents [72, 73]. Since Holt and Cotton first reported the SERS spectrum of bacteria, the identification and detection of microorganism by SERS have attracted high interest recently due to the spectroscopic fingerprint and nondestructive data acquisition in aqueous environment [74]. To date, there have been many SERS biosensors developed, especially based on a "magnetic separation" approach, which focus on bacterial pathogen detection. Wang et al. [75] reported a magnetically assisted SERS biosensor for single-cell detection of *Staphylococcus aureus* on the basis of aptamer recognition. The biosensor consists of two basic elements including a SERS substrate (Ag-coated magnetic nanoparticles) and a novel SERS tag (Au nanorod-5,5-dithiobis-(2-nitrobenzoic acid) (AuNR-DTNB)@Ag-DTNB core-shell plasmonic NPs or DTNB-labeled inside-and-outside plasmonic NPs (DioPNPs)). Based on these, the LOD of 10 cells/mL can be achieved for *Staphylococcus aureus* detection. Similarly, through combined gold NPs (GNPs) modified with Raman molecules and Fe_3O_4 magnetic GNPs immobilized with aptamer, Zhang et al. [76] successfully fabricated GNP-enhanced SERS aptasensor for the simultaneous detection of *Salmonella typhimurium* and *Staphylococcus aureus*. In comparison with these label-based SERS methods, label-free methods do not require a secondary label dye and can directly obtain the intrinsic fingerprint of bacteria, which relies on the mutual interaction of bacteria cell with the SERS substrate [77]. With this regard, a lot of label-free methods have been developed for the detection of pathogens. For example, Gao's group [78] successfully achieved intuitive label-free SERS detection of bacteria using aptamer-based in situ Ag NP synthesis. The biosensor as prepared can recognize bacteria quickly and directly by SERS with the formation of well-defined bacteria-aptamer@Ag NPs. The detection limit is down to 1.5 CFU/mL.

As another typical spectroscopic method, fluorescence resonance energy transfer (FRET, a homogeneous signal transduction technique), has been gradually employed for the determination of pathogenic bacteria. Yu et al. [79] presented a universal and facile one-step strategy for sensitive and selective detection of pathogenic bacteria using a dual-molecular affinity-based FRET platform based on the recognition of bacterial cell walls by antibiotic and aptamer molecules, respectively. Within 30 min, the FRET signal shows a linear variation with the concentration of *Staphylococcus aureus* in the range from 20 to 10^8 CFU/mL with a detection limit of 10 CFU/mL. Moreover, Duan's group [80] further achieved simultaneous detection of *Vibrio parahaemolyticus*, *Staphylococcus aureus*, and *Salmonella typhimurium* through using multicolor dyes as donors and carbon NPs as a sole acceptor in FRET.

2.3.2. *Electrochemical strategies*

Compared with optical-based biosensors, electrochemical methods, in general, show the potential for construction of fast, simple, low-cost, sensitive, and high-throughput biosensors that can be miniaturized [81–84]. To date, electrochemical aptasensors are widely used for identification and quantification of pathogens. For example, Labib et al. [85] developed an impedimetric sensor *via* assembling their selected highly specific DNA aptamers onto a gold NP-modified screen-printed carbon electrode for the highly sensitive detection of live *Salmonella typhimurium*. This aptasensor is very simple and highly selective. It can successfully detect *Salmonella typhimurium* down to 600 CFU/mL (equivalent to 18 live cells in 30 μL of assay volume). Moreover, to further improve the sensitivity, Abbaspour et al. [86] innovatively combined the magnetic beads' fast separation with the Ag NPs' signal amplification. They successfully fabricated an electrochemical dual-aptamer-based sandwich detection method for *Staphylococcus aureus*. The aptasensor as prepared shows an extended dynamic range from 10 to 1×10^6 CFU/mL with a low detection limit of 1.0 CFU/mL ($S/N = 3$). Despite much progress has been made, these methods always require probe labeling and aptamer immobilization, which may affect the binding affinities between bacteria and their aptamers. With this respect, Ding's group [87] constructed a label-free potentiometric aptasensor for rapid, sensitive, and selective detection of *Listeria monocytogenes*. In this strategy, the target-binding event prevents the aptamer from electrostatically interacting with protamine, which can be sensitively detected using a polycation-sensitive membrane electrode.

2.4. Conclusion

Culture-based foodborne pathogen detection methods, although sensitive enough, are often too time-consuming to reduce foodborne disease occurrence. Therefore, a large number of innovative methods have been developed to overcome this performance limitation. These rapid detection methods can be classified into nucleic acid-based methods, antibody-based methods, and aptamer-based methods. All these rapid methods for foodborne pathogen detection are superior to culture-based methods. However, some of them still require improvement in sensitivity, selectivity, simplicity, or accuracy to be of any practical use. Nucleic acid-based methods, as a replacement method for culture-based methods, have high sensitivity and require a shorter time than conventional culture-based techniques for foodborne pathogen detection. Most of them still require highly trained personnel and expensive instruments, which limit their use in a practical environment. The development of antibody-based methods helped improve the time required to yield results. The specific binding of antibody to its antigen results in its high specificity and sensitivity of antibody-based methods, and they work well in food matrices without being interfered by other DNAs, proteins, or nontarget cells. Aptamer-based methods are similar to antibody-based methods, which also exhibit high sensitivity and selectivity. However, they still need to be improved for food matrix detection. Increasing detection accuracy and decreasing detection time are the eternal themes in rapid detection. In the future, new nanomaterials and rational biosensing strategies would be developed to approach the goal.

Author details

Lingwen Zeng*, Lihua Wang and Jiao Hu

*Address all correspondence to: zeng6@yahoo.com

Institute of Environment and Safety, Wuhan Academy of Agricultural Sciences, China

References

[1] Tian F, Lyu J, Shi JY, Tan F, Yang M. A polymeric microfluidic device integrated with nanoporous alumina membranes for simultaneous detection of multiple foodborne pathogens. Sensors & Actuators, B: Chemical. 2016;**225**:312-318

[2] Gould LH, Mungai EA, Johnson SD, Richardson LC, Williams IT, Griffin PM, Cole DJ, Hall AJ. Surveillance for foodborne disease outbreaks-United States, 2009–2010. Morbidity and Mortality Weekly Report. 2013;**62**

[3] Gould LH, Nisler AL, Herman KM, Cole DJ, Williams IT, Mahon BE, Griffin PM, Hall AJ. Surveillance for foodborne disease outbreaks-United States, 2008. JAMA, Journal of the American Medical Association. 2011;**306**:2212-2214

[4] Law JWF, Mutalib NSA, Chan KG, Lee LH. Rapid methods for the detection of foodborne bacterial pathogens: Principles, applications, advantages and limitations. Frontiers in Microbiology. 2015;**5**

[5] Chao GX, Zhou XH, Jiao XN, Qian XQ, Xu L. Prevalence and antimicrobial resistance of foodborne pathogens isolated from food products in China. Foodborne Pathogens and Disease. 2007;**4**:277-284

[6] Henao-Herreño LX, López-Tamayo AM, Ramos-Bonilla JP, Haas CN, Husserl J. Risk of illness with *Salmonella* due to consumption of raw unwashed vegetables irrigated with water from the Bogota River. Risk Analysis. 2017;**37**:733-743

[7] Crim SM, Iwamoto M, Huang JY, Griffin PM, Gilliss D, Cronquist AB, Cartter M, Tobin-D'Angelo M, Blythe D, Smith K, et al. Incidence and trends of infection with pathogens transmitted commonly through food-Foodborne Diseases Active Surveillance Network, 10 US Sites, 2006–2013. Morbidity and Mortality Weekly Report. 2014;**63**:328-332

[8] Vinothkumar K, Bhardwaj AK, Ramamurthy T, Niyogi SK. Triplex PCR assay for the rapid identification of 3 major *Vibrio* species, *Vibrio cholerae, Vibrio parahaemolyticus*, and *Vibrio fluvialis*. Diagnostic Microbiology and Infectious Disease. 2013;**76**:526-528

[9] Oliver SP, Jayarao BM, Almeida RA. Foodborne pathogens in milk and the dairy farm environment: Food safety and public health implications. Foodborne Pathogens and Disease. 2005;**2**:115-129

[10] Andrews JR, Ryan ET. Diagnostics for invasive *Salmonella* infections: Current challenges and future directions. Vaccine. 2015;**33**:C8-C15

[11] Zhao X, Lin CW, Wang J, Oh DH. Advances in rapid detection methods for foodborne pathogens. Journal of Microbiology and Biotechnology. 2014;**24**:297-312

[12] Kawasaki S, Fratamico PM, Horikoshi N, Okada Y, Takeshita K, Sameshima T, Kawamoto S. Evaluation of a multiplex PCR system for simultaneous detection of *Salmonella spp., Listeria monocytogenes*, and *Escherichia coli* O157:H7 in foods and in food subjected to freezing. Foodborne Pathogens and Disease. 2009;**6**:81-89

[13] Velusamy V, Arshak K, Korostynska O, Oliwa K, Adley C. An overview of foodborne pathogen detection: In the perspective of biosensors. Biotechnology Advances. 2010;**28**: 232-254

[14] Alizadeh N, Memar MY, Moaddab SR, Kafil HS. Aptamer-assisted novel technologies for detecting bacterial pathogens. Biomedicine & Pharmacotherapy. 2017;**93**:737-745

[15] Park J, Shin JH, Park JK. Pressed paper-based dipstick for detection of foodborne pathogens with multistep reactions. Analytical Chemistry. 2016;**88**:3781-3788

[16] Shan S, Lai W, Xiong Y, Wei H, Xu H. Novel strategies to enhance lateral flow immunoassay sensitivity for detecting foodborne pathogens. Journal of Agricultural and Food Chemistry. 2015;**63**:745-753

[17] Wei T, Du D, Zhu MJ, Lin Y, Dai Z. An improved ultrasensitive enzyme-linked immunosorbent assay using hydrangea-like antibody–enzyme–inorganic three-in-one nanocomposites. ACS Applied Materials & Interfaces. 2016;**8**:6329-6335

[18] Mustafa F, Hassan R, Andreescu S. Multifunctional nanotechnology-enabled sensors for rapid capture and detection of pathogens. Sensors. 2017;**17**:2121

[19] Park SH, Aydin M, Khatiwara A, Dolan MC, Gilmore DF, Bouldin JL, Ahn S, Ricke SC. Current and emerging technologies for rapid detection and characterization of *Salmonella* in poultry and poultry products. Food Microbiology. 2014;**38**:250-262

[20] Wu W, Zeng L. Current and emerging innovations for detection of food-borne *Salmonella*. Current topics in *Salmonella* and *Salmonellosis*. Associate Prof. Mihai Mares (Ed.), INTECH. DOI: 10.5772/67264

[21] De BE, Beumer RR. Methodology for detection and typing of foodborne microorganisms. International Journal of Food Microbiology. 1999;**50**:119-130

[22] Gyawali P, Sidhu JPS, Ahmed W, Jagals P, Toze S. Rapid concentration and sensitive detection of *Hookworm ova* from wastewater matrices using a real-time PCR method. Experimental Parasitology. 2015;**159**:5-12

[23] Mackay IM. Real-time PCR in the microbiology laboratory. Clinical Microbiology and Infection. 2004;**10**:190-212

[24] Malorny B, Lofstrom C, Wagner M, Kramer N, Hoorfar J. Enumeration of *Salmonella* bacteria in food and feed samples by real-time PCR for quantitative microbial risk assessment. Applied and Environmental Microbiology. 2008;**74**:1299-1304

[25] Gokduman K, Avsaroglu MD, Cakiris A, Ustek D, Gurakan GC. Recombinant plasmid-based quantitative real-time PCR analysis of *Salmonella enterica serotypes* and its application to milk samples. Journal of Microbiological Methods. 2016;**122**:50-58

[26] Touron A, Berthe T, Pawlak B, Petit F. Detection of *Salmonella* in environmental water and sediment by a nested-multiplex polymerase chain reaction assay. Research in Microbiology. 2005;**156**:541-553

[27] Kim JS, Lee GG, Park JS, Jung YH, Kwak HS, Kim SB, Nam YS, Kwon ST. A novel multiplex PCR assay for rapid and simultaneous detection of five pathogenic bacteria: *Escherichia coli* O157:H7, *Salmonella, Staphylococcus aureus, Listeria monocytogenes,* and *Vibrio parahaemolyticus*. Journal of Food Protection. 2007;**70**:1656-1662

[28] Chen Y, Zhang W, Knabel SJ. Multi-virulence-locus sequence typing identifies single nucleotide polymorphisms which differentiate epidemic clones and outbreak strains of *Listeria monocytogenes*. Journal of Clinical Microbiology. 2007;**45**:835-846

[29] Mukhopadhyay A, Mukhopadhyay UK. Novel multiplex PCR approaches for the simultaneous detection of human pathogens: *Escherichia coli* O157:H7 and *Listeria monocytogenes*. Journal of Microbiological Methods. 2007;**68**:193-200

[30] Lehmann LE, Hunfeld KP, Emrich T, Haberhausen G, Wissing H, Hoeft A, Stuber F. A multiplex real-time PCR assay for rapid detection and differentiation of 25 bacterial and fungal pathogens from whole blood samples. Medical Microbiology and Immunology. 2008;**197**:313-324

[31] Farka Z, Juriik T, Kovaar D, Trnkova L, Sklaadal P. Nanoparticle-based immunochemical biosensors and assays: Recent advances and challenges. Chemical Reviews. 2017;**117**: 9973-10042

[32] Mandal TK, Parvin N. Rapid detection of bacteria by carbon quantum dots. Journal of Biomedical Nanotechnology. 2011;**7**:846-848

[33] Maciorowski KG, Herrera P, Jones FT, Pillai SD, Ricke SC. Cultural and immunological detection methods for *Salmonella spp.* in animal feeds–A review. Veterinary Research Communications. 2006;**30**:127-137

[34] Chen R, Huang XL, Xu HY, Xiong YH, Li YB. Plasmonic enzyme-linked immunosorbent assay using nanospherical brushes as a catalase container for colorimetric detection of ultralow concentrations of *Listeria monocytogenes*. ACS Applied Materials & Interfaces. 2015;**7**:28632-28639

[35] Ye R, Zhu C, Song Y, Lu Q, Ge X, Yang X, Zhu MJ, Du D, Li H, Lin Y. Bioinspired synthesis of all-in-one organic-inorganic hybrid nanoflowers combined with a hand-held pH meter for on-site detection of food pathogen. Small. 2016;**12**:3094-3100

[36] Bahadır EB, Sezgintürk MK. Lateral flow assays: Principles, designs and labels. TrAC Trends in Analytical Chemistry. 2016;**82**:286-306

[37] Dzantiev BB, Byzova NA, Urusov AE, Zherdev AV. Immunochromatographic methods in food analysis. TrAC Trends in Analytical Chemistry. 2014;**55**:81-93

[38] Singh J, Sharma S, Nara S. Evaluation of gold nanoparticle based lateral flow assays for diagnosis of *Enterobacteriaceae* members in food and water. Food Chemistry. 2015;**170**:470-483

[39] Sajid M, Kawde AN, Daud M. Designs, formats and applications of lateral flow assay: A literature review. Journal of Saudi Chemical Society. 2015;**19**:689-705

[40] Huang X, Aguilar ZP, Xu H, Lai W, Xiong Y. Membrane-based lateral flow immunochromatographic strip with nanoparticles as reporters for detection: A review. Biosensors & Bioelectronics. 2016;**75**:166-180

[41] Song CM, Liu C, Wu SY, Li HL, Guo HQ, Yang B, Qiu S, Li JW, Liu L, Zeng HJ, et al. Development of a lateral flow colloidal gold immunoassay strip for the simultaneous detection of *Shigella boydii* and *Escherichia coli* O157:H7 in bread, milk and jelly samples. Food Control. 2016;**59**:345-351

[42] Pyo D, Yoo J. New trends in fluorescence immunochromatography. Journal of Immunoassay and Immunochemistry. 2012;**33**:203-222

[43] Ju Q, Noor MO, Krull UJ. Paper-based biodetection using luminescent nanoparticles. Analyst. 2016;**141**:2838-2860

[44] Cordeiro M, Carlos FF, Pedrosa P, Lopez A, Baptista PV. Gold nanoparticles for diagnostics: Advances towards points of care. Diagnostics. 2016;**6**:43

[45] Jung BY, Jung SC, Kweon CH. Development of a rapid immunochromatographic strip for detection of *Escherichia coli* O157. Journal of Food Protection. 2005;**68**:2140-2143

[46] Bautista DA, Elankumaran S, Arking JA, Heckert RA. Evaluation of an immunochromatography strip assay for the detection of *Salmonella sp* from poultry. Journal of Veterinary Diagnostic Investigation. 2002;**14**:427-430

[47] Huang SH, Wei HC, Lee YC. One-step immunochromatographic assay for the detection of *Staphylococcus aureus*. Food Control. 2007;**18**:893-897

[48] Shim WB, Choi JG, Kim JY, Yang ZY, Lee KH, Kim MG, Ha SD, Kim KS, Kim KY, Kim CH, et al. Production of monoclonal antibody against *Listeria monocytogenes* and its application to immunochromatography strip test. Journal of Microbiology and Biotechnology. 2007;**17**:1152-1161

[49] Preechakasedkit P, Pinwattana K, Dungchai W, Siangproh W, Chaicumpa W, Tongtawe P, Chailapakul O. Development of a one-step immunochromatographic strip test using gold nanoparticles for the rapid detection of *Salmonella typhi* in human serum. Biosensors & Bioelectronics. 2012;**31**:562-566

[50] Li XP, Lu DL, Sheng ZH, Chen K, Guo XB, Jin ML, Han HY. A fast and sensitive immunoassay of avian influenza virus based on label-free quantum dot probe and lateral flow test strip. Talanta. 2012;**100**:1-6

[51] Yang Q, Gong X, Song T, Yang J, Zhu S, Li Y, Cui Y, Zhang B, Chang J. Quantum dot-based immunochromatography test strip for rapid, quantitative and sensitive detection of alpha fetoprotein. Biosensors & Bioelectronics. 2011;**30**:145-150

[52] Li X, Li W, Yang Q, Gong X, Guo W, Dong C, Liu J, Xuan L, Chang J. Rapid and quantitative detection of prostate specific antigen with a quantum dot nanobeads-based immunochromatography test strip. ACS Applied Materials & Interfaces. 2014;**6**:6406-6414

[53] Medintz IL, Uyeda HT, Goldman ER, Mattoussi H. Quantum dot bioconjugates for imaging, labelling and sensing. Nature Materials. 2005;**4**:435-446

[54] Alivisatos AP. Semiconductor clusters, nanocrystals, and quantum dots. Science. 1996; **271**:933-937

[55] Resch-Genger U, Grabolle M, Cavaliere-Jaricot S, Nitschke R, Nann T. Quantum dots versus organic dyes as fluorescent labels. Nature Methods. 2008;**5**:763-775

[56] Bruno J. Application of DNA aptamers and quantum dots to lateral flow test strips for detection of foodborne pathogens with improved sensitivity versus colloidal gold. Pathogens. 2014;**3**:341-355

[57] Quesada-González D, Merkoçi A. Nanoparticle-based lateral flow biosensors. Biosensors & Bioelectronics. 2015;**73**:47-63

[58] Chen XX, Gan M, Xu H, Chen F, Ming X, Xu HY, Wei H, Xu F, Liu CW. Development of a rapid and sensitive quantum dot-based immunochromatographic strip by double labeling PCR products for detection of *Staphylococcus aureus* in food. Food Control. 2014;**46**: 225-232

[59] Liu CY, Jia QJ, Yang CH, Qiao RR, Jing LH, Wang LB, Xu CL, Gao MY. Lateral flow immunochromatographic assay for sensitive pesticide detection by using Fe_3O_4 nanoparticle aggregates as color reagents. Analytical Chemistry. 2011;**83**:6778-6784

[60] Wang DB, Tian B, Zhang ZP, Wang XY, Fleming J, Bi LJ, Yang RF, Zhang XE. Detection of *Bacillus anthracis* spores by super-paramagnetic lateral-flow immunoassays based on "road closure". Biosensors & Bioelectronics. 2015;**67**:608-614

[61] Qiao ZH, Lei CY, Fu YC, Li YB. Rapid and sensitive detection of *E-coli* O157:H7 based on antimicrobial peptide functionalized magnetic nanoparticles and urease-catalyzed signal amplification. Analytical Methods. 2017;**9**:5204-5210

[62] Ren W, Cho H, Zhou Z, Irudayaraj J. Ultrasensitive detection of microbial cells using magnetic focus enhanced lateral flow sensors. Chemical Communications. 2016;**52**:4930-4933

[63] Suaifan G, Alhogail S, Zourob M. Paper-based magnetic nanoparticle-peptide probe for rapid and quantitative colorimetric detection of *Escherichia coli* O157:H7. Biosensors & Bioelectronics. 2017;**92**:702-708

[64] Xia SQ, Yu ZB, Liu DF, Xu CL, Lai WH. Developing a novel immunochromatographic test strip with gold magnetic bifunctional nanobeads (GMBN) for efficient detection of *Salmonella choleraesuis* in milk. Food Control. 2016;**59**:507-512

[65] Jyoti A, Vajpayee P, Singh G, Patel CB, Gupta KC, Shanker R. Identification of environmental reservoirs of nontyphoidal *Salmonellosis*: Aptamer-assisted bioconcentration and subsequent detection of *Salmonella typhimurium* by quantitative polymerase chain reaction. Environmental Science & Technology. 2011;**45**:8996-9002

[66] Lorsch JR, Szostak JW. In-vitro selection of RNA aptamers specific for cyanocobalamin. Biochemistry. 1994;**33**:973-982

[67] Wrzesinski J, Ciesiolka J. Characterization of structure and metal ions specificity of Co^{2+}-binding RNA aptamers. Biochemistry. 2005;**44**:6257-6268

[68] Bock LC, Griffin LC, Latham JA, Vermaas EH, Toole JJ. Selection of single-stranded-DNA molecules that bind and inhibit human thrombin. Nature. 1992;**355**:564-566

[69] Gao FL, Lei JP, Ju HX. Label-free surface-enhanced Raman spectroscopy for sensitive DNA detection by DNA-mediated silver nanoparticle growth. Analytical Chemistry. 2013;**85**:11788-11793

[70] Jiang XH, Yang M, Meng YJ, Jiang W, Zhan JH. Cysteamine-modified silver nanoparticle aggregates for quantitative SERS sensing of pentachlorophenol with a portable Raman spectrometer. ACS Applied Materials & Interfaces. 2013;**5**:6902-6908

[71] Shi ML, Zheng J, Tan YJ, Tan GX, Li JS, Li YH, Li X, Zhou ZG, Yang RH. Ultrasensitive detection of single nucleotide polymorphism in human mitochondrial DNA utilizing ion-mediated cascade surface-enhanced Raman spectroscopy amplification. Analytical Chemistry. 2015;**87**:2734-2740

[72] Gao FL, Du LL, Tang DQ, Lu Y, Zhang YZ, Zhang LX. A cascade signal amplification strategy for surface enhanced Raman spectroscopy detection of thrombin based on DNAzyme assistant DNA recycling and rolling circle amplification. Biosensors & Bioelectronics. 2015;**66**:423-430

[73] Xu LJ, Lei ZC, Li JX, Zong C, Yang CJ, Ren B. Label-free surface-enhanced Raman spectroscopy detection of DNA with single-base sensitivity. Journal of the American Chemical Society. 2015;**137**:5149-5154

[74] Liu Y, Zhou HB, Hu ZW, Yu GX, Yang DT, Zhao JS. Label and label-free based surface-enhanced Raman scattering for pathogen bacteria detection: a review. Biosensors & Bioelectronics. 2017;**94**:131-140

[75] Wang JF, Wu XZ, Wang CW, Shao NS, Dong PT, Xiao R, Wang SQ. Magnetically assisted surface-enhanced Raman spectroscopy for the detection of *Staphylococcus aureus* based on aptamer recognition. ACS Applied Materials & Interfaces. 2015;**7**:20919-20929

[76] Zhang H, Ma X, Liu Y, Duan N, Wu S, Wang Z, Xu B. Gold nanoparticles enhanced SERS aptasensor for the simultaneous detection of *Salmonella typhimurium* and *Staphylococcus aureus*. Biosensors & Bioelectronics. 2015;**74**:872-877

[77] Pahlow S, Meisel S, Cialla-May D, Weber K, Rosch P, Popp J. Isolation and identification of bacteria by means of Raman spectroscopy. Advanced Drug Delivery Reviews. 2015;**89**: 105-120

[78] Gao WC, Li B, Yao RZ, Li ZP, Wang XW, Dong XL, Qu H, Li QX, Li N, Chi H, et al. Intuitive label-free SERS detection of bacteria using aptamer-based *in situ* silver nanoparticles synthesis. Analytical Chemistry. 2017;**89**:9836-9842

[79] Yu MQ, Wang H, Fu F, Li LY, Li J, Li G, Song Y, Swihart MT, Song EQ. Dual-recognition förster resonance energy transfer based platform for one-step sensitive detection of pathogenic bacteria using fluorescent vancomycin-gold nanoclusters and aptamer-gold nanoparticles. Analytical Chemistry. 2017;**89**:4085-4090

[80] Duan N, Gong WH, Wang ZP, Wu SJ. An aptasensor based on fluorescence resonance energy transfer for multiplexed pathogenic bacteria determination. Analytical Methods. 2016;**8**:1390-1395

[81] Duan N, Ding XY, He LX, Wu SJ, Wei YX, Wang ZP. Selection, identification and application of a DNA aptamer against *Listeria monocytogenes*. Food Control. 2013;**33**:239-243

[82] Lian Y, He FJ, Wang H, Tong FF. A new aptamer/graphene interdigitated gold electrode piezoelectric sensor for rapid and specific detection of *Staphylococcus aureus*. Biosensors & Bioelectronics. 2015;**65**:314-319

[83] Jiang DN, Liu F, Zhang LQ, Liu LL, Liu C, Pu XY. An electrochemical strategy with molecular beacon and hemin/G-quadruplex for the detection of Clostridium perfringens DNA on screen-printed electrodes. RSC Advances. 2014;**4**:57064-57070

[84] Wu SJ, Duan N, Shi Z, Fang CC, Wang ZP. Simultaneous aptasensor for multiplex pathogenic bacteria detection based on multicolor upconversion nanoparticles labels. Analytical Chemistry. 2014;**86**:3100-3107

[85] Labib M, Zamay AS, Koloyskaya OS, Reshetneva IT, Zamay GS, Kibbee RJ, Sattar SA, Zamay TN, Berezovski MV. Aptamer-based viability impedimetric sensor for bacteria. Analytical Chemistry. 2012;**84**:8966-8969

[86] Abbaspour A, Norouz-Sarvestani F, Noon A, Soltani N. Aptamer-conjugated silver nanoparticles for electrochemical dual-aptamer-based sandwich detection of *Staphylococcus aureus*. Biosensors & Bioelectronics. 2015;**68**:149-155

[87] Ding JW, Lei JH, Ma X, Gong J, Qin W. Potentiometric aptasensing of *Listeria monocytogenes* using protamine as an indicator. Analytical Chemistry. 2014;**86**:9412-9416

Chapter 3

Volatile Organic Compound and Metabolite Signatures as Pathogen Identifiers and Biomarkers of Infectious Disease

Elizabeth Hong-Geller and Samantha Adikari

Additional information is available at the end of the chapter

http://dx.doi.org/10.5772/intechopen.72398

Abstract

Volatile organic compound (VOC)-based diagnostics have great potential to be the next generation of screening tools for pathogen identification and infectious disease management. VOCs are low molecular weight metabolic compounds that have high vapor pressures and low boiling points, both of which facilitate evaporation at ambient temperatures. There is increasing evidence that particular VOCs, or profiles of VOCs, are unique to various disease states. Different pathogenic species have been found to produce characteristic profiles of VOCs by virtue of their distinct metabolisms. The detection of these metabolite profiles from patient samples could provide an effective means of rapid, non-invasive pathogen identification, thus enabling early diagnosis and treatment. In this review, we will discuss the potential of VOC profiles to be utilized as biomarkers of pathogenic infection, with a focus on bacterial pathogens. Herein we describe the common methods for clinical VOC sample collection, provide an overview of the various instruments and techniques used for VOC detection and analysis, and summarize the key findings of recent studies that have investigated VOC biomarkers in various infectious diseases. We will also discuss the challenges associated with translating VOC analysis into a clinical diagnostic tool.

Keywords: volatile organic compounds, VOCs, metabolites, signatures, biomarkers, profiles, pathogen identification, infectious diseases, clinical diagnostics, non-invasive tools, antibiotic resistance

1. Introduction

Although VOC identification has only been enabled by the development of sophisticated analytical techniques in the last two decades, the premise that VOC profiles can be used as biomarkers for disease can be traced back to ancient times, when physicians diagnosed diseases based on their senses. The ancient Greek physician Hippocrates (460–370 BC) is said to have poured human sputum over hot coals to liberate the distinct odors indicative of tuberculosis infection. In the early 20th century, it was postulated that bad breath in many mammalian species may be sexually unattractive precisely because it is indicative of disease [1]. Currently, there is a great public health need to develop rapid, non-invasive methods of identifying pathogens and determining their antibiotic resistance or susceptibility status in order to effectively treat infectious diseases. Conventional diagnostic methods offer limited sensitivity and specificity, and can be expensive, invasive for patients, and time-consuming, often requiring several days for cell culture and low-throughput microscopy assays. Delays and limitations in diagnostic results often lead to the initiation of untargeted therapies, such as treatment with broad-spectrum antibiotics, which contribute to the evolution of antibiotic-resistant pathogens.

VOCs represent a diverse group of carbon-based molecules, including alcohols, ketones, aldehydes, hydrocarbons, isocyanates, amines, terpenes and sulfides [2]. VOCs are generally short-lived and become rapidly diluted in microenvironments. Altering growth conditions can modulate VOC profiles, reflecting the unique metabolic state of an organism in specific environments. Many animals, plants, and microbes have evolved chemical sensing mechanisms that can detect minute quantities of VOCs released during growth to protect against antagonists and to act as signaling molecules for intercellular communication. For example, plants use volatiles to communicate with pollinators and to coordinate growth with their own kind to out-compete foreign species.

As a result of normal metabolic functions, the healthy human body produces a vast number of VOCs that are liberated in exhaled breath, skin secretions, saliva, blood, urine and feces. Many of these VOCs likely derive from commensal microbes in the body and are often detectable by odor [3]. Pathogenic infection in humans alters both the quantity and composition of VOCs produced. As a result of their distinct metabolisms, different pathogens produce characteristic VOC profiles, which can often be detected in the headspace of cultures grown *in vitro* [4, 5]. Upon pathogen infection, VOCs released by both the pathogen and infected host can potentially be used as a diagnostic signature of the infection state. Analysis of the VOC profiles released from clinical samples have yielded VOC biomarkers indicative of specific diseases and infections [6–8]. Exhaled breath tests in particular have already proven useful in the diagnosis of a broad range of pathologies, including lung disorders, diabetes, gastrointestinal and liver disease, cancer, and pathogen infection [9–11].

VOC signatures uniquely associated with specific pathogens can be clinically relevant for diagnosing various infectious diseases, elucidating antibiotic resistance versus susceptibility, designing treatment regimens, and monitoring disease progression. The ability to reliably distinguish between different pathogenic species, based on their VOC signatures, will facilitate the development of rapid, highly-sensitive, and non-invasive diagnostic methods and tools, ultimately leading to improved patient outcomes.

2. Overview of clinical sample collection for VOC analysis

There are potential advantages to employing VOC signatures for disease diagnostics, such as ease of collection from all patients, including the critically ill, children, and the elderly.

http://dx.doi.org/10.5772/intechopen.72398

Furthermore, longitudinal samples from patients could be more easily obtained to track disease progression and monitor therapeutic interventions during follow-up studies. The following section describes VOC collection and detection from various types of clinical samples.

2.1. Breath

The vast majority of studies on VOC biomarkers have been conducted using exhaled breath samples, as they are the most easily obtained [12]. VOC analysis from breath samples has proven useful for diagnosing a wide range of diseases and various infections [11, 13]. Exhaled breath contains hundreds of VOCs that can be attributed to either exogenous or endogenous sources. Exogenous volatiles include compounds inhaled from the external environment, such as the ingestion of food or smoking cigarettes. Endogenous volatiles consist of compounds derived from the body. These may include compounds produced by the human body's assortment of commensal bacteria, or in the case of infectious disease, compounds released by pathogenic microbes. Endogenous volatiles are transported from different organs via the bloodstream to the lungs, excreted via diffusion across the pulmonary alveolar membrane, and subsequently exhaled via breath. Distinguishing exogenously derived VOCs from the endogenous compounds in a breath sample is a significant challenge in elucidating VOC signatures related to disease. The detection of exogenous VOCs in a breath sample may suggest exposure to a drug or environmental toxin, which can confound the search for disease biomarkers [14].

VOCs contained in clinical breath samples and bacterial culture headspace samples are present at very low levels. To concentrate and analyze breath VOCs, several methods have been developed, such as chemical trapping, sorbent trapping, cold trapping, or condensate trapping, followed by thermal desorption to analyze the VOC content [15]. Pre-concentration of breath VOCs can further be achieved by solid-phase micro-extraction (SPME), in which different VOCs in a sample are adsorbed by a coated microfiber. These VOCs are then delivered directly into the mass spectrometer or other instrument for analysis. A more recently developed method is membrane extraction with a sorbent interface, which combines sampling and pre-concentration in a single step [16]. Exhaled breath condensate (EBC) is another new technique in which aerosolized micro-droplets from the lower respiratory tract are captured by directing the exhaled air through a cooling device, resulting in the accumulation of EBC in the collection chamber. In general, EBC collection is an inefficient VOC capture method, due to the abundance of non-volatile components in the micro-droplets [11].

2.2. Saliva

Human saliva from healthy subjects is a complex secretion containing peptides, proteins and metabolites. Saliva is not a homogenous fluid, but a mixture of different fluids made from three distinct salivary glands (the parotid, the submandibular, and the sublingual glands). The protein composition of these fluids varies significantly depending on the gland sampled. A small amount of saliva is also secreted through hundreds of minor glands located within the mouth. As such, when sampling saliva, it is essential to characterize the sample in terms of its location. Most studies utilizing saliva samples collect the whole saliva mixture comprised of all the various glandular saliva types produced in the mouth [17]. While the protein composition arising from each salivary gland is well characterized, the metabolite composition is not well understood. However, it has been determined that saliva contains numerous VOCs including alcohols, aldehydes, ketones, carboxylic acids, esters, amines, amides, lactones and hydrocarbons [18]. The various bacterial species found in the oral cavity also contribute to the chemical composition of saliva through secretion of their metabolic by-products. Analysis of sulfur-containing volatile compounds in exhaled breath has linked malodorous breath to anaerobic bacterial activity in the oral cavity [19]. Furthermore, exogenous VOCs inhaled through the lungs or absorbed through the skin can be excreted into saliva. Other considerations for saliva sampling include time since brushing teeth, time since ingesting sugary or acidic foods, evidence of oral injury, and the presence of contaminating fluids such as blood [20]. The endogenous VOC profile of human saliva is of particular interest in medical forensics, where oral fluids are routinely analyzed for the presence of drugs or toxins.

2.3. Skin

VOCs emitted from the skin surface are mainly derived from a combination of sweat secreted by the sweat glands and sebum, an oily substance secreted by the sebaceous glands. Although some of these VOCs result from internal hormonal or metabolic changes, many VOCs appear to be derived from commensal skin bacteria that metabolize compounds secreted in sweat and sebum. Samples are easily obtained by wiping the patient's skin with an organic solvent (e.g. acetone), or by collecting the VOCs directly from the affected skin onto an absorbent SPME fiber. However, care must be taken to avoid contaminating the sample with cosmetics, perfumes, or compounds present in the ambient air. This may be especially difficult given that even trace VOCs associated with the preservatives found in skin creams and gels are detectable in skin swab samples [21].

2.4. Blood

Blood directly reflects the internal environment of the body, including nutritional, metabolic, and immune status. Given that most endogenous VOCs are secreted from cells directly into the bloodstream, as the main conduit of communication between different parts of the body, the analysis of plasma-derived VOCs has garnered much interest from researchers and clinicians alike. Recent work has focused on building up a compendium of blood-borne VOCs in healthy human subjects to compare these profiles with patient samples, and thereby identify VOC biomarkers unique to disease states [22]. However, acquiring blood samples is more invasive than either breath or skin, and the requisite pre-treatment of blood to remove red and white blood cells has the disadvantage of being very time-consuming. The SPME method has been shown to detect a range of volatiles at very low concentrations in human blood, including hydrocarbons (pentane and isoprene), ketones (acetone), halogenated compounds (isoflurane), and thioethers (dimethyl sulfide). Since blood-borne VOCs can also be liberated in exhaled breath, a greater understanding of blood VOCs will also contribute to the diagnostic potential of breath analysis [23].

2.5. Urine

Given that urine samples are routinely used for diagnosis of disease, urine components and urine profiles have been well characterized [24]. The compounds predominantly found in urine are intermediate products or end-products of many metabolic pathways. These substances contain a variety of chemical motifs, such as ketone, alcohol, furan, pyrrole and sulfide, which often generate specific odors. Since there are many components present in urine samples, VOC patterns will only be evident after statistical analysis of many patient samples. In addition, considerable variation among individuals has been found in profiles of urine-derived VOCs [7]. Importantly, urine components are affected not only by the metabolic status of the body, but also significantly by ingested foods and drinks. Therefore, caution must be taken when determining whether or not any particular VOC biomarker is the result of disease-related changes in metabolism or an exogenous cause.

2.6. Feces

Fecal samples contain dietary end-products resulting from intestinal bacterial metabolism and digestive and excretory processes. The composition of a patient's gut microbiota is reflected in their fecal sample [25]. As such, fecal VOCs may provide the best non-invasive means of diagnosing gastrointestinal and liver diseases. Although many volatile compounds might be easily detected in fecal samples, they are still influenced by a range of confounding factors, such as diet, gender, age, smoking and certain medications. Also, a large number of VOCs in healthy patients is derived from the breakdown of food by intestinal normal flora, and is not indicative of any disease. Nevertheless, distinct patterns of VOCs have been discovered in the fecal samples of patients with certain bacterial infections, including *V. cholerae*, *C. jejuni* and *C. difficile* infections [8, 26].

3. Overview of VOC detection methods and analytical instruments

Over the last two decades, significant advances in analytical chemical techniques and instruments have facilitated the identification of VOCs with improved sensitivity and accuracy. Here we summarize the various methods used for VOC detection. The advantages and limitations associated with these techniques and instruments are summarized in **Table 1**, and reviewed in detail elsewhere (see [17, 21, 27, 28]).

Gas chromatography–mass spectrometry (GC–MS) is currently considered the gold standard for separation, detection, identification and quantification of VOCs. Samples for GC–MS must be in the gaseous phase such that a pure inert carrier gas can transport the sample through the chromatographic column. Depending on the VOC concentration, sample pre-concentration may be required [21]. Compound resolution improves as the length of the chromatographic column increases. Each unique compound is eluted from the column at a different time (termed the retention time) and detected by the mass spectrometer via compound ionization and measurement of the mass to charge ratio of each ion, thereby generating a unique mass spectrum for each compound. The class of volatile that can be detected by GC depends on the type of detector used. Examples include time of flight (TOF), plasma ionization, photoionization and electron capture detectors [17].

There are also several analytical methods that can be coupled with GC to achieve different outputs. As mentioned earlier, SPME followed by GC–MS can provide a solvent-free and easily automated system for quantifying trace amounts of VOCs [29]. However, it is important

Technique	Description	Advantages	Limitations
GC–MS	GC–MS combines separation, GC and MS. Separation is typically performed by a capillary column, with compounds being separated by their boiling point and polarity. As compounds are eluted, they are detected by the mass spectrometer as a function of their mass to charge ratio. Different MS detectors are available, with Time Of Flight (TOF) and tandem quadrupoles (MS–MS) being the most common.	• Good sensitivity (ppm-ppb) • Separates, identifies and quantifies VOCs all in one • High chromatographic resolution achievable • Highly reproducible results • Can analyze VOCs from complex mixtures • Can tentatively identify unknown compounds based on comparison to known mass spectra	• Often requires sample pre-concentration • Lengthy processing and analysis times • Unsuitable for screening unknown compounds • Requires a supply of pure inert carrier gas
GC-IMS	GC-IMS combines separation, GC and IMS. Separation may be performed using standard GC capillary columns or multi-capillary columns. Dual separation occurs first through the column and then in the detector according to the compound's gas-phase ion mobility. Ionized molecules are accelerated by an electric field towards a Faraday plate, where the impact of single ions is detected.	• High sensitivity (ppb-ppt) • Rapid results • Best for identifying differences between non-identical samples • Simple to use on site • Can use ambient air as the carrier gas	• Detection is compound-specific and depends on the ion's mass and charge • Limited dynamic range for quantitation • Unsuitable for screening unknown compounds • Confusing mass spectra can arise when high levels of solvents are present
Direct detection	These methods include SIFT-MS, IMR-MS, PTR-MS. They are popular for their sensitivity, rapid analysis times, and ability to extract target compounds from samples with little or no pre-separation.	• High sensitivity (sub-ppb) • Rapid results • Absolute quantification • Can detect trace compounds in mixtures	• Very expensive • Unsuitable for screening unknown compounds • PTR-MS only suitable for compounds with higher proton affinity than water
E-nose	A variety of E-nose detectors exist today. They generally consist of a micro-array of sensors which differ from each other in polarity. The sample passes through the array, and compounds adsorb to varying degrees on the different sensors depending on their composition. Compound adsorption on sensors changes the mass or resistance of each sensor, and this change is detected to provide different outputs.	• Best for identifying the differences between non-identical samples • Rapid results • Does not require sample separation or pre-concentration. • Relatively small, portable, and simple to use on site	• Cannot quantify VOCs • Can only identify known patterns of VOCs stored in its database • Unsuitable for screening unknown compounds • Sensitive to high ambient temperature and humidity

Table 1. Summary of most common VOC analytical techniques and their advantages and limitations.

to note that SPMEs are coated with different materials for selective compound adsorption. Therefore, individual SPMEs may not trap all VOCs present in a sample. GC ion mobility spectrometry (GC-IMS), based on separation of ions relative to their gas phase mobility, is highly sensitive and enables rapid quantification of separated VOCs, but is not suitable for identifying unknown compounds. The advantage of GC-IMS over GC–MS stems from its ability to use ambient air as the carrier gas, which negates the need for a pure inert gas supply and allows GC-IMS devices to be portable and particularly useful for breath sample analysis [30]. GC flame ionization detection (GC-FID), which is also widely used for breath analysis, detects VOCs with high sensitivity and low background noise.

Optical spectroscopic methods, such as laser absorption spectrometry, are also useful for the detection and quantification of specific VOCs in a mixture. These methods are highly selective and sensitive, and can be connected to different types of spectroscopic sensors, such as conductive polymer sensors and acoustic wave sensors, to detect the specific VOCs of interest [31]. Non-optical direct-injection methods for VOC measurement include Ion Molecule Reaction mass spectrometry (IMR-MS), Selected Ion Flow Tube mass spectrometry (SIFT-MS) and Proton Transfer Reaction mass spectrometry (PTR-MS). These methods do not require pre-concentration and little or no pre-separation. However, unknown compound identification is not possible. SIFT-MS provides real-time absolute quantification of several VOCs simultaneously, and therefore is well suited for analyzing clinical samples. A small SIFT-MS-based analytical instrument has been developed for routine use in a clinical setting [32]. Both GC and PTR ionization technology can be coupled to a Time Of Flight mass spectrometer (GC-TOF-MS, PTR-TOF-MS), thereby making real-time VOC analysis possible [33, 34].

Finally, devices that electronically mimic the human olfactory system, termed electronic noses or 'e-noses', have been developed and improved upon since the 1980s [28]. E-noses employ several gas sensors combined with pattern recognition software to detect overall odor fingerprints rather than specific compounds. This may be considered a limitation of the technology, as it cannot identify individual biomarkers. On the other hand, unlike GC–MS, e-noses have the advantage of being able to differentiate between non-identical samples without the need to separate the mixture into its individual components, a process which can be highly variable based on the technique(s) used. E-noses provide rapid results, but are limited by the VOC patterns they are programmed to detect, and thus cannot be used for screening unknown compounds. Before e-noses can be used routinely for practical diagnosis, it will be necessary to improve their accuracy and sensitivity to enable reliable recognition of a large number of VOC profiles.

While the informatics approaches used in conjunction with the aforementioned instruments can vary, three main methods are typically used, alone or concurrently, to confirm VOC identification: (1) comparing mass spectra data obtained to those in reference libraries and databases, (2) comparing mass spectra and peak retention times to those obtained from pure standard compounds, and (3) comparing mass spectra data obtained to those characterized in the literature.

4. VOC analysis for detecting infectious diseases

A growing number of studies clearly demonstrate the efficacy of VOC analysis in identifying a wide range of non-infectious diseases, including inflammatory disease [35], diabetes [36], lung cancer [37], and even Alzheimer's disease [38]. In the context of infectious diseases, VOC detection has clinical value in three aspects of diagnostics: (1) identifying the absence of pathogens (i.e. no antibiotic treatment), (2) identifying the presence of a specific pathogen (i.e. start appropriate antibiotic treatment), and (3) distinguishing between pathogenic species (i.e. determine antibiotic resistance versus sensitivity for the pathogen to guide treatment regimens). Examples of candidate VOCs identified as being associated with specific pathogens are summarized in **Table 2**. It should be noted here that many researchers emphasize the importance of considering the entire VOC profile of a pathogen and how it differs from another pathogen, rather than relying on any single VOC biomarker to reveal an association.

4.1. Respiratory infections

Although pathogens are capable of producing a large variety of VOCs, very few metabolites are produced exclusively by only one bacterial species. Particularly in cases of polymicrobial pulmonary infections, such as cystic fibrosis (CF), identification of the specific bacterial species responsible for the pathology is critical for correct diagnosis and treatment. Since patient prognoses can decline rapidly following these types of opportunistic infections, particularly in children, early detection is vital for the timely initiation of appropriate therapies [48]. GC-TOF-MS analysis of breath samples from CF patients has demonstrated that a distinctive VOC profile consisting of 22 compounds can discriminate CF patients from healthy controls with 100% accuracy. Furthermore, within the CF patients analyzed, a profile of 14 VOCs was able to correctly discriminate between patients with *Pseudomonas aeruginosa* positive cultures compared to those with negative cultures [49]. Interestingly, genotypically diverse strains of *P. aeruginosa* under the same culture conditions have been shown to exhibit a high degree of variability in detectable VOCs [50], indicating that additional CF patients need to be studied to determine which VOCs are truly discriminatory. In another study, distinct VOCs were characterized in the culture headspaces of four different opportunistic pathogens (*P. aeruginosa, Staphylococcus aureus, Stenotrophomonas maltophilia* and the *Burkholderia cepacia* complex) that cause lung and airway infection in CF patients, providing additional VOC signatures to test in infected host systems [51].

Pathogen	Infectious disease(s)	VOC candidates for disease biomarkers	Reference(s)
M. tuberculosis	Active pulmonary tuberculosis	1-methyl-naphthalene, methyl nicotinate, 1,4-dimethyl-cyclohexane	[13, 39, 40]
C. jejuni	Ulcerative colitis, diarrhea	Butanoic acid, 1-octen-3-ol, 1-butoxy-2-propanol	[8]
C. difficile	Ulcerative colitis, diarrhea	Ethanol, Butanol, Isopropanol	[8]
V. cholera	Cholera	Dimethyl disulfide, p-menth-1-en-8-ol	[9, 26]
H. pylori	Peptic ulcers	Hydrogen cyanide	[41]
S. aureus	Sinusitis, pneumonia	acetoin, hydroxyacetone, acetic acid, isovaleric acid, acetaldehyde, 2-propanol, 3-methyl-1-butanol	[42, 43]
P. aeruginosa	Sinusitis, pneumonia	2-aminoacetophenone, pyrrole, 1-vinylaziridine, 3-methylpyrrole, 1-undecene, 2-nonanone, methyl thiocyanate	[43–46]
K. pneumoniae	Bronchitis, pneumonia	butyraldehyde, octyl acetate, tridecanol, dodecenal, butanoic acid	[47]

Table 2. Examples of VOCs associated with specific pathogens and infectious diseases.

Mycobacterium tuberculosis infection is another respiratory disease that has been the focus of much VOC research. GC–MS analysis of urine sample headspaces was used to identify and distinguish VOC profiles from tuberculosis (TB) patients and healthy controls. Five biomarker compounds were able to discriminate between these two groups with 98.8% accuracy: alpha-xylene, isopropyl acetate, 3-pentanol, dimethylstyrene, and cymol. These compounds also served to discriminate TB patients from patients with lung cancer and COPD [52]. In another study using GC–MS analysis of exhaled breath, active pulmonary TB could be distinguished from non-active TB with 85% accuracy. 1,3,5-Trimethylbenzene was identified in active pulmonary TB, whereas 1,2,3,4-tetramethylbenzene was a biomarker for the non-active state. Exhaled breath samples from all the TB patients contained the *M. tuberculosis*-associated biomarkers 1-methyl-naphthalene and 1,4-dimethyl-cyclohexane, which were also observed in *in vitro* cultures [39]. Other studies focusing on headspace VOCs from *in vitro* cultured *Mycobacterium* species have revealed several metabolites of nicotinic acid, four of which are considered specific for *M. tuberculosis* and *M. bovis* strains: methyl phenylacetate, methyl p-anisate, methyl nicotinate, and o-phenylanisole [53]. Methyl nicotinate has also been detected at high levels in the exhaled breath of smear-positive TB patients [40]. VOCs derived from *in vitro M. tuberculosis* cultures are distinct from those VOCs produced by an infected host, as a result of oxidative stress. Volatiles related to oxidative stress include alkanes and methylated alkane derivatives, whereas *in vitro*-defined VOCs of *M. tuberculosis* origin include cyclohexane, benzene, decane, and heptane derivatives [13].

4.2. Gastrointestinal infections

Fecal samples taken from patients suffering from various forms of infectious diarrhea have revealed characteristic VOC profiles depending on the causative pathogen. For example, the absence of hydrocarbons and terpenes indicated a *Campylobacter* infection, whereas the absence of furans and indoles indicated a *Clostridium difficile* infection [54]. Another study focusing on ulcerative colitis, a disease marked by inflammation of the colonic mucosa, found that while hundreds of volatiles were detectable in donor fecal samples, distinct VOC patterns could discriminate between healthy controls and patients infected with *C. jejuni* and *C. difficile* [8]. Typhoid fever is caused by *Salmonella typhi* infection and is spread by consuming contaminated water or food. VOC metabolite profiles specific to *S. typhi* can be detected by GC–MS from the blood samples of typhoid patients. Importantly, such metabolite profiles can also differentiate between *Salmonella typhi* and *Salmonella paratyphi A* infections, enabling targeted therapies [55].

4.3. Urinary tract infections

In cases of urinary tract infection (UTI), appropriate and effective therapy is heavily dependent on early diagnosis. UTIs are most frequently caused by *Escherichia coli* and other enteric pathogens such as *Enterococci, Klebsiella, Staphylococci,* and *Proteus* species, and also fungal pathogens such as *Candida albicans* [56]. Volatile metabolites released by these pathogens are detectable in the headspace of urine samples [56–58]. E-noses have proven particularly useful in recognizing the VOC patterns of healthy versus infected urine samples, though sample pre-concentration is often required. The relative efficacies of the various types of e-noses currently in use were compared in a recent review [57]. Since urine contains a complex mixture of VOCs that is relatively well-defined

[24], significant changes to the VOC profile of patients with UTIs may serve as diagnostic biomarkers of infection. To this end, more sensitive methodologies that do not require sample preincubation are needed to enable the efficient routine diagnosis of UTIs using VOC profiling.

4.4. Blood infections

A review of multiple studies revealed that distinct VOC signatures are produced by each of the six most abundant and pathogenic bacteria in sepsis (*Staphylococcus aureus, Streptococcus pneumoniae, Enterococcus faecalis, Pseudomonas aeruginosa, Klebsiella pneumoniae,* and *Escherichia coli*). While all six species produced isopentanol, formaldehyde, methyl mercaptan, and trimethylamine, each species also produced unique key compounds that can be used as specific VOC signatures [59]. Another blood-borne disease, malaria, is transmitted by mosquitoes that introduce the *Plasmodium falciparum* parasite into the blood of the host. Breath-based VOC analysis offers a rapid and non-invasive alternative to the current approach of visualizing *P. falciparum* on stained blood films. A recent study identified nine malaria-associated VOCs: carbon dioxide, isoprene, acetone, benzene, cyclohexanone, and four types of thioethers. The concentrations of these compounds varied significantly as the disease progressed. Following antimalarial drug treatment, parasite clearance correlated strongly with a decline in VOC levels [60]. Notably, another recent study found that blood cultures of *E. coli* and *S. aureus* yielded different VOC profiles before and after exposure to gentamicin or flucloxacillin, demonstrating that antibiotic susceptibility status can also be rapidly evaluated by VOC analysis [61].

5. Challenges in the clinical application of VOC analysis

There remain both logistical and technical challenges to the translation of VOC analysis from the research laboratory to the clinical setting. On the logistical side, the analytical instruments required for VOC detection are very expensive and require a large footprint and specialized training to operate and analyze the data. Furthermore, the methods are time-consuming and not readily scalable for high-throughput sample processing. There remains a lack of standardization for procedures in sample collection, pre-concentration, and storage, which are essential for effective clinical implementation.

From a technical standpoint, it is important to emphasize that the presence of a unique pattern of VOCs (constituting a complete VOC signature), rather than a single VOC biomarker, will be necessary for bacterial species identification [34]. Diagnostic tests based on a single VOC biomarker do not appear possible, given the fact that all pathogens produce a wide range of overlapping volatile metabolites. It should also be noted that the conspicuous absence of certain volatile compounds from a culture or sample actually forms part of the distinct VOC signature for a particular pathogen [36]. Furthermore, the specific profile of VOCs detectable *in vitro* is largely dependent on the bacterial growth state and density (e.g. logarithmic versus stationary phase), sample storage conditions (e.g. short-term versus long-term), and the type of culture media used [34, 62, 63]. To confound analysis further, patient samples are far less well-defined than laboratory cultures of reference strains, and therefore vary greatly in terms of growth phase, host response, viscosity, confounding co-morbidities, and medications (including antibiotics)

[43, 61, 64]. Therefore, reproducibility of VOC signatures, even in patients infected with the same pathogen, remains a challenge given the variability between individual patient samples.

If VOCs from primary patient samples are to be used effectively for clinical diagnostic purposes, we must recognize the confounding factors associated with VOC analysis. Firstly, the environment of the human body is entirely different from *in vitro* growth media for pathogen and human cell culture, thereby resulting in a completely different set of metabolic by-products [43]. Secondly, genotypic variability between different strains of a pathogen can strongly influence the types and concentrations of volatile metabolites detected [50]. Thirdly, the human body mounts an inflammatory response against pathogen infection, potentially leading to a change in bacterial and host metabolism. Future studies should address the metabolic differences between infectious and non-infectious inflammatory responses [65]. Fourthly, VOCs derived from exogenous sources, such as the host environment and diet, can easily contaminate a sample [66]. Before diagnostic tests based on endogenously produced VOCs can be routinely used on patient samples, it is necessary to definitively separate true biomarkers from contaminating components. Lastly, the human body plays host to an entire microbiome unique to each individual. It may be that these commensal bacteria produce many metabolites that are indistinguishable from those generated by disease-causing pathogens, and therefore may interfere with a VOC-based diagnostic test [67].

6. Conclusions and future perspectives

In the last two decades, diverse studies have used emerging and established technologies to assess the applicability of the VOC profiling approach to the diagnosis and treatment of pathogenic infections. At present, numerous studies have identified VOC profiles and candidate biomarkers for certain infectious diseases, which allow researchers to discriminate between different pathogenic species and between healthy and diseased individuals. VOC analysis continues to be a rapidly expanding field of inquiry. However, as outlined in the previous section, VOC-based diagnostics will require further development and vetting of reproducibility before transition from the laboratory to the clinic.

Existing VOC profiles and candidate biomarkers must still be corroborated across several coordinated studies before there can be sufficient confidence in their diagnostic efficacy. For example, independent *in vitro* studies that investigate the same organism, but subjected to different sampling methods and analytical techniques, have led to identification of different VOC patterns. Similarly, direct comparisons of independent clinical studies are difficult, given that experimental design and parameters differ between studies. In addition, very few studies to date have compared individuals with active disease to individuals at other disease stages (e.g. comparison of active TB and latent TB). Likewise, little data exists on the effect that comorbidities or co-infections (e.g. TB co-infection with HIV) may have on the range and type of detectable VOCs. Targeted studies are still required to fully characterize VOC disease signatures and to further evaluate the diagnostic accuracy of these biomarkers in patient samples. It is clear that before this approach can become integrated into routine clinical practice, it must first be validated by clinical trials using sufficiently large numbers of test subjects across a range of infections.

Despite the challenges, it is foreseeable that continued research in this area may pave the way for the design of unique diagnostic tools, such as disease-specific sensor arrays and targeted metabolite breathalyzers, that could also have potential applications in forensics, pharmacokinetics, and toxicology. Furthermore, the development of portable, sensor-based devices for the personalized monitoring of disease states and therapy progress would represent a clear advancement beyond the current state-of-the-art in clinical practice. In the long term, such tools could enable a more selective approach to antimicrobial drug use, while also opening up the possibility of individually tailored treatments.

Acknowledgements

The writing of this review was supported by a Defense Threat Reduction Agency (DTRA) grant to EH-G to study the potential for VOC profiling to discriminate between antibiotic sensitive and resistant strains of bacterial pathogens.

Author details

Elizabeth Hong-Geller* and Samantha Adikari

*Address all correspondence to: ehong@lanl.gov

Los Alamos National Laboratory, Bioscience Division, Los Alamos, NM, USA

References

[1] Fisher RA. The evolution of sexual preference. The Eugenics Review. 1915;**7**(3):184-192

[2] Cicolella A. Volatile organic compounds (VOC): Definition, classification and properties. Revue des Maladies Respiratoires. 2008;**25**(2):155-163

[3] Liddell K. Smell as a diagnostic marker. Postgraduate Medical Journal. 1976;**52**(605): 136-138

[4] Thorn RM, Reynolds DM, Greenman J. Multivariate analysis of bacterial volatile compound profiles for discrimination between selected species and strains in vitro. Journal of Microbiological Methods. 2011;**84**(2):258-264

[5] Korpi AJ, Jarnberg ALP. Microbial volatile organic compounds. Critical Reviews in Toxicology. 2009;**39**(2):139-193

[6] Cao WQ, Duan YX. Breath analysis: Potential for clinical diagnosis and exposure assessment. Clinical Chemistry. 2006;**52**(5):800-811

[7] Guernion N et al. Identifying bacteria in human urine: Current practice and the potential for rapid, near-patient diagnosis by sensing volatile organic compounds. Clinical Chemistry and Laboratory Medicine. 2001;**39**(10):893-906

[8] Garner CE et al. Volatile organic compounds from feces and their potential for diagnosis of gastrointestinal disease. Faseb Journal. 2007;**21**(8):1675-1688

[9] Probert CSJ et al. Volatile organic compounds as diagnostic biomarkers in gastrointestinal and liver diseases. Journal of Gastrointestinal and Liver Diseases. 2009;**18**(3):337-343

[10] Horvath I et al. Exhaled biomarkers in lung cancer. European Respiratory Journal. 2009; **34**(1):261-275

[11] Chambers ST, Scott-Thomas A, Epton M. Developments in novel breath tests for bacterial and fungal pulmonary infection. Current Opinion in Pulmonary Medicine. 2012; **18**(3):228-232

[12] Boots AW et al. The versatile use of exhaled volatile organic compounds in human health and disease. Journal of Breath Research. 2012;**6**(2):027108

[13] Phillips M et al. Breath biomarkers of active pulmonary tuberculosis. Tuberculosis (Edinburgh, Scotland). 2010;**90**(2):145-151

[14] Kataoka H et al. Noninvasive analysis of volatile biomarkers in human emanations for health and early disease diagnosis. Bioanalysis. 2013;**5**(11):1443-1459

[15] Phillips M. Method for the collection and assay of volatile organic compounds in breath. Analytical Biochemistry. 1997;**247**(2):272-278

[16] Lord H et al. Breath analysis and monitoring by membrane extraction with sorbent interface. Analytical Chemistry. 2002;**74**(21):5650-5657

[17] Beale DJ et al. A review of analytical techniques and their application in disease diagnosis in Breathomics and Salivaomics research. International Journal of Molecular Sciences. 2016;**18**(1)

[18] Soini HA et al. Analysis of volatile organic compounds in human saliva by a static sorptive extraction method and gas chromatography-mass spectrometry. Journal of Chemical Ecology. 2010;**36**(9):1035-1042

[19] van den Velde S et al. Halitosis associated volatiles in breath of healthy subjects. Journal of Chromatography. B, Analytical Technologies in the Biomedical and Life Sciences. 2007; **853**(1-2):54-61

[20] Granger DA et al. Integration of salivary biomarkers into developmental and behaviorally-oriented research: Problems and solutions for collecting specimens. Physiology & Behavior. 2007;**92**(4):583-590

[21] Ashrafi M et al. Volatile Organic Compound Detection as a Potential Means of Diagnosing Cutaneous Wound Infections. Wound Repair Regen; 2017

[22] Mochalski P et al. Blood and breath levels of selected volatile organic compounds in healthy volunteers. The Analyst. 2013;**138**(7):2134-2145

[23] Miekisch W et al. Analysis of volatile disease markers in blood. Clinical Chemistry. 2001;**47**(6):1053-1060

[24] Pauling L et al. Quantitative analysis of urine vapor and breath by gas-liquid partition chromatography. Proceedings of the National Academy of Sciences of the United States of America. 1971;**68**(10):2374-2376

[25] van Gaal N et al. Faecal volatile organic compounds analysis using field asymmetric ion mobility spectrometry: Non-invasive diagnostics in paediatric inflammatory bowel disease. Journal of Breath Research; 2017

[26] Garner CE et al. A pilot study of faecal volatile organic compounds in faeces from cholera patients in Bangladesh to determine their utility in disease diagnosis. Transactions of the Royal Society of Tropical Medicine and Hygiene. 2009;**103**(11):1171-1173

[27] Smith D, Spanel P. Pitfalls in the analysis of volatile breath biomarkers: Suggested solutions and SIFT-MS quantification of single metabolites. Journal of Breath Research. 2015;**9**(2):022001

[28] Arasaradnam RP et al. Insights into 'fermentonomics': Evaluation of volatile organic compounds (VOCs) in human disease using an electronic 'e-nose'. Journal of Medical Engineering & Technology. 2011;**35**(2):87-91

[29] Miekisch WJ, Schubert K, Noeldge-Schomburg GF. Diagnostic potential of breath analysis--focus on volatile organic compounds. Clinica Chimica Acta. 2004;**347**(1-2):25-39

[30] Sethi S, Nanda R, Chakraborty T. Clinical application of volatile organic compound analysis for detecting infectious diseases. Clinical Microbiology Reviews. 2013;**26**(3):462-475

[31] Wojtas J et al. Ultrasensitive laser spectroscopy for breath analysis. Opto-Electronics Review. 2012;**20**(1):26-39

[32] Spanel P, Smith D. Progress in SIFT-MS: Breath analysis and other applications. Mass Spectrometry Reviews. 2011;**30**(2):236-267

[33] Herbig J et al. On-line breath analysis with PTR-TOF. Journal of Breath Research. 2009; **3**(2):027004

[34] Nizio KD et al. In vitro volatile organic compound profiling using GCxGC-TOFMS to differentiate bacteria associated with lung infections: A proof-of-concept study. Journal of Breath Research. 2016;**10**(2):026008

[35] Smolinska A et al. The potential of volatile organic compounds for the detection of active disease in patients with ulcerative colitis. Alimentary Pharmacology & Therapeutics. 2017;**45**(9):1244-1254

[36] Buljubasic F, Buchbauer G. The scent of human diseases: A review on specific volatile organic compounds as diagnostic biomarkers. Flavour and Fragrance Journal. 2015;**30**(1): 5-25

[37] Chan HP, Lewis C, Thomas PS. Exhaled breath analysis: Novel approach for early detection of lung cancer. Lung Cancer. 2009;**63**(2):164-168

[38] Mazzatenta A et al. Volatile organic compounds (VOCs) fingerprint of Alzheimer's disease. Respiratory Physiology & Neurobiology. 2015;**209**:81-84

[39] Phillips M et al. Volatile biomarkers of pulmonary tuberculosis in the breath. Tuberculosis (Edinburgh, Scotland). 2007;**87**(1):44-52

[40] Syhre M et al. The scent of mycobacterium tuberculosis--part II breath. Tuberculosis (Edinburgh, Scotland). 2009;**89**(4):263-266

[41] Lechner MH, Tilg J. Rieder. Analysis of volatile compounds emitted by the Helicobacter pylori reference strain NCTC 11637 in vitro. Helicobacter. 2006;**11**(1):66

[42] Filipiak W et al. Molecular analysis of volatile metabolites released specifically by Staphylococcus Aureus and Pseudomonas Aeruginosa. BMC Microbiology. 2012;**12**:113

[43] Preti G et al. Volatile compounds characteristic of sinus-related bacteria and infected sinus mucus: Analysis by solid-phase microextraction and gas chromatography-mass spectrometry. Journal of Chromatography. B, Analytical Technologies in the Biomedical and Life Sciences. 2009;**877**(22):2011-2018

[44] Scott-Thomas AJ et al. 2-Aminoacetophenone as a potential breath biomarker for Pseudomonas Aeruginosa in the cystic fibrosis lung. BMC Pulmonary Medicine. 2010; **10**:56

[45] Shestivska V et al. Quantification of methyl thiocyanate in the headspace of Pseudomonas Aeruginosa cultures and in the breath of cystic fibrosis patients by selected ion flow tube mass spectrometry. Rapid Communications in Mass Spectrometry. 2011;**25**(17):2459-2467

[46] Savelev SU et al. Volatile biomarkers of Pseudomonas Aeruginosa in cystic fibrosis and noncystic fibrosis bronchiectasis. Letters in Applied Microbiology. 2011;**52**(6):610-613

[47] Karami N et al. Identification of bacteria using volatile organic compounds. Cellular and Molecular Biology (Noisy-le-Grand, France). 2017;**63**(2):112-121

[48] Gibson RL, Burns JL, Ramsey BW. Pathophysiology and management of pulmonary infections in cystic fibrosis. American Journal of Respiratory and Critical Care Medicine 2003;**168**(8):918-951

[49] Robroeks CM et al. Metabolomics of volatile organic compounds in cystic fibrosis patients and controls. Pediatric Research. 2010;**68**(1):75-80

[50] Shestivska V et al. Variability in the concentrations of volatile metabolites emitted by genotypically different strains of Pseudomonas Aeruginosa. Journal of Applied Microbiology. 2012;**113**(3):701-713

[51] Dryahina K et al. Differentiation of pulmonary bacterial pathogens in cystic fibrosis by volatile metabolites emitted by their in vitro cultures: Pseudomonas Aeruginosa, Staphylococcus Aureus, Stenotrophomonas maltophilia and the Burkholderia cepacia complex. Journal of Breath Research. 2016;**10**(3):037102

[52] Banday KM et al. Use of urine volatile organic compounds to discriminate tuberculosis patients from healthy subjects. Analytical Chemistry. 2011;**83**(14):5526-5534

[53] Syhre M, Chambers ST. The scent of mycobacterium tuberculosis. Tuberculosis (Edinburgh, Scotland). 2008;**88**(4):317-323

[54] Probert CS, Jones PR, Ratcliffe NM. A novel method for rapidly diagnosing the causes of diarrhoea. Gut. 2004;**53**(1):58-61

[55] Nasstrom E et al. Salmonella Typhi and salmonella Paratyphi a elaborate distinct systemic metabolite signatures during enteric fever. eLife. 2014;**3**

[56] Storer MK et al. Detection of volatile compounds produced by microbial growth in urine by selected ion flow tube mass spectrometry (SIFT-MS). Journal of Microbiological Methods. 2011;**87**(1):111-113

[57] Capelli L et al. Application and uses of electronic noses for clinical diagnosis on urine samples: A review. Sensors (Basel). 2016;**16**(10)

[58] Pavlou AK et al. Use of an electronic nose system for diagnoses of urinary tract infections. Biosensors & Bioelectronics. 2002;**17**(10):893-899

[59] Bos LD, Sterk PJ, Schultz MJ. Volatile metabolites of pathogens: A systematic review. PLoS Pathogens. 2013;**9**(5):e1003311

[60] Berna AZ et al. Analysis of breath specimens for biomarkers of plasmodium falciparum infection. The Journal of Infectious Diseases. 2015;**212**(7):1120-1128

[61] Allardyce RAHill AL, Murdoch DR. The rapid evaluation of bacterial growth and antibiotic susceptibility in blood cultures by selected ion flow tube mass spectrometry. Diagnostic Microbiology and Infectious Disease. 2006;**55**(4):255-261

[62] Trefz P et al. Volatile emissions from Mycobacterium avium subsp. paratuberculosis mirror bacterial growth and enable distinction of different strains. PLoS One. 2013;**8**(10): e76868

[63] Tait E et al. Identification of volatile organic compounds produced by bacteria using HS-SPME-GC-MS. Journal of Chromatographic Science. 2014;**52**(4):363-373

[64] Fend R et al. Prospects for clinical application of electronic-nose technology to early detection of mycobacterium tuberculosis in culture and sputum. Journal of Clinical Microbiology. 2006;**44**(6):2039-2045

[65] Scholpp J et al. Breath markers and soluble lipid peroxidation markers in critically ill patients. Clinical Chemistry and Laboratory Medicine. 2002;**40**(6):587-594

[66] Filipiak W et al. Dependence of exhaled breath composition on exogenous factors, smoking habits and exposure to air pollutants. Journal of Breath Research. 2012;**6**(3):036008

[67] Human Microbiome Project C. Structure, function and diversity of the healthy human microbiome. Nature. 2012;**486**(7402):207-214

Chapter 4

Biosensors: A Fast-Growing Technology for Pathogen Detection in Agriculture and Food Sector

Adetunji Charles Oluwaseun,
Paomipem Phazang and Neera Bhalla Sarin

Additional information is available at the end of the chapter

http://dx.doi.org/ 10.5772/intechopen.74668

Abstract

Agriculture and food have a greater role to play in order to achieve sustainable development goals. Therefore, there is a need to put an end to the effect of pathogens on food quality and safety. Pathogens have been recognized as one of the major factors causing a reduction in profitable food production. The conventional methods of detecting pathogens are time-consuming and expensive for the farmers in rural areas. In view of this, this chapter reviews the biosensors that have been developed for the detection of biological hazards in food and agricultural sectors. This chapter also lays emphasis on the impact of nanotechnology on building a fast, reliable, more sensitive, accessible, user-friendly and easily adaptable technology for illiterate farmers in the rural communities. On the whole, we have addressed the past and most recent biosensors that could ensure the quick delivery of vision 2030 which aims to end hunger and poverty.

Keywords: agriculture, food safety, pathogen, biosensor, nanotechnology

1. Introduction

Biosensor could be defined as an analytical device that produces a quantifiable signal proportional to the concentration of an analyte (i.e., pathogen or its cellular component or toxin molecule). The device comprises a transducer and biologically active elements or materials such as nucleic acids, enzyme, and an antibody that allows detection of an analyte by specific interactions [1]. Biosensors symbolize the end product of a quickly growing field, integrating fundamental and engineering and computer sciences to meet the urgent demands in various areas where its application is required [2–4]. There are different types of biosensors: acoustic, amperometric, electrochemical, optoelectric, calorimetric, potentiometric, immuno and piezoelectric. In this chapter, we report the earlier and recent trends in the usage of biosensors in the identification of pathogens that are responsible for biological hazards in food and agricultural sectors.

2. Traditional methods for pathogen detection in food and agricultural sectors

2.1. Polymerase chain reaction

The discovery and the development of polymerase chain reaction (PCR) have been a boon in the identification and characterization of pathogens [5–7] . PCR employs the following steps: isolation and purification of genomic DNA from plants or food-based pathogens, amplification of the target sequences followed by application of agarose gel electrophoresis for resolving the amplified products, and approximation of their fragment size by comparing with a standard DNA molecular mass marker [8].

The PCR is a nucleic-acid-based detection method. It is preferable than the other culture dependent techniques in the determination of microbial pathogens. The reasons being rapidity, accuracy, specificity, sensitivity, and the ability to identify small quantities of target nucleic acid in a given sample. It can also detect different pathogens in a single multiplex reaction. In addition, the detection of pathogens is not limited to the laboratory alone. Some portable PCR machines have been made available. The Smart Cycler is an example of portable PCR. It was developed to perform PCR for field identification of *Phytophthora ramorum* [9, 10]. Another example is the detection of *Sharka* virus in crude plant extracts of stone fruit trees, such as apricot, peach, and plum [11]. The International Plant Protection Convention has adapted this technique for the early detection of this devastating and destructive virus [12–14]. RT-PCR-based method has also been utilized to manage the emergence or presence of *Citrus tristeza* virus (a harmful virus causing tristeza syndrome in citrus) without any necessity for preparation of plant extracts or purifying nucleic acids [14–16]. This technique allows large-scale diagnoses thereby reducing the time and cost of analyses [12, 14].

Random amplified polymorphic DNA (RAPD) assays have been carried out on different isolates of *Fusarium poae* so as to discover the strain responsible for the head blight disease [17]. This method enabled them to identify markers common to all isolates. Turner et al. also performed RAPD profiling to screen and differentiate two different isolates of *Fusarium tricinctum* [18]. In another discovery, Schilling et al. utilized polymerase chain reaction to amplify, sequence and identify fungal pathogens *F. culmorum, F. graminearum,* and *F. avenaceum* [19]. Fraaije et al. invented a multiplex PCR assay that can sense and quantify pathogenic fungi, *S. tritici* causing leaf blotch; and *S. nodorum* causing leaf and glume blot, in wheat [20]. A TaqMan real-time PCR method has also been used to evaluate different species of *Fusarium* in wheat kernels [21, 22].

2.2. Culture and colony counting

The culture methods of identifying pathogens from food and agricultural based products involve the morphological and biochemical identification by staining and studying the metabolic profile of the pathogens. These methods require determination of the most suitable media that would favor their growth at different conditions. This may involve pre-enrichment, selective enrichment, biochemical screening, and serological confirmation. The major problems associated with using cultures for identifying pathogens are the high cost of media and the laborious and time-consuming techniques. In addition, they are not feasible for on the spot and real-time or rapid sensoring/identification of threat agents [23].

2.3. Immunology-based method

The immunological approaches for the detection of pathogens work on the principle of specific affinity between microbial antigens and monoclonal or polyclonal antibodies. They are used for rapid detection and identification of pathogens, including bacteria, viruses, fungus as well as their toxins. This method is very sensitive, rapid, selective and cost-effective. Latex agglutination and enzyme-linked immunosorbent assay (ELISA) are the techniques majorly used in food industry for identification of food pathogens like *Listeria monocytogenes, Salmonella, Campylobacter, Escherichia coli* O157: H7, *Listeria* and *Shigella, Staphylococcus aureus* [24].

2.4. Hand-held immunochromatographic assays (HHIA)

The hand-held immunochromatographic assays (test strips) are normally used for tentative or preliminary identification, both on-site and in laboratories. The test strips consist of nitrocellulose membrane immobilized with specific antibodies followed by a second antibody that is coupled to the colored particle. The liquid sample containing the analyte is then allowed to mix with the antibody-coupled colored particle. The analyte binds to the antibody-coupled particle and this complex migrate by capillary action along the nitrocellulose strip until it meets the immobilized antibody. The interaction produces a visible colored line indicating a positive result and vice versa. This type of assay takes only about 15 min to perform and the result can be read visually without any instruments. Therefore this detection technique is especially suitable for on-site identification. However, HHIA have two major limitations; limitation in the number of biological hazards that can be detected per strip and display of varying sensitivity levels with their respective target agents [25].

3. Biosensors used for pathogen detection in food and agricultural sector

3.1. Detection of food pathogens

Liébana et al. have developed a quick and simple biosensor based on electrochemical magnet immunosensing with *magnetic graphite-epoxy composite* (m-GEC) electrodes for the recognition of *Salmonella* in milk. The graphite-epoxy composite maintains a unique hybridization property that allows immediate immobilization of the DNA of the pathogens. This technique has a greater advantage over the cultural and biochemical/serological methods of detecting pathogens, as they do not require reagents and offers quick detection [26–30]. Based on this principle, Pividori and Alegret have also invented a biosensor that can detect the presence of b-lactamase resistance in *Staphylococcus aureus* [31]. Oliveira Marques et al. invented a gold nanoparticle-based biosensor with graphite-epoxy composite electrodes for the identification of *Salmonella* IS200 [32]. A double-tagged PCR strategy had been used for the detection of pathogenic bacteria, enterohemorrhagic *E. coli* O157: H7. The biosensor works on electrochemical magnet genosensing and allows electrochemical real-time quantification of an amplicon [33]. Ricci et al. have developed an electrochemical biosensor that can detect pathogens such as *Escherichia coli, Salmonella typhimurium,* and *Listeria monocytogenes* in milk [34].

Majumdar et al. developed an amperometric biosensor which was able to detect *Staphylococcus aureus* in food samples such as milk, cheese, and meat [35]. Banada et al. utilized light scattering sensors for the detection of microorganisms in vegetable and meat samples [36]. Shriver-Lake et al. also used an optical (fluorescence)-based portable Naval Research Laboratory (NRL) array biosensor that can sense the presence of *Salmonella typhimurium* in milk and apple juice within 45 min [37]. Karsunke et al. invented a multiplexing optical (luminescence) biosensor which can sense the presence of *E. coli* O157: H7, *S. typhimurium* and *Legionella pneumophila* in any sample in a disposable microarray format. In their discovery, immunospecific antibodies were immobilized in a microarray format [38]. Several authors have described many multiplexing biosensors that make use of polymerase chain reaction. Koets et al. in their study developed the use of magnetoresistance biosensor that can sense the presence of *E. coli* and four different antibiotic-resistant genes in *Salmonella* spp. along with a double-tagged PCR amplification step [39]. Bai et al. used a biosensor that has a microarray approach with biospecific DNA probes immobilized on a sensor surface for the sensing of 11 food-borne pathogens present in beef and pork meat [40]. Schütz et al. developed a biosensor that can detect the volatile compounds emitted by the pathogenic fungus *Phytophthora infestans* that is responsible for spoilage in potatoes [41].

3.2. Detection of animal, poultry, and dairy pathogens

Ellis et al. were able to develop a sensor that could detect breath-derived 500 volatile organic compounds. The analysis helped in identifying Bovine tuberculosis (*M. bovis*) in affected cattles [42]. Tarasov et al. developed a direct potentiometric biosensor that could detect Bovine Herpes Virus-1 viral protein. The biosensor is sensitive and selective to anti-IgE present in commercially available anti-Bovine Herpes Virus-1 antiserum as well as in real serum samples from cattle. The biosensor can also be easily used with *point-of-care* devices and ELISA [43]. ELISA and PCR-based methods have been utilized for quick detection of bovine viral diarrhea virus, especially for the onsite monitoring and early diagnosis of the bovine viral diarrhea virus infection in animals [44, 45]. In addition, Luo et al. have established an electrospun biosensor which works on the principle of capillary separation and conductometric immunoassay for the early sensing of bovine viral antibodies where the sensing time takes 8 minutes [46]. Microparticle immunoagglutination assay on a microfluidic chip using forward light scattering measurements have also been developed to sense the presence of bovine virus particles [47]. A new biosensor with a miniaturized gold electrode which works on impedance spectroscopy that can detect the presence of H7N1 has also been developed [48, 49]. Xu et al. have developed an interferometric biosensor immunoassay which can sense different avian influenza strains, especially H7 and H8 [50]. Bai et al. also developed a simple and portable biosensor with DNA aptamers as recognition elements in portable surface plasmon resonance (SPR) which can sense the presence of H5N1 available in poultry swab samples [51]. Ye et al. have also developed a biosensor that is based on the principle of Luminescence 645 resonance energy transfer for the quick detection of H7 strain [52], while Guo et al. developed a biosensor which consists of an indium-tin-oxide thin-film transistors built on a glass substrate for immune detection of H5N1 antibodies [53]. Lum et al. developed a nano-based biosensor that works on the principles of immune magnetic nanoparticles for the detection of H5 subtype virus [54].

Neitzel et al. have developed a biosensor that can detect the presence of mastitis in any milk product [55]. Duarte et al. had also developed a biosensor that couples immune assay with magnetic nanoparticles [56]. Fűtő et al. developed selective amperometric methods that could sense the presence of spoilt and affected milk [57]. The spore-based biosensor is another novel strategy that has been developed to detect the presence of contaminants, including aflatoxins, antibiotics and microbial pathogens in milk. Balhara et al. developed a biosensor that can detect the presence of *L. monocytogenes* and *Listeria* spp. in milk products. This sensor employs the enzyme-substrate reaction that produces a color change and can be easily visualized [58]. Kumar et al. had also developed a biosensor that utilized two-stage enzyme assay for the detection of *Enterococci* spp. in milk [59].

3.3. Detection of pathogens in plants

A high-density microelectrode array biosensor was developed by Radke and Alocilja [60]. The biosensor can detect *E. coli* O157: H7 bacteria in food materials. They discovered that change in impedance of the biosensor is directly proportional to the number of bacteria on the biosensor surface. They detected up to 10 cells of *E. coli* O157: H7 by testing the biosensor in different concentrations of bacteria in lettuce. The advantage of this sensor is that it is field-deployable, easy to use, portable, and reagent-less and provides result in minutes compared to hours or days in conventional methods. Kim and Park developed a flow-type antibody sensor using quartz crystal microbalance chip as biological component and transducer to detect *E. coli* in drinking water, beef, pork, and dumpling. The developed sensor measures frequency changes due to mass deposits which are produced by antigen-antibody interaction [61]. Mendes et al. developed a biosensor that can detect the pathogenic fungus *Phakopsora pachyrhizi* that had been reported to cause Soybean rust [62]. Papadakis et al. also had developed an acoustic-based biosensor (the Quartz Crystal Microbalance) that could sense three out of the most reported plant pathogens, i.e., *Ralstonia solanacearum, Pseudomonas syringae pv tomato* and *Xanthomonas campestris pv. Vesicatoria* [63].

3.4. Detection of mycotoxins

Carlson et al. developed a fluorometric biosensor to detect and quantify aflatoxins. These toxins are produced by a family of fungi and are commonly found in a variety of agricultural products. The device developed by Carlson et al. operates on the principle of immunoaffinity for specificity and fluorescence for a quantitative assay [64]. Pohanka et al. and Ben Rejeb et al. used Electrochemical (amperometric) antibody-based biosensor to detect the presence of Aflatoxin B1 in spices and olive oil respectively [65, 66]. Wang et al. used an electrochemical (amperometric) antibody/enzyme biosensor to detect Aflatoxin M1 in milk [67]. Asuncion

Alonso-Lomillo et al. used an electrochemiluminescent aptamer biosensor to detect the presence of Ochratoxin A in beer and coffee samples [68]. Panini et al. used electrochemical (amperometric) antibody biosensor to detect the presence of zearalenone in corn silage [69]. The presence of deoxynivalenol, T-2, and HT-2 toxins was also detected in cereals and baby food with the help of optical (SPR) antibody biosensor [70, 71].

4. Application of nanotechnology-based sensors in agriculture and food sectors

4.1. Nanomaterial-based sensors for food industry

The food industry as mentioned earlier is continuously challenged by the occurrences of foodborne diseases. WHO in its report for the year (2015) estimated 420,000 deaths occurring every year due to consumption of contaminated food, of which 125,000 deaths are of children under the age of 5, bearing a 40% burden of foodborne diseases [72]. Foodborne disease can be defined as "any disease usually either infectious or toxic in nature, caused by agents that enter the body through ingestion of food." The causal agents are bacteria, viruses, and protozoa, fungal or bacterial toxins, metal ions, and pesticides. Some of the important pathogenic organisms categorized are *Staphylococcus aureus, Bacillus cereus, Campylobacter jejuni, Clostridium botulinum, Clostridium perfringens, Escherichia coli, Brucella, Listeria monocytogenes, Salmonella typhi* and *paratyphi, Shigella* spp., *Vibrio cholerae, Vibrio parahaemolyticus* [73]. In spite of the advances in healthcare, food-borne diseases are likely to remain a global phenomenon even in the next decade. The contributing factors are urbanization and changes in consumer habits, increased demand for food varieties resulting in a global food cuisine trade, changes in agricultural practices and food processing methods and climate change. The WHO has thus placed food safety as one of its top 11 priorities [74]. In order to manage and contain foodborne diseases, it is important to develop low cost ready to use tests for immediate detection of pathogenic contamination or presence of toxins that would replace the conventional methods. Some of the conventional methods that are routinely used are PCR based methods and immunoassay-based techniques.

These methods are robust and sensitive as they allow the detection of pathogens by targeting specific nucleic acids or proteins. However, the requirement of an expensive instrument and chemical reagents, experienced personnel, large sample preparation and slow generation time prevent the immediate detection of pathogens thus delaying preventive treatment in patients [75, 76]. Thus, the shift has been to the development of easy to use, rapid and sensitive on the site detection and also stable and portable detecting kits. Nanotechnology has paved way for such developments in the last decade. The versatility of nanomaterials has made possible the development of sensors in the food industry for monitoring the environment and food quality [77]. Some of the advancements in the design and development of nanoparticle-based sensors for food safety are discussed below.

4.1.1. Gold nanoparticle (AuNP)-based sensors

E. coli O157: H7 is the serotype among *E. coli* strains associated with foodborne diseases. A circulating flow piezoelectric biosensor (PEB) was developed to detect *E. coli* O157: H7. The

PEB has *E. coli* O157: H7 *eaeA* gene specific AuNP-conjugated thiolated probe that acts as mass enhancer and sequence verifier. The detection limit obtained in PEB is 1.2×10^2 CFU/mL in the linear working range of 10^2–10^6 CFU/mL [78]. The AuNP conjugated with *E. coli* O157: H7 antibodies were also developed for detecting *E. coli* O157: H7 in milk. Screen printed carbon electrodes (SPCE) having 13 nm AuNP were fabricated with *E. coli* O157: H7 specific antibodies conjugated with horseradish. Hydrogen peroxide and ferrocene dicarboxylic acid (FeDC) were used as substrates. AuNP and FeDC enhance the detection limit to 10^2–10^7 CFU/mL [79]. The AuNP based electrochemical immunoassay was also developed for detecting *S. typhimurium* [80]. Polystyrene immobilized with *S. typhimurium* specific monoclonal antibodies that were further layered with AuNP-conjugated polyclonal antibodies were used as the probe. In the presence of copper enhancer solution and ascorbic acid, the bacteria bind to the AuNP-conjugated polyclonal antibodies. The copper released upon reduction, bind to the AuNP thus allowing direct detection of *S. typhimurium* by anodic stripping voltammetry. The detection limit for this AuNP based immunoassay is 98.9 CFU/mL. Colorimetric based AuNP-conjugated with anti-Salmonella antibody has also been developed for detecting and selectively targeting *S. typhimurium* [81]. The AuNP based sensors were also developed for detecting mycotoxins in food products. AuNP-aptasensor for detecting aflatoxinB1 was developed by Hosseini et al. [82]. The presence of aflatoxin destabilizes the AuNP-aptamer and causes aggregation of AuNP. The color change from yellow to purple allows the detection of the presence of the toxins. Similar AuNP-aptasensor for detecting Aflatoxin B2 was developed by Luan et al. The detection here was also based on colorimetric method [83].

4.1.2. Magnetic nanoparticle (MNP)-based sensors

Magnetic nanoparticle-derived sensors are one of the widely used sensors for detecting and removing food contaminants. The large surface area of MNPs makes them one of the best supports for immobilization of functionalized surface groups thereby improving the loading control and immobilization efficiency [84]. D-mannose functionalized MNPs were used for detecting *E. coli* cells at 10^4 cells/mL. These modified MNPs when incubated with fluorescently labeled concanavalin allowed the magnetic separation and visualization of the cells [85]. Antibody conjugated MNPs were developed to detect *Salmonella* in milk. The immobilized antibodies allowed the capturing of the bacteria that are further separated by application of magnetic field. The separated cells are then exposed to antibody immobilized TiO_2 nanocrystals. Thus, the antibody-MNP-TiO_2 nanocrystals are magnetically separated and the unbound TiO_2 nanocrystals are determined using the UV-visible spectrophotometer. A detection limit of 100 CFU/mL was obtained from milk samples [86]. Amine functionalized MNPs were also developed for rapid detection and capturing of both gram-positive and gram-negative bacteria from water and food matrices. Organisms that showed high adsorption affinity are *Sarcina lutea, S. aureus, E. coli, B. cereus, B. subtilis, Salmonella, P. vulgaris,* and *P. aeruginosa.* It was shown that the amount of amine functionalized MNPs and the ionic strength of the buffer was crucial for mediating fast and effective interaction [87].

4.1.3. Quantum dots (QD)-based sensors

Semiconductor QDs show size-dependent optical and electronic properties making them most suitable for fluorometric-based sensors [88]. The most commonly used are the CdSe quantum dots [89]. The QD-derived fluorescent biosensor was developed for detecting *S. typhimurium* in chicken carcass wash water. Magnetic beads coated with anti-Salmonella antibody was used for capturing the bacteria that was further made to react with a biotin-labeled anti-Salmonella antibody. This facilitated the reaction of biotin to the streptavidin-coated QDs. The fluorescence intensity is a direct measure of the cell number in the sample. The detection limit obtained was about 10^3 CFU/mL [90]. The CdSe QDs derived sensors were also developed for detection of *Cholera*, *Shiga* toxin and *Staphylococcal* enterotoxin A.

4.2. Nanomaterial-based biosensors for agriculture

The use of nanobiosensors has been regarded as the more advantageous approach for detecting pathogens in healthcare and food industry as mentioned above. Their rapid and high sensitivity further extends their application in agriculture for disease assessment. Fluorescent silica nanoparticles (FSNP) conjugated with antibodies were successfully used for detecting plant pathogens such as *Xanthomonas axonopodis pv. vesicatoria* which causes bacterial spot disease in tomatoes and peppers [91]. Copper oxide (CuO) nanoparticles have been used in the detection of the *A. niger* fungi [92]. In addition, silver-based nanoparticles, AgNPs are commonly used for detecting contaminants and microbial pathogens in the soil and water bodies. Thus the use of nanosensors has allowed plant disease forecasting and disease management in agriculture to an admissible level [93].

5. Recommendations and future trends

There is a need to develop biosensors that would be effective and reliable for the routine utilization especially in the area of food and agriculture. Therefore, there is a need to develop biosensor that has the following characteristics in one device: hand-held, and portable, viable cell countability, single button device, easy utilization, accurate strain and species determination, selectivity and short detection time. And most importantly, the biosensor must be inexpensive with simple configuration for access to the illiterate farmers in developing countries.

6. Conclusions

Because of the useful features of biosensors, their utilization in the bio-monitoring of biological hazards, commonly recorded in agriculture and food sectors has been necessitated. The constant application of pesticides in controlling pathogens has led not only to pathogen resistance but also, bioaccumulation and biomagnification of the chemicals with subsequent health hazards and environmental pollution. Therefore, the demand for biosensors in the market has increased tremendously. Biosensors should be within the reach of food handlers and agro-allied industries to enable them to monitor and determine the presence of pathogens in their food and agricultural products.

http://dx.doi.org/ 10.5772/intechopen.74668

Acknowledgements

The authors are grateful to the Department of Biotechnology (DBT), New Delhi, India, The World Academy of Science (TWAS) for TWAS-DBT post-doctoral given to Dr. Adetunji. FR number: 3240293141.

Conflict of interest

The authors declare no conflict of interest.

Author details

Adetunji Charles Oluwaseun[1,2*], Paomipem Phazang[2] and Neera Bhalla Sarin[2]

*Address all correspondence to: charliguitar@yahoo.com; adetunjicharles@gmail.com

1 Department of Biological Sciences, Applied Microbiology, Biotechnology and Nanotechnology Laboratory, Landmark University, Omu Aran, Kwara State, Nigeria

2 School of Life Sciences, Laboratory of Genetic Manipulation for Stress Alleviation and Value Addition in Plants, Jawaharlal Nehru University, New Delhi, India

References

[1] Songa EA, Vernon SS, Tesfaye W, Priscilla GLB, Emmanuel II. Amperometric nanobiosensor for determination of glyphosate and glufosinate residues in corn and soya bean samples. Pure and Applied Chemistry. 2009;**81**:123-139

[2] Belkin S. Microbial whole-cell sensing systems of environmental pollutants. Current Opinion in Microbiology. 2003;**6**:206-212

[3] Eggins BR. Chemical Sensors and Biosensors. Chichester: John Wiley; 2002

[4] Wilson JS. Sensor Technology Handbook. Amsterdam/Boston: Elsevier; 2005

[5] Louws FJ, Rademaker JLW, de Bruijn FJ. The three ds of PCR-based genomic analysis of phytobacteria: Diversity, detection, and disease diagnosis. Annual Review of Phytopathology. 1999;**37**:81-125

[6] López MM, Bertolini E, Olmos A, Caruso P, Gorris MT, Llop P, Penyalver R, Cambra M. Innovative tools for detection of plant pathogenic viruses and bacteria. International Microbiology. 2003;**6**:233-43

[7] Palacio-Bielsa A, Cambra MA, Lypez MM. PCR detection and identification of plant pathogenic bacteria: Updated review of protocols (1989-2007). Journal of Plant Pathology. 2009;**91**:249-97

[8] Greiner R, Konietzny U. Presence of genetically modified maize and soy in food products sold commercially in Brazil from 2000 to 2005. Food Control. 2008;**19**:499-505

[9] Higgins JA, Nasarabadi S, Karns JS, Shelton DR, Cooper M, Gbakima A, Koopman RP. A handheld real time thermal cycler for bacterial pathogen detection. Biosensors and Bioelectronics. 2003;**18**:1115

[10] Tomlinsson JA, Boonham N, Hughes KJD, Griffin RL, Barker I. On-site DNA extraction and real-time PCR for detection of *Phytophthora ramorum* in the field. Applied and Environmental Microbiology. 2005;**71**:6702-6710

[11] García JA, Cambra M. *Plum pox virus* and sharka disease. Plant Viruses. 2007;**1**:69-79

[12] Capote N, Bertolini E, Olmos A, Vidal E, Martinez C, Cambra M. Direct sample preparation methods for the detection of plum pox virus by real-time RT-PCR, validation and practice parameters. International Microbiology. 2009;**12**:1-6

[13] IPPC-FAO. Diagnostics protocols for regulated pests. Plum pox virus. International Standards for Phytosanitary Measures. (ISPM). 2010;**27**:2011

[14] Vidal E, Moreno A, Bertolini E, Cambra M. Estimation of the accuracy of two diagnostic methods for the detection of plum pox virus in nursery blocks by latent class models. Plant Pathology. 2012;**61**:413-422

[15] Bertolini E, Moreno A, Capote N, Olmos A, de Luis A. Quantitative detection of citrus tristeza virus in plant tissues and single aphids by real-time RT-PCR. European Journal of Plant Pathology. 2008;**120**:177-188

[16] Cambra M, Bertolini E, Olmos A, Capote N. Molecular methods for detection and quantitation of virus in aphids. In: Cooper I, Kuehne T, Polischuk V, editors. Virus Diseases and Crop Biosecurity. Springer: Dordrecht, The Netherlands; 2006. pp. 81-88

[17] Parry DW, Nicholson P. Development of a PCR assay to Detect *F .poae* in wheat. Plant Pathology. 1996;**45**:383-391

[18] Turner AS, Leesb AK, Rezanoora HN, Nicholsona P. Refinement of PCR-detection of *Fusarium avenaceum* and evidence from DNA marker studies for phonetic relatedness to *Fusarium tricinctum*. Plant Pathology. 1998;**47**:278-288

[19] Schilling AG, Moller EM, Geiger HH. Polymerase chain reaction-based assays for species specific detection of *Fusarium culmorum, F. graminearum* and *F. avenaceum*. Molecular Plant Pathology. 1996;**86**:515-522

[20] Fraaije BA, Lovell DJ, Coelho JM, Baldwin S, Hollomon DW. PCR-based assays to assess wheat varietal resistance to blotch (*Septoria tritici* and *Stagonospora nodorum*) and rust (*Puccinia striiformis* and *Puccinia recondita*) diseases. European Journal of Plant Pathology. 2001;**107**:905-917

[21] Heid CA, Stevens J, Livak KJ, Williams PM. Real time quantitative PCR. Genome Research. 1996;**6**:986-994

[22] Waalwijk C, van der Heide R, de Vries I, van der Lee T, Schoen C, Costrel-Decorainville G, Haeuser-Hahn I, Kastelein P, Kohl J, Lonnet P, Demarquet T, GHJ K. Quantitative detection of Fusarium species in wheat using TaqMan. European Journal of Plant Pathology. 2004;**110**(5-6):481-494

[23] Tietjen M, Fung DYC. Salmonellae and food safety. Critical Reviews in Microbiology. 1995;**21**:53-83

[24] Crowther JR. ELISA, Theory and Practice. Totowa, NJ: Human Press Inc; 1995

[25] Zhang G, Guo J, Wang X. Immunochromatographic lateral flow strip tests. Methods in Molecular Biology. 2009;**504**:169-183

[26] Liébana S, Lermo A, Campoy S, Cortés M-P, Alegret S, Pividori MI. Rapid detection of salmonella in milk by electrochemical magneto-immunosensing. Biosensors and Bioelectronics. 2009;**25**:510-513

[27] Pividori MI, Alegret S. Graphite-epoxy platforms for electrochemical genosensing. Analytical Letters. 2003;**36**:1669-1695

[28] Pividori MI, Merkoçi A, Alegret S. Graphite-epoxy composites as a new transducing material for electrochemical genosensing. Biosensors and Bioelectronics. 2003;**19**:473

[29] Pividori MI, Merkoçi A, Barbé J, Alegret S. PCR genosensor rapid test for detecting salmonella. Electroanalysis. 2003;**15**:1815-1823

[30] Pividori MI, Alegret S. DNA adsorption on carbonaceous materials. In: Wittman C, editor. Topics in Current Chemistry. Vol. 260. Berlin: Springer; 2005. pp. 1-36

[31] Pividori MI, Alegret S. Electrochemical genosensing based on rigid carbon composites. A review. Analytical Letters. 2005;**38**:2541-2565

[32] Oliveira Marques PRB, Lermo A, Campoy S, Yamanaka H, Barbé J, Alegret S, Pividori MI. Double-tagging polymerase chain reaction with a thiolated primer and electrochemical genosensing based on gold nanocomposite sensor for food safety. Analytical Chemistry. 2009;**81**:1332-1339

[33] Lermo A, Zacco E, Barak J, Delwiche M, Campoy S, Barbé J, Alegret S, Pividori MI. Towards Q-PCR of pathogenic bacteria with improved electrochemical double-tagged genosensing detection. Biosensors and Bioelectronics. 2008;**23**:1805-1811

[34] Ricci F, Volpe G, Micheli L, Palleschi G. A review on novel developments and applications of immunosensors in food analysis. Analytica Chimica Acta. 2007;**605**:111-129

[35] Majumdar T, Agarwal S, Chakraborty R, Raychaudhuri U. Study on electrochemical immunoassay methodology for protein a: A modified approach towards detection and quantification of Staphylococcus Aureus in food samples. Research Journal of chemical Sciences. 2012;**2**:62-68

[36] Banada PP, Huff K, Bae E, Rajwa B, Aroonnual A, Bayraktar B, Adil A, Robinson JP, Hirleman ED, Bhunia AK. Label-free detection of multiple bacterial pathogenusing light-scattering sensor. Biosensors and Bioelectronics. 2009;**24**:1685-1692

[37] Shriver-Lake LC, Erickson JS, Sapsford KE, Ngundi MM, Shaffer KM, Kulagina NV, Hu JE, Gray SA, Golden JP, Ligler FS, Taitt CR. Blind laboratory trials for multiple pathogens in spiked food matrices. Analytical Letters. 2007;**40**(16-18):3219-3231

[38] Karsunke XYZ, Niessner R, Seidel M. Development of a multichannel flow-through chemiluminescence microarray chip for parallel calibration and detection of pathogenic bacteria. Analytical and Bioanalytical Chemistry. 2009;**395**:1623-1630

[39] Koets M, van der Wijk T, van Eemeren JTWM, van Amerongen A, Prins MWJ. Rapid DNA multi-analyte immunoassay on a magneto-resistance biosensor. Biosensors & Bioelectronics. 2009;**24**:1893-1898

[40] Bai S, Zhao J, Zhang Y, Huang W, Xu S, Chen H, Fan LM, Chen Y, Deng XW. Rapid and reliable detection of 11 food-borne pathogens using thin-film biosensor chips. Applied Microbiology and Biotechnology. 2010;**86**:983-990

[41] Schütz S, Weißbecker B, Koch UT, Hummel HE. Detection of volatiles released by diseased potato tubers using a biosensor on the basis of intact insect antennae. Biosensors & Bioelectronics. 1999;**14**:221-228

[42] Ellis CK, Stahl RS, Nol P, Waters WR, Palmer MV, Rhyan JC, Ver Cauteren KC, McCollum M, Salman MD. A pilot study exploring the use of breath analysis to differentiate healthy cattle from cattle experimentally infected with *Mycobacterium bovis*. PLoS One. 2014;**9**(2):e89280

[43] Tarasov A, Gray DW, Tsai MY, Shields N, Montrose A, Creedon N, Lovera P, O'Riordan A, Mooney MH, Vogel EM. Biosensors and Bioelectronics. 2016;**79**:669-678. DOI: 10.1016/j.bios.2015.12.086. Epub 2015 Dec 24

[44] Da Silva N, Zardoya R, Santurde G, Solana A, Castro J. Rapid and sensitive detection of the bovine viral diarrhea virus genome in semen. Journal of Virological Methods. 1995;**55**(2):209-218

[45] Pritchard G, Kirkwood G, Sayers A. Detecting antibodies to infectious bovine Rhinotracheitis and BVD virus infections using milk samples from individual cows. Veterinary Record. 2002;**150**(6):182-183

[46] Luo Y, Nartker S, Miller H, Hochhalter D, Wiederoder M, Wiederoder S, Setterington E, Drzal LT, Alocilja EC. Surface functionalization of electrospun nanofibers for detecting *E. coli* O157:H7 and BVDV cells in a direct-charge transfer biosensor. Biosensors and Bioelectronics. 2010;**26**(4):1612-1617

[47] Heinze BC, Song JY, Lee CH, Najam A, Yoon JY. Microfluidic immunosensor for rapid and sensitive detection of bovine viral diarrhea virus. Sensors and Actuators B: Chemical. 2009;**138**(2):491-496

[48] Diouani MF, Helali S, Hafaid I, Hassen WM, Snoussi MA, Ghram A, Jaffrezic-Renault N, Abdelghani A. Miniaturized biosensor for avian influenza virus detection. Materials Science and Engineering. 2008;**C28**(5-6):580-583

[49] Wang R, Wang Y, Lassiter K, Li Y, Hargis B, Tung S, Berghman L, Bottje W. Interdigitated array microelectrode based impedance immunosensor for detection of avian influenza virus H5N1. Talanta. 2009;**79**(2):159-164

[50] Xu J, Suarez D, Gottfried DS. Detection of avian influenza virus using and interferometric biosensor. Analytical and Bioanalytical Chemistry. 2007;**389**(4):1193-1199

[51] Bai H, Wang R, Hargis B, Lu H, Li Y. A SPR Aptasensor for detection of avian influenza virus H5N1. Sensors. 2012;**12**(9):12506-12518

[52] Ye WW, Tsang MK, Liu X, Yang M, Hao J. Upconversion luminescence resonance energy transfer (LRET)-based biosensor for rapid and ultrasensitive detection of avian influenza virus H7 subtype. Small. 2014;**10**(12):2390-2397

[53] Guo D, Zhuo M, Zhang X, Xu C, Jiang J, Gao F, Wan Q, Li Q, Wang T. Indium-tin-oxide thin film transistor biosensors for label-free detection of avian influenza virus H5N1. Analytica Chimica Acta. 2013;**773**:83-88

[54] Lum J, Wang R, Lassiter K, Srinivasan B, Abi-Ghanem D, Berghman L, Hargis B, Tung S, Lu H, Li Y. Rapid detection of avian influenza H5N1 virus using impedance measurement of immuno-reaction coupled with RBC amplification. Biosensors and Bioelectronics. 2012;**38**(1):67-73

[55] Neitzel AC, Stamer E, Junge W, Thaller G. Calibration of an automated California mastitis test with focus on the device-dependent variation. Springer Plus. 2014;**3**:760

[56] Duarte C, Costa T, Carneiro C, Soares R, Jitariu A, Cardoso S, Piedade M, Bexiga R, Freitas P. Semi-quantitative method for streptococci magnetic detection in raw milk. Biosensors. 2016;**6**:19

[57] Fűtő P, Markus G, Kiss A, Adányi N. Development of a catalase-based amperometric biosensor for the determination of increased catalase content in milk samples. Electroanalysis. 2015;**24**(1):107-113. DOI: 10.1002/elan.201100399

[58] Balhara M, Kumar N, Thakur G, Raghu HV, Singh VK, Lawania R, Khan AS. Novel enzyme substrate based bio-assay for real time detection of *L. monocytogenes* in milk system. Indian Patent reg. No. 1357/DEL/2014. Published in Indian patent Journal Publication no. 50/2014 date 12th Dec 2014. 2014

[59] Kumar N, Kaur G, Thakur G, Raghu H V, Singh NA, Raghav N, Singh VK. Real-time detection of Enterococci in dairy foods using spore germination based bioassay. Indian patent publication no. 19/2015 Date: 08/05/2015 (119/DEL/2012). 2012

[60] Radke SM, Alocilja EC. A high density microelectrode array biosensor for detection of *E. coil* O157:H7. Biosensors & Bioelectronics. 2005;**20**:1662-1667

[61] Kim N, Park I. Application of a flow-type antibody sensor to the detection of *Escherichia coli* in various foods. Biosensors & Bioelectronics. 2003;**18**:1101-1107

[62] Mendes RK, Carvalhal RF, Machado SDR, Kubota LT. Surface plasmon resonance immunosensor for early diagnosis of Asian rust on soybean leaves. Biosensors and Bioelectronics. 2009;**24**:2483-2487

[63] Papadakis G, Skandalis N, Dimopoulou A, Glynos P, Gizeli E. Bacteria murmur: Application of an acoustic biosensor for plant pathogen detection. PLoS One. 2015;**10**(7):e0132773

[64] Carlson MA, Bargeron CB, Benson RC, Fraser AB, Phillips TE, Velky JT, Groopman JD, Strickland PT, Ko HW. An automated, handheld biosensor for aflatoxin. Biosensors & Bioelectronics. 2000;**14**:841-848

[65] Pohanka M, Malir F, Roubal T, Kuca K. Detection of aflatoxins in capsicum spice using an electrochemical immunosensor. Analytical Letters. 2008;**41**:2344-2353

[66] Ben Rejeb I, Arduini F, Arvinte A, Amine A, Gargouri M, Micheli L, Bala C, Moscone M, Palleschi G. Development of a bio-electrochemical assay for AFB detection in olive oil. Biosensors & Bioelectronics. 2009;**24**:1962-1968

[67] Wang Y, Dostalek J, Knoll W. Long range surface plasmon-enhanced fluorescence spectroscopy for the detection of aflatoxin M-1 in milk. Biosensors & Bioelectronics. 2009;**24**: 2264-2267

[68] Asuncion Alonso-Lomillo M, Dominguez-Renedo O, Ferreira-Goncalves L, Julia Arcos-Martinez M. Sensitive enzyme-biosensor based on screen-printed electrodes for ochratoxin a. Biosensors & Bioelectronics. 2010;**25**:1333-1337

[69] Panini NV, Bertolino FA, Salinas E, Messina GA, Raba J. Zearalenone determination in corn silage samples using an immunosensor in a continuous-flow/stopped-flow systems. Biochemical Engineering Journal. 2010;**51**:7-13

[70] Meneely J, Fodey T, Armstrong L, Sulyok M, Krska R, Elliott C. Rapid surface plasmon resonance immunoassay for the determination of deoxynivalenol in wheat, wheat products, and maize-based baby food. Journal of Agricultural and Food Chemistry. 2010;**58**:8936-8941

[71] Meneely JP, Sulyok M, Baumgartner S, Krska R, Elliott CT. A rapid optical immunoassay for the screening of T-2 and HT-2 toxin in cereals and maize-based baby food. Talanta. 2010;**81**:630-636

[72] WHO. WHO estimates the burden of food borne diseases. 2015. http://www.who.int/foodsafety/areas_work/foodborne-diseases/ferg/en/

[73] Kaittanis C, Santra S, Perez JM. Emerging nanotechnology-based strategies for the identification of microbial pathogenesis. Advanced Drug Delivery Reviews. 2010;**62**: 408-423

[74] Salyers AA, Whitt DD. Bacterial Pathogenesis: A Molecular Approach. 2nd ed. Washington DC: ASM Press; 2002

[75] Valdes MG, ACV G, JAG C, Díaz-García ME. Analytical nanotechnology for food analysis. Microchimica Acta. 2009;**166**:1-19

[76] Cheng WC, Kuo CW, Chi TY, Lin LC, Lee CH, Feng RL, Tsai SJ. Investigation on the trend of food-borne disease outbreaks in Taiwan (1991-2010). Journal of Food and Drug Analysis. 2013;**21**:261-267

[77] Pérez-López B, Merkoçi A. Nanomaterials based biosensors for food analysis applications. Trends in Food Science and Technology. 2011;**2**:625-639

[78] Chen SH, Wu VC, Chuang YC. Using oligonucleotide-functionalized Au nanoparticles to rapidly detect foodborne pathogens on a piezoelectric biosensor. Journal of Microbiological Methods. 2008;**73**:7-17

[79] Lin YH, Chen SH, Chuang YC, Lu YC, Shen TY, Chang CA, Lin CS. Disposable amperometric immunosensing strips fabricated by au nanoparticles-modified screen-printed carbon electrodes for the detection of foodborne pathogen *Escherichia coli* O157:H7. Biosensors & Bioelectronics. 2008;**23**:1832-1837

[80] Dungchai W, Siangproh W, Chaicumpa W, Tongtawe P, Chailapakul O. Salmonella typhi determination using voltammetric amplification of nanoparticles: A highly sensitive strategy for metalloimmunoassay based on a copper-enhanced gold label. Talanta. 2008;**77**:727-732

[81] Wang SG, Singh AK, Senapati D, Neely A, Yu HT, Ray PC. Rapid colorimetric identification and targeted photothermal lysis of salmonella bacteria by using bioconjugated oval-shaped gold nanoparticles. Chemistry: A European Journal. 2010;**16**:5600-5606

[82] Hosseini M, Khabbaz H, Dadmehr M, Ganjali MR, Mohamadneja J. Aptamer-based colorimetric and chemiluminescence detection of aflatoxin B1 in foods samples. Acta Chimica Slovenica. 2015;**62**:721-728. DOI: 10.17344/acsi.2015.1358

[83] Luan Y, Chen J, Xie G, Li C, Ping H, Ma Z, Lu A. Visual and microplate detection of aflatoxin B2 based on NaCl-induced aggregation of aptamer-modified gold nanoparticles. Microchimica Acta. 2015;**182**:995-1001

[84] Hayat A, Yang C, Rhouati A, Marty JL. Recent advances and achievements in nanomaterial-based, and structure switchable aptasensing platforms for ochratoxin A detection. Sensors. 2013;**13**:15187-15208

[85] El-Boubbou K, Zhu DC, Vasileiou C, Borhan B, Prosperi D, Li W, Huang X. Magnetic glycol-nanoparticles: A tool to detect, differentiate and unlock the glyco-codes of cancer via magnetic resonance imaging. Journal of the American Chemical Society. 2010;**132**:4490-4499

[86] Huang YF, Wang YF, Yan XP. Amine-functionalized magnetic nanoparticles for rapid capture and removal of bacterial pathogens. Environmental Science & Technology. 2010; **44**:7908-7913

[87] Joo J, Yim C, Kwon D, Lee J, Shin HH, Cha HJ, Jeon S. A facile and sensitive detection of pathogenic bacteria using magnetic nanoparticles and optical nanocrystal probes. The Analyst. 2012;**137**:3609-3612

[88] Michalet X, Pinaud FF, Bentolila LA, Tsay JM, Doose S, Li JJ, Sundaresan G, Wu AM, Gambhir SS, Weiss S. Quantum dots for live cells, in vivo imaging, and diagnostics. Science. 2005;**307**:538-544

[89] Yang L, Li Y. Quantum dots as fluorescent labels for quantitative detection of *Salmonella typhimurium* in chicken carcass wash water. Journal of Food Protection. 2005;**68**:1241-1245

[90] Yao KS, Li SJ, Tzeng KC, Cheng TC, Chang CY, Chiu CY, Liao CY, Hsu JJ, Lin ZP. Fluorescence silica nanoprobe as a biomarker for rapid detection of plant pathogens. Advanced Materials Research. 2009;**79**:513-516. DOI: 10.4028/www.scientific.net/AMR.79-82.513

[91] Etefagh R, Azhir E, Shahtahmasebi N. Synthesis of CuO nanoparticles and fabrication of nanostructural layer bio-sensors for detecting *Aspergillus niger* fungi. Scientia Iranica. 2013;**20**(3):1055-1058

[92] Dubertret B, Calame M, Libchaber AJ. Single-mis-match detection using gold-quenched fluorescent oligonucleotides. Nature Biotechnology. 2001;**19**(4):365-370

[93] Bogue B. Nanosensors: A Review of Recent Progress. UK: Emerald Group Publishing Limited; 2008

Chapter 5

Foodborne Pathogens Detection: Persevering Worldwide Challenge

Amina Baraketi, Stephane Salmieri and
Monique Lacroix

Additional information is available at the end of the chapter

http://dx.doi.org/10.5772/intechopen.74421

Abstract

According to Health Canada, foodborne disease is responsible of more than 4 million cases per year. In United States, more than 48 million people get sick, 128,000 are hospitalized and 3000 die every year in United States due to foodborne diseases according to the Center for Disease Control and Prevention. Cross-contamination from the raw materials, during the process or on working surface has to be rapidly detected. Good manufacturing practices (GMP) and hazard analysis critical control point (HACCP) can help to reduce the incidence of contamination. However, the development of sensitive and rapid methods of detection is still an important need. Standard culture-based methods request the consumption of large amounts of media, are time-consuming and interferences can occur when samplings are done in complex food matrices. The polymerase chain reaction (PCR)-based methods are new technologies. These methods show high level of specificity and sensitivity because they can detect nucleic acid sequences of target bacteria. However, they require an expensive instrumentation and trained scientific technicians. This review is focusing on the development of new simple, sensitive, specific, and time-saving technologies in order to detect quickly foodborne pathogens for application in food industries.

Keywords: foodborne pathogens, rapid technologies, food industries, food safety

1. Introduction

Large-scale of foodborne outbreaks is still an ever-present threat to public health, particularly, for very young and elderly people as well as pregnant women, and people susceptible to a weakened immune system [1]. The global incidence of foodborne disease is difficult to estimate, but it has been reported that every year, foodborne pathogens cause millions of infections and intoxications as well as thousands of deceases. Moreover, outbreaks generate billions of dollars in worth of damage, public health problems, and agricultural product losses [2].

The etiology was determined in the United States in the period from 1993 to 1997 and reported outbreaks showing that bacteria caused 75% of outbreaks and 86% of cases [3]. Furthermore, among the 31 pathogens identified as causing foodborne illnesses, *Salmonella, Campylobacter, Staphylococcus aureus, Listeria monocytogenes, Clostridium perfringens,* and *Escherichia coli* O157:H7 have been incriminated for the large majority of illnesses, hospitalizations, and deaths [4]. Indeed, *Salmonella* spp., *L. monocytogenes, E. coli* O157:H7, and *S. aureus* are on the top of list for the largest number of outbreaks, cases, and deaths [5, 6].

The frequent occurrence of foodborne diseases in previous years is mainly based on five factors, inter-related, and difficult to control to a large degree involving environmental conditions, health system including infrastructure social situation, behavior and lifestyles, health and demographic situation, and food supply system [7]. Although pathogen detection is a growing concern for three main application areas including water, environment quality control [8, 9], and clinical diagnosis, food industry still remains the major area concerned with 38% of the relative number of works appeared in the literature about the detection of pathogenic bacteria [10].

In industrialized countries, the public health authorities set up strict measures and regulations for food control systems such as hazard analysis critical control point system (HACCP) and good manufacturing practice (GMP) in order to overpower the spread of these diseases at the level of the food processing and the food supply system. HACCP is a method of food safety assurance based on the application of good hygiene practices. The HACCP system identifies any additional or more specific control measures necessary in food operations, places an additional emphasis on those points of good hygienic practices, foresees corrective measures if monitoring results indicate a loss of control, and finally provides more training and responsibility to operators [7]. Thus, the detection of foodborne pathogenic bacteria is an important key to the prevention and the control of some hazardous points in food processing or supply systems. Traditional detection methods may take up to a week to yield a confirmed result, challenging many researchers to gear their efforts toward the development of rapid methods for obtaining analytical results in the shortest time. The present chapter attempts to compare the different methods of pathogens detection currently used in food industry as measures of prevention from foodborne diseases. Certainly, it is essential to be well informed about the different methods of pathogens detection but this is as much interesting to find out the possible sources of contamination.

2. Sources of contamination

Foodborne diseases are induced by the consumption of foods or water contaminated by pathogens [11]. **Figure 1** shows most of the pathways leading to the presence of foodborne pathogens in daily food products for nowadays consumers. These food products include fresh produce such as fruits, vegetables, herbs, seeds and nuts, milk and dairy products, meat products as well as poultry and eggs. From the preharvest phase, most of these products go

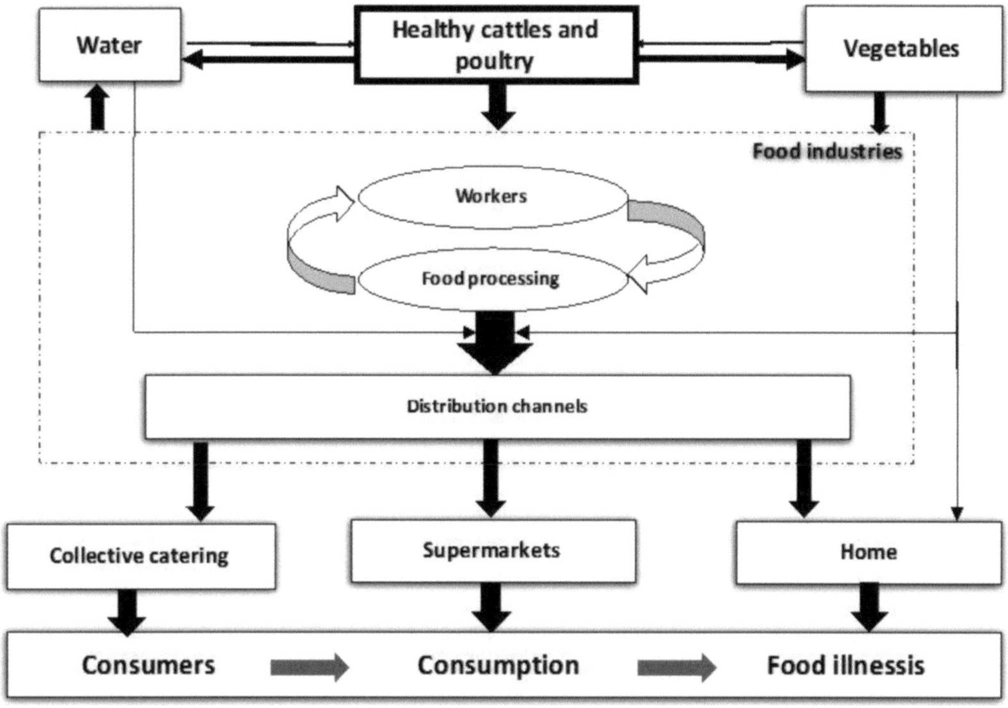

Figure 1. Potential flow of food contamination (adapted from [61]).

through either a local distribution directly from the farmer to the consumer, or a wider distribution to the industry. In industrialized countries, consumers get these raw materials for home use through the supermarkets. In all cases, food is an excellent source of energy and nutrition, not only for human and animals but also for the proliferation of microorganisms.

The contamination by the fresh produce has been well discussed by [2]. Food manufacturing mostly relies on fresh produce, as raw materials that offer to consumers a wide range of benefits such as nutrients, vitamins, and fibers. From farm to fork, the contamination of fresh produce by pathogens may occur at any stage during transformation process from the preharvest to the postharvest phase. In the field, contamination can occur through some elements of nature (water, soil, seeds, insects, dust, etc.) whereas the central part of contamination during the postharvest phase is related to handlers and equipment during processing, transportation, and preparation [12]. The risk for this kind of products is that they are usually consumed in raw state or not heat-treated, avoiding the elimination of pathogens before consumption [13]. *Salmonella* spp., pathogenic *E. coli*, *L. monocytogenes*, *S. aureus*, *Shigella spp.*, *Yersinia spp.*, and *Clostridium spp.* are the main pathogens contaminating fresh produce.

In another side, as described by [14], healthy cattle may hideaway in their liver, kidneys, lymph nodes, and spleen human pathogenic microorganisms. From slaughtering, the first step in meat processing, carcasses are exposed to microorganisms present in animal intestinal tracts and consequently contaminate other cut surfaces and carcasses. Thus, carcass contact surfaces, water, air, and staff during processing and distribution channels are potential sources of contamination in meat and meat products. Concerning poultry products, critical steps that may lead to contamination are defeathering and evisceration with higher probability in case of contaminated hands and toll workers. The pathogens that threaten these products are *Salmonella* and *Campylobacter*. *L. monocytogenes* is the most incriminated pathogen in the contamination of dairy products, which are vulnerable to the risks from udders of cows and milk equipment.

It is obvious that the high volume of food production may lead to a greater likelihood of a cross-contamination as previously described and consequently a high spread of the disease. This finding was also supported by [15] mentioning that in industrialized countries, the amounts of outside food consumption including international travels as well as the increasing demand for minimally processed ready-to-eat (RTE) products increase the risk of foodborne diseases. In a large case-control, 20% of infections with *E. coli* O157:H7 was associated to eating at a table-service restaurant, 35% of infections with *S. enteritidis* with egg consumption in a restaurant, and 35% were attributed to eating chicken prepared out of home.

Although fresh produce, red meat, poultry and milk are the raw materials not only for food industry and restaurants, but also for supermarkets. However, supermarket RTE food products themselves are the raw materials for consumers' homemade meals [16]. To avoid cross-contamination from raw materials, it is essential to wash hands, tools, and prepare surfaces before and after processing. Also, food products that are already prepared/cooked have to be refrigerated at 4°C. However, hot foods should be kept above 60°C. Besides, it is recommended to split large volumes of food into small portions for rapid cooling in the refrigerator as well as heating whole canned foods before tasting. Otherwise, there is a high increase in the consumption of street food and consequently in the need of more food service establishments [7].

The large number of interconnected factors increases the risks of cross-contaminations. To control the spread of these pathogens, first there is a need for monitoring the contamination of raw materials from suspected sources to the end of the supply chain by applying hygiene and sanitation practices and also the advent of new rapid technologies of detection.

3. Conventional methods

According to [17], conventional microbiological methods are usually performed for the isolation and enumeration of pathogens in food samples. Nowadays, these standard culture methods are still considered as the "gold standard" as they are sensitive, inexpensive, and give both qualitative and quantitative information on the number and the nature of microorganisms present in food samples.

On the other side, conventional methods are time-consuming considering all basic pre-enrichment, enrichment, and plating steps needed. They mainly rely on specific media to enumerate and isolate viable bacterial cells in food. The pre-enrichment of the food samples, in a non-selective or selective broth culture, can be used to increase the number of injured but viable bacteria that can be a potential threat to human health, to a detectable level [18]. Pre-enrichment recover a larger proportion of bacteria from food matrices and is usually followed by sublethal stressors such as heating, cooling, acids, or osmotic shocks [19]. In addition to that, the occurrence of toxin production in food requires that the cell pathogen concentration reaches a specific level as much as 5 log CFU/g of *Staphylococcus aureus and Bacillus cereus*, 3 log CFU/g of *Clostridium botulinum* (CFU referring to colony-forming unit). Thus, all existing detection technologies have to be preceded by an enrichment step [20].

Enrichment steps (selective enrichment and selective plating) may require an additional period of 8–24 h before the enumeration or the detection can be completed and mostly they will be followed by biochemical screening and serological confirmation [21]. A variety of chromogenic and fluorogenic culture media are available for selective isolation and differentiation of food-associated spoilage bacteria by incorporation of enzyme substrates. As no single microbiological test, among these standard culture methods, provides a confirmed identification of any unknown microorganism, there is a need for several additional series of analysis [22].

Conventional methods can be laborious too as they usually require the preparation of culture media and colony counting with the most probable number (MPN) method [23]. The duration of these methods depends on the ability of the microorganisms to grow in pre-enrichment, selective enrichment, and selective plating media. This process is often slow and takes 48–72 hours for preliminary identification and more than a week for the confirmation of the pathogen species [4].

Qualitative culture methods are only used to determine the absence or presence of microorganisms in food samples. However, the quantitative ones are preferred for enumeration. The limit of detection (LOD) or sensitivity, the minimum amount of detectable cells, is defined by the presence of microorganisms in 25 g of food examined for qualitative methods and a concentration of <10–100 MPN of bacteria per gram or >10–100 viable counts for quantitative methods [24] considering that the LOD for plating methods is 1 CFU/g.

Regarding the high spread of foodborne pathogens illness, the inspection regulations are very strict with the requirements for process control. The LOD for food pathogens is restricted to 1 cell per unit of food sample [25]. Depending on the target pathogen and the food sample, the analytical unit may be considered from 25 to 325 g.

These methods are recognized for their low cost and ease of use that are relatively interesting compared to alternative methods [21]. Despite these traditional methods are still used due to their high selectivity [10], they are laborious, time-consuming, and may be limited by their low sensitivity [26] compared to other rapid methods. In addition, there is a probability that false negative results may occur due to viable but nonculturable (VBNC) cells.

The challenge of pathogen detection in food matrix, as reported by [23, 17], resides in the presence of pathogens in low numbers and uniformly distributed in a food heterogenic matrix with the presence of non-pathogenic microorganisms that may interfere with the identification step. Food matrices can be found in different physical states (powder, liquid, gel, or semi-solid) and contain a wide range of ingredients that may interfere with the detection.

4. Alternative methods for the detection of foodborne pathogens

To overcome the limitations of conventional methods, various rapid methods have been developed and are commercially available to meet the needs of food industry. Considering that commercialized rapid detection methods should be validated from a recognized organization such as the Association Française de Normalisation (AFNOR) in the European Union or the Association of Analytical Communities (AOAC International) in the United States, most kits of detection are validated according to their the sensitivity and specificity [27]. Ideally for industrial applications, rapid methods should be characterized by their specificity, high sensitivity, and fast performance. Nowadays, current rapid methods are able to detect pathogens in raw and processed foods in low numbers to avoid the risk of infection, which are more time-efficient, labor-saving, and prevent human errors [28]. Currently, the range of detection time for available rapid methods is estimated from a few minutes to a few hours. Nevertheless, the sensitivity and specificity still have to be improved for testing foods samples without the needs to be pre-enriched before analysis [29]. Indeed, the enrichment step is considered as the main limitation in most of the methods but remains essential for the revival of stressed or injured cells, the differentiation of viable from nonculturable cells and the dilution of inhibitors present in the food sample [30].

Rapid detection methods can be categorized into biosensors, immunological methods, and nucleic acid-based methods (**Figure 2**). Simple polymerase chain reaction (PCR), multiplex PCR, real-time PCR, nucleic acid sequence-based amplification (NASBA), loop-mediated isothermal amplification (LAMP), and oligonucleotide DNA microarray are classified as nucleic-based methods. Biosensors-based methods include optical, electrochemical, and mass-based biosensors. Finally, enzyme-linked immunosorbent assay (ELISA) and lateral flow immunoassay are

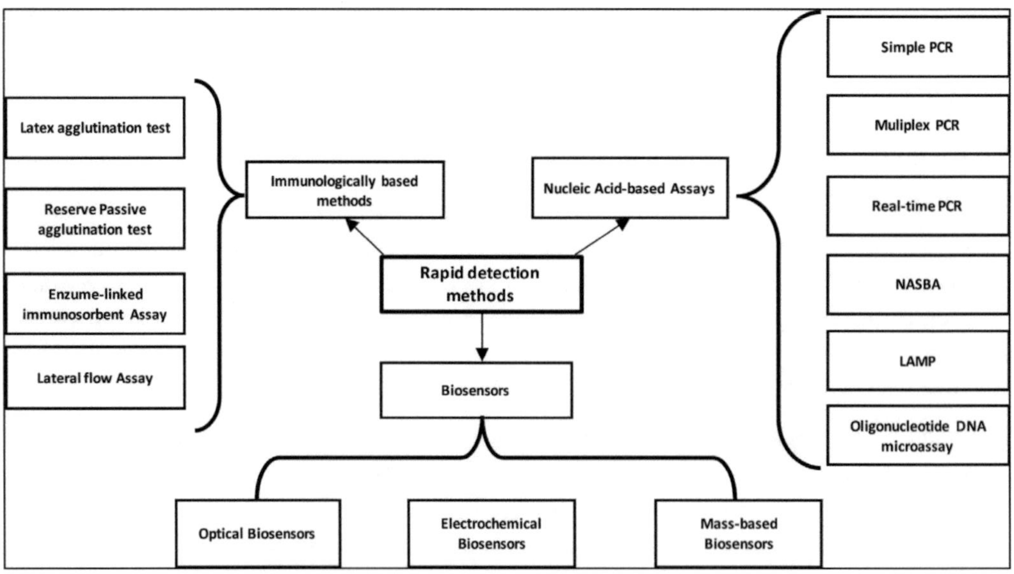

Figure 2. Mapping of rapid detection technologies for foodborne pathogens [32].

recognized as immunology-based methods [31]. Several publications have already detailed the principle of each of these methods [4, 28, 31–33]. However, the aim of this work is to focus on the advantages and limitations of these methods for application in food industry. With the development of new methods, immunology-based methods and PCR become categorized as conventional techniques for the detection of pathogens [34].

4.1. Nucleic acid-based methods

Nucleic acid-based methods prevent ambiguous or wrongly interpreted results. They operate by detecting specific deoxyribonucleic acid (DNA) or ribonucleic acid (RNA) sequences in the target pathogen and hybridizing the target nucleic acid sequence to a synthetic oligonucleotide, which is complementary to the target sequence [4]. Invented 20 years ago, simple PCR [35] is widely used for the detection of *L. monocytogenes* [36], *E. coli* O157:H7 [37], *S. aureus* [38], *Campylobacter jejuni* [39], *Salmonella spp.* [40], and *Shigella spp.* [41]. The presence of sufficient numbers of target molecules, the purity of the target template, the complexity of food matrices containing potential inhibitory compounds may affect the reliability of PCR amplification [42].

Through the years, PCR techniques have undergone significant improvements for faster detection with the development of real-time PCR for monitoring PCR amplification products, in addition to the methods of simultaneous detection such as multiplex PCR and oligonucleotide DNA microarray that can detect up to five or more pathogens simultaneously [43] such as *Salmonella enteritidis, S. aureus, Shigella flexneri, L. monocytogenes*, and *E. coli* O157:H7 [44].

Presently, as shown in **Table 1**, there is an important selection of commercially available kits based on nucleic acid methods for the detection of foodborne pathogens. However, although these techniques are automated for reliable results and characterized with high sensitivity and specificity, they induce some disadvantages such as difficulties to differentiate viable from non-culturable cells and the design of the primers. In some case, they require trained staff in order to minimize the occurrence of cross-contamination. According to [45], the isothermal amplification method for nucleic acids, NASBA, and an amplification system for RNA analytes (e.g., viral genomic RNA, mRNA, or rRNA) could be extended from viral diagnostics to the gene expression and cell viability. Despite, the low cost of these methods and the non-requirement of thermal cycling system, post-NASBA product detection is still considered labor-intensive.

Otherwise, the LAMP method, can provide a large amount, usually 10^3 higher to simple PCR, of DNA with rapidity under isothermal conditions [4], lower detection limits compared to conventional PCR [46, 47] and higher specificity due to the use of four primers targeting six specific regions [48].

4.2. Immunology-based methods

The most successful and popular technology in the field of the detection of bacterial cells, spores, viruses, and toxins is represented by immunological methods. This technology is faster, more robust, and has the ability to detect contaminating organisms as well as their biotoxins. However, they are less specific and less sensitive than nucleic acid-based detection [49]. Compared to traditional counting methods, antibody-based methods generate less assay time

Pathogen	Method	Commercially available kits	Sensitivity	Catalog number	Sample matrix	Company
Staphylococcus	PCR	BAX® System Real-time PCR assay	10^4 CFU/mL, after enrichment	D12762689	Powdered infant formula, ground beef, soy protein isolate	HYGIENA
Salmonella spp.	PCR	BAX® System Standard PCR assays for *Salmonella*	10^4 CFU/mL, after enrichment	D11000133–D14368501	Poultry, dairy, fruits, vegetables, bakery products, pet food and environmentals	HYGIENA
Salmonella spp.	Real-Time PCR	BAX® System Real-time PCR assay for *Salmonella*	10^4 CFU/mL, after enrichment	D14306040	Meat, poultry, dairy, fruits, vegetables, bakery products, pet food and environmentals	HYGIENA
E. coli O157:H7	Multiplex PCR	BAX® System PCR assay for *E. coli* O157:H7 MP	10^4 CFU/mL, after enrichment	D12404903	Raw ground beef, beef trim, produce	HYGIENA
Salmonella	DNA hybridization test	GeneQuence® for *Salmonella*	1–5 CFU/25 g	6700 -	Food and environmental samples	NEOGEN
stx and eae genes – STEC Screening	Real-time PCR assay	BAX® System Real-Time PCR STEC Assay	10^4 CFU/mL, after enrichment	D14642964	Raw ground beef, beef trim, produce	HYGIENA
E. coli O26, O111, O121 -	Real-time PCR assay		10^4 CFU/mL, after enrichment	D14642970	Raw ground beef, beef trim, produce	HYGIENA
E. coli O45, O103, O145	Real-time PCR assay		10^4 CFU/mL, after enrichment	D14642987	Raw ground beef, beef trim, produce	HYGIENA
E. coli O157:H7	Real-time PCR assay	BAX® System Real-Time PCR Assay for *E. coli* O157:H7	10^4 CFU/mL, after enrichment	D14203648	Raw ground beef, beef trim, produce	HYGIENA
Listeria spp.	PCR	BAX® System *Listeria* spp	10^5 CFU/mL, after enrichment	D11000147	Food and environmentals	HYGIENA
Listeria spp. (except L. grayii)	PCR	BAX® System PCR Assay for Genus *Listeria* 24E	10^4 CFU/mL, after enrichment	D13608135	Dairy, meat, fish, vegetables, environmentals	HYGIENA
Listeria species	Real-time PCR assay	BAX® System Real-Time PCR Assay for Genus *Listeria*	10^4 CFU/mL, after enrichment	D15131113	Dairy, ready-to-eat meat, seafood, vegetables, environmentals	HYGIENA
Listeria monocytogenes	PCR	BAX® System PCR Assay for *L. monocytogenes*	10^5 CFU/mL, after enrichment	D11000157	Variety of food types	HYGIENA

Pathogen	Method	Commercially available kits	Sensitivity	Catalog number	Sample matrix	Company
Listeria monocytogenes	PCR	BAX® System PCR Assay for *L. monocytogenes* 24E	10^4 CFU/mL, after enrichment	D13608125	Dairy, meat, fish, vegetables, environmentals	HYGIENA
Listeria monocytogenes	Real-time PCR assay	BAX® System Real-Time PCR Assay for *L. monocytogenes*	10^4 CFU/mL, after enrichment	D15134303	Dairy, ready-to-eat meat, seafood, vegetables, environmentals	HYGIENA
Listeria spp.	DNA hybridization test	GeneQuence® for *Listeria*	1–5 CFU/25 g	6708	Food and environmental samples	NEOGEN
Listeria monocytogenes	DNA hybridization test	GeneQuence® for *L. monocytogenes*	1–5 CFU/26 g	6709	Food and environmental samples	NEOGEN

Table 1. Commercially available nucleic acid-based methods for the detection of foodborne pathogens (adapted from [32]).

but present a lack of ability to detect microorganisms in "real-time" mode if the quantity of pathogens is not high enough to provide real-time information. As reported by [50], problems that may emerge are the low sensitivity of the assays, low affinity of the antibody to the pathogen or other analytes being measured, and potential interference from contaminants.

Among other immunological methods, both of ELISA and lateral flow immunoassay are mainly used for the detection of foodborne pathogens. ELISA is specific and labor-saving as it allows the detection of bacterial toxins and can handle large number of samples. However, this technology presents several disadvantages such as the need of trained staff and the possibility of false negative results due to the cross-reactivity with closely related antigens. As immunoassays rely on the specific binding of an antibody to an antigen, the response of the test depends on the amount of the antigen in the sample and the availability of the binding sites. Thus, the low sensitivity of this technology, in the field of the detection of foodborne pathogens, requires a pre-enrichment step to reach a detectable level of antigen in the sample as well as a labeling of antigens and antibodies [51, 52]. On the other hand, lateral flow assay is low cost, reliable, easy-to-operate, sensitive, specific, and allows the detection of bacterial toxins but still requires labeling of antigens and antibodies [4]. Commercialized kits of these two techniques are summarized in **Table 2**. Toward the progress of rapid methods, new antibody-based methods have been coupled with other methods for pathogen detection, such as immunomagnetic separation on magnetic beads coupled with matrix-assisted laser desorption/ionization time-of-flight mass spectrometry (MALDI-TOF) for detection of staphylococcal enterotoxin B [53] and combination of immunomagnetic separation with flow cytometry for the detection of *L. monocytogenes* [54].

4.3. Biosensors

Nowadays, the use of biosensors is increasing in the field of food pathogen detection using nucleic acid- and immunology-based methods considered as conventional ones. In recent years, there has been much research activity in the area of biosensors development for detecting pathogenic microorganisms. Compared to standard methods, biosensors are more favorable for checking food safety, throughout the production process, due to their real-time response [55]. Biosensors are powerful analysis tools covering a wide range of applications particularly food quality monitoring, disease detection, toxins of defense interest, environmental monitoring, soil quality monitoring, drug discovery, and prosthetic devices [56].

As defined by [35], biosensor devices are constituted with two main parts: the bioreceptor (biological material recognizing the analyte) and the transducer (converting the bio-recognition energy into optical or electrical signals). A bioreceptor can be a microorganism, cell, enzyme, antibody, nucleic acid, aptamers, or biomimic. However, the transduction may be optical, electrochemical, thermometric, piezoelectric, magnetic and micromechanical, or combinations of the above techniques.

The classification of the several types of biosensors is based on their bioreceptors or transducers, as described by [35]. Electrochemical, mass-based, and optical biosensors are the mainly used biosensors for the detection of foodborne pathogens [51], especially surface plasmon

http://dx.doi.org/10.5772/intechopen.74421

Pathogen	Method	Commercially available kits	Sensitivity	Catalog number	Sample matrix	Company
Shiga Toxin-producing *E. coli* (STEC) including	Lateral flow Assay	Food check *E.coli* O157 test kit, Carcass Sponge Kit, Assay Cassettes	1 CFU/375 g of ground beef	FCEC-001, FCEC-005, FCEC-006	Raw ground beef, beef trims and carcass	Foodchek Systems Inc
E.coli O157:H7 and Verotoxin		RapidChekO *E. coli* O157 (including H7) Test Kit	1 CFU/25 g of food.	7,000,157, 7,000,158, 7,000,161, 7,000,165	Boneless beef trim and ground beef	Romer Labs
		Transia Card *E.coli* O157	—	—	Raw ground beef Raw beef product	Raisio Diagnostics
		Reveal® for *E. coli* O157:H7	1 CFU/25 g; 1 CFU/375 g	9714		NEOGEN
	Enzyme-Linked Immuno Sorbent Assay	3MTM TecraTM *E. coli* O157 VIA	1–5 CFU/25 g sample	ECOVIA48 ECOVIA96	NR	3 M Canada
		Assurance® EIA EHEC	—	4000 01	Meat, dairy, poultry, fruit, nuts, and more	BioControl
Listeria	Enzyme-Linked Immuno Sorbent Assay	3MTM TecraTM *Listeria* VIA	1–5 CFU/25 g sample or 1–5 CFU/swab	LISVIA48	NR	3 M Canada
		Assurance *Listeria* EIA	—	67,000–96	Environmental surfaces and food samples.	BioControl
	Lateral flow Assay	Reveal®2.0 for *Listeria*	1 CFU/analytical unit	9707	Food and environmental samples	NEOGEN

Pathogen	Method	Commercially available kits	Sensitivity	Catalog number	Sample matrix	Company
Salmonella spp	Enzyme-Linked Immuno Sorbent Assay	3MTM TecraTM *Salmonella* Visual Immunoassay (VIA)	1–5 CFU/25 g sample	SALVIA48	All Foods	3 M Canada
		3MTM TecraTM *Salmonella* ULTIMA VIA	1–5 CFU/25 g sample	SALULT96	All Foods	3 M Canada
		MaxSignal® *Salmonella* Test Strip Kit	$1x10^5$ CFU - $1x10^6$ CFU/mL	BO_1063–01	Food and Feed Products	Bioo Scientific
	Lateral flow Assay	RapidChek® *Salmonella*	—	7,000,183–7,000,167	Raw ground beef (25 g, 375 g), raw ground chicken, chicken carcass rinsates, liquid eggs, sliced cooked turkey, environmental samples and peanut butter.	SDIX
		RapidChek® SELECT™ *Salmonella*	—	7,000,190–7,000,195 - 7,000,198		SDIX
		RapidChek® SELECT™ *Salmonella enteritidis*	—	7,000,220–7,000,222	Food samples	SDIX
		TRANSIA™ PLATE *Salmonella* gold	—	SA0180	All foods	BioControl
		Reveal® 2.0	1 CFU/analytical unit 10^6 CFU/mL post enrichment	9706	Chicken carcass rinse, raw ground turkey, raw ground beef, hot dogs, raw shrimp, ready-to-eat meal products, dry pet food, ice cream, fresh spinach, cantaloupe, peanut butter, swabs from stainless steel surfaces, and sprout irrigation water	NEOGEN

Pathogen	Method	Commercially available kits	Sensitivity	Catalog number	Sample matrix	Company
Staphylococcus aureus	Enzyme-Linked Immuno Sorbent Assay	3MTM TecraTM *S. aureus* VIA (3 M)	1–5 CFU/25 g sample	STAVIA96	Food samples	3 M Canada
		3MTM TecraTM Staph Enterotoxin VIA (3 M)	1 ng/mL of sample extract	SETVIA48	Food samples	3 M Canada
	Lateral flow Assay	TRANSIA® PlATe Staphylococcal Enterotoxins	0.25 ng S. enterotoxins/g sample	ST0796	Milk and dairy products	BioControl
		TRANSIA™ PLATE Staphylococcal Enterotoxins Plus	0.25 ng S. enterotoxins/g sample	ST0777	Milk and dairy products	BioControl
		TRANSIA™ PLATE Staphylococcal Enterotoxins ID	20–60 pg./mL of each serological group (A-E)	ST0712	Milk and dairy products, Meat, poultry and eggs, Seafood and other foods, Feed products	BioControl
		TRANSIA®IAc Staphylococcal Enterotoxins	0.1 ng S. enterotoxins/g sample	ST0705	Milk and dairy products	BioControl
		TRANSIA® TUBe Staphylococcal Enterotoxins	0.5 ng S. enterotoxins/g	ST724B	Milk and dairy products	BioControl

NR: not reported.

Table 2. Commercially available immunology-based methods for the detection of foodborne pathogens (adapted from [32]).

Pathogen	Method	Commercially available kits	Sensitivity	Sample matrix	Company	References
Escherichia coli O157:H7	*Optical immunosensor based on selective antibody expressed by human cell line*	CANARY™ system	500 CFU/g	Lettuce	Massachusetts Institute of Technology	[62]
Escherichia coli O157:H7 and *Salmonella*	Eectrochemical immunosensor based on the assembly of three nanoparticle	Michigan State Electrochemical Biosensor	10^1 to 10^6 CFU/mL	Fresh produce and meat products	Michigan State University	[63]
Detection of *Salmonella* and *Campylobacter*	Interferometric biosensor	Georgia Tech Interferometric Biosensor	5000 CFU/mL for *Salmonella* 500 CFU/mL for *Campylobacter*	Poultry products	Georgia Research Tech Institute	[62]
Staphylococcal enterotoxin B and Botulinum toxin A	Fluorescencent immunoassay biosensor	Naval Research Laboratory array biosensor	From 20 to 500 ng/mL for Botulinum toxin A From 0.1 to 0.5 ng/ml for Staphylococcal enterotoxin B	Tomatoes, sweet corn, beans and mushrooms	Naval Research Laboratory	[64]
Escherichia coli O157, *Salmonella, Listeria* and *Campylobacter*	Electro-immunoassay biosensor	Detex Pathogen Detection System	NR	Chicken breast	Molecular Circuitry Inc.	[65]

CANARY™: Cellular Analysis and Notification of Antigen Risks and Yields.

Table 3. Commercially available biosensor devices for the detection of foodborne pathogens (adapted from [22]).

resonance (SPR) biosensors due to their high sensitivity [35]. Few commercial biosensors for the detection of foodborne pathogens are nowadays available. **Table 3** presents the rare commercially available devices of biosensors for food analysis [57]. Unlike nucleic-acid based methods and immunological methods, biosensors are easy-to-operate and they do not require any pre-enrichment step [58].

Optical biosensors are very suitable for the detection of pathogens substances in the food as they detect analytes with no need of special sample treatment even in complex matrices, in addition to the less interference and the low loss of signal. As described by [59], optical biosensors are based on the measurement of the change in amplitude, phase, frequency, or polarization of light. Also, optical devices are more specific and more sensitive than the other biosensors, with a compact design minimally invasive. However, the enhancement of stability of immobilized biocomponents is still a challenge. The main inconvenient of these biosensors is that their commercialization is slower than other rapid methods due to several factors such as their high cost in quality assurance, stability, sensitivity issues, and instrumentation design [60].

Electrochemical biosensors, the second type of biosensors, can handle large numbers of samples and are label-free detection devices but they are low sensitive, and analysis may be interfered by food matrices in addition to many required washing steps, which is not suitable for analyzing samples containing low amount of microorganisms. Finally, mass-based biosensors are cost-effective, easy-to-operate, label-free, and real-time detection devices but low specific and low sensitive with long incubation time of bacteria and many required washing/drying steps, in addition to the regeneration of crystal surface that may be problematic [22].

5. Conclusion

The first step to ensure food safety resides in the prevention by raising industry and consumer awareness. Few primary daily actions can prevent food diseases. Despite conventional methods are often regarded as the “Gold standard” for their specificity and reliability, in addition to their low cost and simplicity, they remain time-consuming and laborious. Over the years, many rapid methods for the detection and identification of foodborne pathogens have been developed to overcome the limitations of their conventional counterparts. Several different types of nucleic-based methods, immunology-based methods and biosensors have been developed and discussed in a large number of publications. Each one offers advantages depending on the target pathogen and the food sample. But also, several disadvantages have to be solved for practical applications in the food industry.

Compared to conventional microbiological methods, rapid commercially available technologies are sensitive enough to detect pathogens, which are expected to be more time-efficient, labor-saving, and able to reduce human errors significantly. Although they are expensive and require a trained technical staff, they are not practical for daily industrial uses.

Nowadays, novel detection methods are released regularly but their acceptance by the industry depends not only on speed but also on initial investment, cost, technical support, and usability.

Indeed, advanced researches have converged to rise to the challenge of developing new simple, sensitive, specific, and time-saving technologies of foodborne pathogens detection that could be mostly practical in food industry.

Author details

Amina Baraketi, Stephane Salmieri and Monique Lacroix*

*Address all correspondence to: monique.lacroix@iaf.inrs.ca

Research Laboratories in Sciences Applied to Food, Canadian Irradiation Center, INRS-Institut Armand-Frappier, Institute of Nutraceutical and Functional Foods, Lava, QC, Canada

References

[1] Scallan E, Hoekstra RM, Angulo FJ, Tauxe RV, Widdowson M-A, Roy SL, et al. Foodborne illness acquired in the United States—Major pathogens. Emerging Infectious Diseases. 2011;**17**(1):7

[2] Yeni F, Yavaş S, Alpas H, Soyer Y. Most common foodborne pathogens and mycotoxins on fresh produce: A review of recent outbreaks. Critical Reviews in Food Science and Nutrition. 2016;**56**(9):1532-1544

[3] Olsen SJ, MacKinnon LC, Goulding JS, Bean NH, Slutsker L. Surveillance for foodborne-disease outbreaks—United States, 1993-1997. MMWR. CDC Surveillance Summaries. 2000;**49**(1):1-62

[4] Zhao X, Lin C-W, Wang J, Oh DH. Advances in rapid detection methods for foodborne pathogens. Journal of Microbiology and Biotechnology. 2014;**24**(3):297-312

[5] Oussalah M, Caillet S, Saucier L, Lacroix M. Inhibitory effects of selected plant essential oils on the growth of four pathogenic bacteria: *E. coli* O157: H7, *Salmonella typhimurium*, *Staphylococcus aureus* and *Listeria monocytogenes*. Food Control. 2007;**18**(5):414-420

[6] Wu S, Duan N, Gu H, Hao L, Ye H, Gong W, et al. A review of the methods for detection of staphylococcus aureus enterotoxins. Toxins. 2016;**8**(7):176

[7] Motarjemi Y, Käferstein F. Food safety, hazard analysis and critical control point and the increase in foodborne diseases: A paradox? Food Control. 1999;**10**(4):325-333

[8] Leonard P, Hearty S, Brennan J, Dunne L, Quinn J, Chakraborty T, et al. Advances in biosensors for detection of pathogens in food and water. Enzyme and Microbial Technology. 2003;**32**(1):3-13

[9] O'Kennedy R, Leonard P, Hearty S, Daly S, Dillon P, Brennan J, et al. Advances in biosensors for detection of pathogens in food and water. In: van Amerongen A, Barug D,

Lauwaars M, editors. Rapid Methods for Biological and Chemical Contaminants in Food and Feed. Wagningen, The Netherlands: Wagningen Academic Publishers; 2005. pp. 85-104

[10] Lazcka O, Del Campo FJ, Munoz FX. Pathogen detection: A perspective of traditional methods and biosensors. Biosensors & Bioelectronics. 2007;**22**(7):1205-1217

[11] Dwivedi HP, Jaykus L-A. Detection of pathogens in foods: The current state-of-the-art and future directions. Critical Reviews in Microbiology. 2011;**37**(1):40-63

[12] Gorny J. Microbial contamination of fresh fruits and vegetables. In: Microbiology of Fruits and Vegetables. Boca Raton, FL: CRC Press; 2006. pp. 3-32

[13] Ribot E, Hyytia-Trees E, Cooper K. PulseNet and emerging foodborne pathogens. In: Microbial Food Contamination. 2nd ed. Boca Raton: CRC Press; 2008

[14] Marriott NG, Gravani RB. Food Contamination Sources. Principles of Food Sanitation; 2006. pp. 76-82

[15] Angulo FJ, Jones TF, Angulo FJ. Eating in restaurants: A risk factor for foodborne disease? Clinical Infectious Diseases. 2006;**43**(10):1324-1328

[16] Goldburn K, editor. Management of E. coli O157 in fresh fruit and vegetables: how can we be safe. Chilled Food Association Conference an *E. coli*: cases, controls and common sense. London, UK; 2009

[17] Doyle MP, Buchanan RL. Food Microbiology: Fundamentals and Frontiers. Washington DC, USA: American Society for Microbiology Press; 2012

[18] Zhao T, Doyle MP. Evaluation of universal preenrichment broth for growth of heat-injured pathogens. Journal of Food Protection. 2001;**64**(11):1751-1755

[19] Harrigan WF. Laboratory Methods in Food Microbiology. London, UK: Gulf Professional Publishing; 1998

[20] Wang Y, Salazar JK. Culture-independent rapid detection methods for bacterial pathogens and toxins in food matrices. Comprehensive Reviews in Food Science and Food Safety. 2016;**15**(1):183-205

[21] Gracias KS, McKillip JL. A review of conventional detection and enumeration methods for pathogenic bacteria in food. Canadian Journal of Microbiology. 2004;**50**(11):883-890

[22] Ivnitski D, Abdel-Hamid I, Atanasov P, Wilkins E. Biosensors for detection of pathogenic bacteria. Biosensors & Bioelectronics. 1999;**14**(7):599-624

[23] Mandal PK, Biswas AK, Choi K, Pal UK. Methods for rapid detection of foodborne pathogens: An overview. American Journal of Food Technology. 2011;**6**(2):87-102

[24] López-Campos G, Martínez-Suárez JV, Aguado-Urda M, López-Alonso V. Detection, identification, and analysis of foodborne pathogens. In: Microarray Detection and Characterization of Bacterial Foodborne Pathogens. New York, USA: Springer; 2012. pp. 13-32

[25] Gill A. The importance of bacterial culture to food microbiology in the age of genomics. Frontiers in Microbiology. 2017;**8**

[26] Lee N, Kwon KY, Oh SK, Chang H-J, Chun HS, Choi S-W. A multiplex PCR assay for simultaneous detection of *Escherichia coli* O157: H7, *Bacillus cereus*, Vibrio Parahaemolyticus, *Salmonella* spp., *Listeria monocytogenes*, and *Staphylococcus aureus* in Korean ready-to-eat food. Foodborne Pathogens and Disease. 2014;**11**(7):574-580

[27] Beumer R, Hazeleger W. Rapid methods: The detection of foodborne pathogens. Food Engineering & Ingredients. 2009:15-17

[28] Mandal P, Biswas A, Choi K, Pal U. Methods for rapid detection of foodborne pathogens: An overview. American Journal Of Food Technology. 2011;**6**(2):87-102

[29] Feng P. Impact of molecular biology on the detection of foodborne pathogens. Molecular Biotechnology. 1997;**7**(3):267-278

[30] Feng P. Rapid methods for detecting foodborne pathogens. FDA, editor Bacteriological Analytical Manual Online. 2001

[31] Law JW-F, Ab Mutalib N-S, Chan K-G, Lee L-H. Rapid methods for the detection of foodborne bacterial pathogens: Principles, applications, advantages and limitations. Frontiers in Microbiology. 2015;**5**:770

[32] Valderrama WB, Dudley EG, Doores S, Cutter CN. Commercially available rapid methods for detection of selected food-borne pathogens. Critical Reviews in Food Science and Nutrition. 2016;**56**(9):1519-1531

[33] Gopinath SC, Tang T-H, Chen Y, Citartan M, Lakshmipriya T. Bacterial detection: From microscope to smartphone. Biosensors and Bioelectronics. 2014;**60**:332-342

[34] Alahi MEE, Mukhopadhyay SC. Detection methodologies for pathogen and toxins: A review. Sensors. 2017;**17**(8):1885

[35] Velusamy V, Arshak K, Korostynska O, Oliwa K, Adley C. An overview of foodborne pathogen detection: In the perspective of biosensors. Biotechnology Advances. 2010; **28**(2):232-254

[36] Manzano M, Cocolin L, Ferroni P, Cantoni C, Comi G. A simple and fast PCR protocol to detect listeria monocytogenes from meat. Journal of the Science of Food and Agriculture. 1997;**74**(1):25-30

[37] Lindqvist R. Preparation of PCR samples from food by a rapid and simple centrifugation technique evaluated by detection of *Escherichia coli* O157: H7. International Journal of Food Microbiology. 1997;**37**(1):73-82

[38] Johnson W, Tyler S, Ewan E, Ashton F, Pollard D, Rozee K. Detection of genes for enterotoxins, exfoliative toxins, and toxic shock syndrome toxin 1 in Staphylococcus Aureus by the polymerase chain reaction. Journal of Clinical Microbiology. 1991;**29**(3):426-430

[39] Wang H, Farber J, Malik N, Sanders G. Improved PCR detection of campylobacter jejuni from chicken rinses by a simple sample preparation procedure. International Journal of Food Microbiology. 1999;**52**(1):39-45

[40] Cheah Y-K, Salleh NA, Lee L-H, Radu S, Sukardi S, Sim J-H. Comparison of PCR fingerprinting techniques for the discrimination of *Salmonella enterica* subsp. enterica serovar Weltevreden isolated from indigenous vegetables in Malaysia. World Journal of Microbiology and Biotechnology. 2008;**24**(3):327

[41] Lindqvist R. Detection of Shigella spp. in food with a nested PCR method–sensitivity and performance compared with a conventional culture method. Journal of Applied Microbiology. 1999;**86**(6):971-978

[42] Lampel KA, Orlandi PA, Kornegay L. Improved template preparation for PCR-based assays for detection of food-borne bacterial pathogens. Applied and Environmental Microbiology. 2000;**66**(10):4539-4542

[43] Chen J, Tang J, Liu J, Cai Z, Bai X. Development and evaluation of a multiplex PCR for simultaneous detection of five foodborne pathogens. Journal of Applied Microbiology. 2012;**112**(4):823-830

[44] Kim JS, Lee GG, Park JS, Jung YH, Kwak HS, Kim SB, et al. A novel multiplex PCR assay for rapid and simultaneous detection of five pathogenic bacteria: *Escherichia coli* O157: H7, *Salmonella*, *Staphylococcus aureus*, *Listeria monocytogenes*, and *Vibrio parahaemolyticus*. Journal of Food Protection. 2007;**70**(7):1656-1662

[45] Leone G, van Gemen B, Schoen CD, van Schijndel H, Kramer FR. Molecular beacon probes combined with amplification by NASBA enable homogeneous, real-time detection of RNA. Nucleic Acids Research 1998;**26**(9):2150-2155

[46] Xu Z, Li L, Chu J, Peters BM, Harris ML, Li B, et al. Development and application of loop-mediated isothermal amplification assays on rapid detection of various types of staphylococci strains. Food Research International. 2012;**47**(2):166-173

[47] Zhao X, Li Y, Wang L, You L, Xu Z, Li L, et al. Development and application of a loop-mediated isothermal amplification method on rapid detection *Escherichia coli* O157 strains from food samples. Molecular Biology Reports. 2010;**37**(5):2183-2188

[48] Hara-Kudo Y, Yoshino M, Kojima T, Ikedo M. Loop-mediated isothermal amplification for the rapid detection of *Salmonella*. FEMS Microbiology Letters. 2005;**253**(1):155-161

[49] Iqbal SS, Mayo MW, Bruno JG, Bronk BV, Batt CA, Chambers JP. A review of molecular recognition technologies for detection of biological threat agents. Biosensors & Bioelectronics. 2000;**15**(11):549-578

[50] Meng J, Doyle MP. Introduction. Microbiological food safety. Microbes and Infection. 2002;**4**(4):395-397

[51] Zhang G. Foodborne pathogenic bacteria detection: An evaluation of current and developing methods. The Meducator. 2013;**1**(24)

[52] Park SH, Aydin M, Khatiwara A, Dolan MC, Gilmore DF, Bouldin JL, et al. Current and emerging technologies for rapid detection and characterization of *Salmonella* in poultry and poultry products. Food Microbiology. 2014;**38**:250-262

[53] Schlosser G, Kačer P, Kuzma M, Szilágyi Z, Sorrentino A, Manzo C, et al. Coupling immunomagnetic separation on magnetic beads with matrix-assisted laser desorption ionization-time of flight mass spectrometry for detection of staphylococcal enterotoxin B. Applied and Environmental Microbiology. 2007;**73**(21):6945-6952

[54] Hibi K, Abe A, Ohashi E, Mitsubayashi K, Ushio H, Hayashi T, et al. Combination of immunomagnetic separation with flow cytometry for detection of listeria monocytogenes. Analytica Chimica Acta 2006;**573**:158-63

[55] Bahadır EB, Sezgintürk MK. Applications of commercial biosensors in clinical, food, environmental, and biothreat/biowarfare analyses. Analytical Biochemistry. 2015;**478**:107-120

[56] Bhalla N, Jolly P, Formisano N, Estrela P. Introduction to biosensors. Essays in Biochemistry. 2016;**60**(1):1-8

[57] da Costa Silva LM, dos Santos VPS, Salgado AM, Pereira KS. Biosensors for contaminants monitoring in food and environment for human and environmental health. State of the Art in Biosensors-Environmental and Medical Applications: InTech; Rijeka. 2013

[58] Singh A, Poshtiban S, Evoy S. Recent advances in bacteriophage based biosensors for food-borne pathogen detection. Sensors. 2013;**13**(2):1763-1786

[59] Narsaiah K, Jha SN, Bhardwaj R, Sharma R, Kumar R. Optical biosensors for food quality and safety assurance—A review. Journal of Food Science and Technology. 2012;**49**(4): 383-406

[60] Velasco-Garcia MN, Mottram T. Biosensor technology addressing agricultural problems. Biosystems Engineering. 2003;**84**(1):1-12

[61] Andral B, Bouve J, Brugere H, Espié E, Leclerc V, Roze S, et al. Epidémiologie environmentale et alimentaire des STEC. Agence française de sécurité sanitaire des aliments Bilan des connaissances relatives aux *Escherichia coli* producteurs de Shiga-toxines (STEC) Maisons-Alfort; 2003. pp. 81-103

[62] Innovative Biosensors Are Opening New Frontiers 2004. Available from: http://www.atrp.gatech.edu/pt16-3/16-3_p1.html

[63] Wang Y, Fewins PA, Alocilja EC. Electrochemical immunosensor using nanoparticle-based signal enhancement for *Escherichia coli* O157: H7 detection. IEEE Sensors Journal. 2015;**15**(8):4692-4699

[64] Sapsford KE, Taitt CR, Loo N, Ligler FS. Biosensor detection of botulinum toxoid a and staphylococcal enterotoxin B in food. Applied and Environmental Microbiology. 2005;**71**(9):5590-5592

[65] Detex Pathogen Detection Technology Ready to Roll; VWR to Distribute 2000 [01/22/2018]. Available from: https://www.dairynetwork.com/doc/detex-pathogen-detection-technology-ready-to-0002

Detection and Control of Indoor Airborne Pathogenic Bacteria by Biosensors Based on Quorum Sensing Chemical Language: Bio-Tools, Connectivity Apps and Intelligent Buildings

Claudia Ibacache-Quiroga, Natalia Romo,
Rodrigo Díaz-Viciedo and M. Alejandro Dinamarca

Additional information is available at the end of the chapter

http://dx.doi.org/10.5772/intechopen.72390

Abstract

Nowadays, lifestyles and climate change lead people to spend long periods in indoors spaces, where reduced ventilation and artificial light favor the concentration and spread of airborne pathogenic microorganisms. Current procedures for microbiological air evaluation are based on air sampling coupled to traditional microbiological culture-dependent methods such as biochemical tests and molecular rDNA 16S sequencing. These techniques generate an important delay in the application of prevention and control measures. This chapter presents whole cell-based biosensors that are able to detect quorum sensing signaling molecules produced by airborne pathogenic bacteria as a tool for indoor air monitoring. Furthermore, a general biosensor model is proposed. In this model, *in vivo* biosensors technology can be connected to online applications (Apps), being part of intelligent buildings, in order to reduce airborne pathogenic bacteria concentration and dissemination.

Keywords: air microbiology, quorum sensing, biosensors, airborne pathogens, hyperconnectivity, pathogen control, intelligent buildings

1. Introduction

Legionnaire's disease outbreak (1976) is a masterpiece that allows us to understand how the interaction between environment, pathogen and host can be influenced by lifestyle and technology [1]. Nowadays, because human population continues to grow and people spend their time in confined and shared spaces, concentration and spread of microorganisms must be controlled to avoid infectious outbreaks produced by airborne pathogens.

In indoor spaces, airborne pathogens can be part of aerosols that are produced and disseminated by heating, ventilation, air conditioning or humidifier systems (HVAC) [2]. These systems can be found in several buildings, including shopping centers, hospitals, hotels, cinemas, supermarkets, educational centers, restaurants, houses, airports, cars, trains and busses. Based on the above building design, HVAC equipment and population density are factors that must be considered to avoid the spread of airborne pathogenic microorganisms. In addition, appropriate air microbial quality controls are necessary to reduce biological risks.

Current procedures for microbiological air quality evaluation (ISO 14698-1:2003) are based on passive or active air sampling methods [3]. Passive methods involve the exposition of a petri dish (containing a selected solid culture media) to the environment during an established period, while active methods consist of automatic air samplers with a culture medium that is exposed to a forced airflow. In both methods, samples are incubated in favorable conditions for microorganism (bacteria, yeasts or molds), during 24–72 h. These methods are suitable for the risk assessment through microbial quantification in air [colony forming units (CFU) count]; however, they are not adequate for pathogen identification, for which biochemical characterization, immunoassays and 16S rDNA amplification and sequencing are more accurate and adequate. Nevertheless, these time-consuming procedures generate a delay in the surveillance of microbial air quality. For this reason, it is necessary to consider other methods that are able to detect and identify pathogenic microorganisms in a more efficient and rapid manner. In this context, biosensors able to detect specific molecules produced by pathogenic microorganisms are a more precise and faster method for the detection of airborne pathogens.

In this chapter, we describe different biosensors (based on whole cell sensing-reporter systems) that are able to detect bacterial signaling molecules produced in a concentration-dependent manner by the quorum sensing (QS) cell-to-cell communication system. These signaling molecules called autoinducers (AI) are present inside bacterial cells as well as in the environment and can be specific according to producer strain. Since QS is present in different pathogenic bacteria like *Acinetobacter baumannii, Klebsiella pneumoniae, Legionella pneumophila, Pseudomonas aeruginosa* and *Streptococcus pyogenes,* it is proposed that biosensors can be applied to develop new technologies for the detection of airborne pathogenic bacteria in indoor spaces. Furthermore, a general model for biosensor technology focused on the development of intelligent buildings is presented. The aim of this model is to reduce airborne pathogenic bacteria concentration and dissemination, in association with online applications (Apps).

2. Airborne pathogens and quorum sensing

2.1. Airborne pathogens and indoor spaces

In confined and shared spaces, the host-environment-pathogen equilibrium can be altered due to inadequate building design that leads to a reduced air renewal, limitation of natural

http://dx.doi.org/10.5772/intechopen.72390

light and favors overcrowding, increasing microbial concentration and dissemination of airborne pathogenic bacteria. **Figure 1** shows four different models of pathogen-environment-host interaction. When environment-host-pathogen interplay is at equilibrium, pathogenic microorganisms exist at low concentration in the environment due to physical-chemical or biological factors such as temperature, ultraviolet light, pH and water activity (A_w) (a). In certain conditions, in which biological risks should be reduced at minimum or eliminated, pathogens should get excluded from the host's environment (b). This includes research facilities with biosafety level 3 or 4, and pharmaceutical facilities for production of vaccines, medical devices or parenteral nutrition. On the other hand, in confined or overcrowded spaces, a major biological risk is expected due to impact of the environment on pathogen-host interaction (c). In this condition, different strategies to reduce microbial concentrations and disseminations should be considered. These strategies include ventilation, heating, air conditioning and humidifiers systems, as well as high efficiency particulate air (HEPA) and ultra-low particulate air (ULPA) filters, UV lamps and sanitizers (aerosol). On the other hand, when all measures for air quality control fail, the loss of host-environment-pathogen equilibrium generates an infectious outbreak (d).

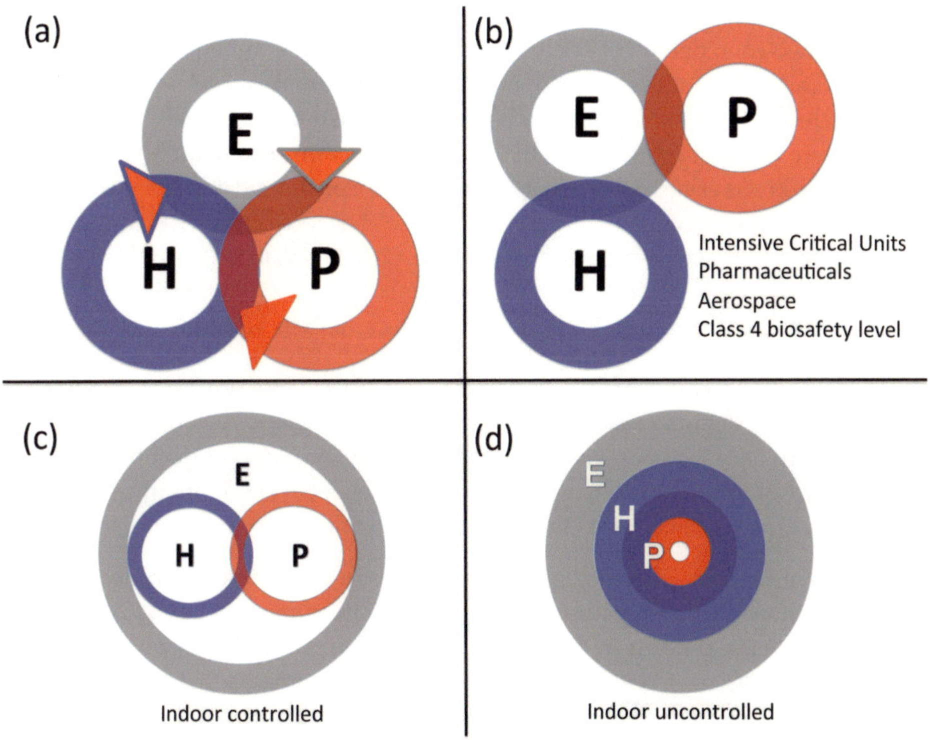

Figure 1. Host (H)-environment (E)-pathogen (P) interplay in different conditions. The schemes show four different interaction conditions between the host and the pathogen. In an ideal condition (a), pathogens have a low interaction with the environment and the host, even though it is circulating in the population and the environment. In (b), there is a restrictive condition in which for biosafety reasons, the pathogen must be excluded from the environment and the host. In (c) and (d), a model is shown for host-environment-pathogen interaction in indoor at low and high biological risk, respectively.

2.2. Quorum sensing and chemical signals

Quorum sensing is a cell-to-cell communication system that allows bacteria to act in a coordinate manner. This mechanism is based on the synthesis, release and detection of signal molecules, called autoinducers (AI), whose increase is in a cell-density dependent mode. When AI reaches a threshold concentration due to an increase in bacterial population, the autoinducer activates a transcriptional regulator that controls gene expression of genetic elements under QS regulation. The first report of QS was in 1979, when Nelson and Hasting described this communication system as a regulatory mechanism of bioluminescence in *Vibrio harveyi* [4]. Nowadays, three parallel quorum sensing mechanisms have been identified in *V. harveyi* as regulators of gene expression [5].

In Gram-negative bacteria, QS consists typically of an autoinducer synthase and transcriptional regulator protein that binds to the AI and regulates gene expression of target genes. The chemical structure of the AI can vary between microorganisms; nevertheless, the main AIs in Gram-negative bacteria are *N*-acyl homoserine lactones (AHL). Other autoinducers identified in Gram-negative bacteria include: autoinducer-2 (AI-2); cholera autoinducer CAI-1, diffusible signal factor (DSF), *Legionella* autoinducer (LAI-1), among others (for review, see Ref. [6]). In Gram-positive bacteria, two types of QS systems have been identified: a one-component system and a two-component QS system. In both systems, the autoinducers correspond to oligopeptides called autoinducer peptide (AIP) that are synthetized and secreted to the environment, where they suffer structural modifications. In the one-component QS system, extracellular AIPs are transported back into the cell through permeases and are recognized by a specific receptor in the cytoplasm that acts as a transcriptional regulator. The two-component system consists of a membrane-bound protein kinase that recognized AIP and activates the transcriptional regulator in the cytoplasm through its phosphorylation (for review, see Ref. [7]).

2.3. Quorum sensing in airborne bacterial pathogens and their autoinducers

Quorum sensing (QS) communication system is present in a diverse group of microorganisms from environmental to human pathogenic bacteria. In pathogenic bacteria, QS regulates the expression of virulence factors such as biofilm formation, enzyme production and secretion and antibiotic resistance [8, 9]. Regarding airborne pathogens, QS communication system is present in several airborne bacteria (**Table 1**), playing a role in virulence and pathogenesis.

Pseudomonas aeruginosa is a Gram-negative opportunistic bacterium that causes healthcare-associated infections, including respiratory infections in immunodeficient patients. These infections are of major concern in patients with cystic fibrosis and severe burn injuries [10, 11]. The Centre for Disease Control and Prevention (CDC) estimated that *P. aeruginosa* causes 51,000 healthcare-associated infections per year in the United States. Due to antibiotic resistance that reaches 13% in the USA, these infections can become chronic and are associated with high mortality rates. In this pathogen, several virulence factors are under QS control: biofilm formation, pyoverdine synthesis and hemolysin production, among others [12, 13]. The major autoinducer molecules identified in *P. aeruginosa* QS are *N*-butyryl-L-homoserine lactone and *N*-(3-oxododecanoyl)-L-homoserine lactone [14, 15].

Airborne pathogen	Pathology	Main autoinducer(s) type	Refs.
Pseudomonas aeruginosa	Opportunistic infections	AHL*	[14, 15]
		3-oxo-AHL*	
Klebsiella pneumoniae	Pneumonia, bronchitis	AI-2**	[19]
Acinetobacter baumannii	Opportunistic infections	3-hydroxy-AHL*	[18]
Streptococcus pyogenes	Pharyngitis, cellulitis	AI-2**	[22]
Legionella pneumophila	Legionnaire's disease	LAI-1*** (3-hydroxypentadecane-4-one)	[20]

*AHL: acyl homoserine lactone.
**AI-2: autoinducer-2.
***LAI-1: *Legionella* autoinducer.

Table 1. Selected airborne pathogens with quorum sensing communication system.

Acinetobacter baumannii is a Gram-negative pathogen associated with hospital-acquired infections. The ability of this pathogen to develop antibiotic resistance is a public health issue worldwide. Its main QS signaling molecule has been identified as *N*-3-hydroxy-dodecanoyl-homoserine lactone, and in this pathogen, QS regulates biofilm formation and the expression of drug-resistance genes [16–18].

Klebsiella pneumoniae is also a Gram-negative bacterium that causes nosocomial infections. This pathogen presents type 2 QS system and uses AI-2 (furanosyl borate diester) as autoinducer, and this system is involved in biofilm formation [19].

Legionella pneumophila is a Gram-negative opportunistic pathogen that, through inhalation, can cause Legionnaires′ disease, which is a severe type of pneumonia. This pathogen uses LAI-1 (3-hydroxypentadecane-4-one) as autoinducers for *Legionella* quorum sensing (Lqs) system [20]. In *L. pneumophila,* QS system regulates biofilm formation, and LAI-1 has been described to be involved in inter-kingdom communication with eukaryotic cells [21].

Streptococcus pyogenes is a Gram-positive microorganism that causes pharyngitis and other respiratory tract infections. In this pathogen, QS has been related to protease production, among other phonotypical characteristics. Despite *S. pyogenes* is a Gram-positive bacterium, recent studies have identified that it uses AI-2 as a signaling molecule in QS [22].

3. Biosensors for detections of quorum sensing signals molecules

Due to quorum sensing (QS), communication system allows bacteria to act in a coordinate manner, to coordinate gene expression and to have a greater impact on their host, and this system has become a new target for the development of antimicrobial therapies as well as for bacterial diagnosis and therapeutic purposes [23, 24]. In this context, a diverse number of biosensors have been designed and developed to identify QS communication signals called autoinducers (AIs).

3.1. Diversity of quorum sensing biosensors: accuracy, precision and sensibility for autoinducers detection

Biosensors are analytical bio-physicochemical-electronic devices that are able to detect and quantify analytes from a sample (for review, see Ref. [25]). The physical-chemical-electronic component of a biosensor is a detector and transducer able to capture a specific signal generated by the biological component when it is associated with its cognate analyte. The biological component of a biosensor can be whole cells (genetically modified microorganisms containing a genic construct based on a sensing-reporter system); proteins (enzymes, antibodies and antigens) or nucleic acids. To enhance the interaction with the analyte and detector-transducer unit, the biosensor can be encapsulated or adsorbed on inert supports. This chapter focuses on whole cell genetically modified microorganisms designed to detect chemical analytes that are produced by specific bacteria, specifically to detect chemical signals called autoinducers (AIs) produced by the cell-to-cell QS communication system.

3.1.1. Accuracy, precision and sensibility of quorum sensing whole cell biosensors

Accuracy of QS biosensors for pathogen detection depends on the specificity of each molecular sensor (regulatory protein) in response to its autoinducer (AI). In this context, there exist QS whole cell detection systems for acylated homoserine lactones (AHL) and their 3-oxo-AHL and 3-hydroxy-AHL derivatives that are able to differentiate between the length of the acyl chain. For example, *Chromobacterium violaceum* CV026 and pSB536 can detect short-chain AHL, while pSB1075 detects long-chain AHL. On the other hand, other biosensors detect furanosyl borate diester (AI-2) using genetically modified *Vibrio harveyi* strains that do not produce this autoinducer and do not present receptors for other QS systems. From this point of view, QS biosensors can be considered an accurate method; however, it should be noted that it is an indirect detection method for pathogens.

Regarding QS biosensor precision and sensibility, whole cell biosensors can be classified according to their reporter system, which are activated by the transcriptional regulator associated to the AI. **Table 2** shows different biosensors, their phenotypes and detection methods. From these detection systems, luminescence (fluorescence or chemiluminescence) is considered a precise and highly sensitive method [26]. Both, signal and detection methods (luminometer or spectrofluorimeter), allow to detect low concentrations of its AI, which is of special interest due to AI and can activate QS system at low concentrations. For example, threshold concentration of 3-oxo-N-acyl homoserine lactone for the activation of QS system in *P. aeruginosa* is 10 nM [27]; therefore, it is of extreme importance that biosensors can detect AI concentrations of this order of magnitude. In this context, QS biosensor can detect QS signaling molecules at concentrations ranging from pM to μM [28].

Table 2 shows different types of biosensors for the detection of quorum sensing signaling molecules and the reporter systems used in each case.

As previously described, AIs can diffuse outside the cell into culture medium (environment) and be sensed by other microorganisms. **Figure 2** shows *C. violaceum* CV026 (A) exposed to AHL

Biosensor	Host	Detected signaling molecule	Reporter system		Detection method	Refs.
			Genotype	Phenotype		
Chromobacterium violaceum CV026		C4-AHL C6-AHL* C6–3-oxo-AHL C8-AHL C8–3-oxo-AHL	*vioABCD*	Violacein synthesis, Color	Colorimetric	[29]
pSB401	*Escherichia coli* JM109	C6-AHL C6–3-oxo-AHL* C8-AHL C8–3-oxo-AHL	*luxCDABE*	Luciferase synthesis, Luminiscence	Luminiscence	[30]
pSB536	*Escherichia coli* JM109	C4-AHL*	*luxCDABE*	Luciferase synthesis, Luminiscence	Luminiscence	[31]
pSB1075	*Escherichia coli* JM109	C10–3-oxo-AHL C12–3-oxo-AHL* C12-AHL	*luxCDABE*	Luciferase synthesis, Luminiscence	Luminiscence	[30]
pZLR4	*Agrobacterium tumefaciens* NT1	C8–3-oxo-AHL* All 3-oxo-AHL C6-AHL C8-AHL C10-AHL C12-AHL C14-AHL C6–3-hydroxy-AHL C8–3-hydroxy-AHL C10–3-hydroxy-AHL	*lacZ*	β-galactosidase activity, Color	Colorimetric	[32]
pAS-C8	Broad host range	C8-AHL C10-AHL	*gfp*	GFP synthesis, Fluorescence	Fluorescence	[33]
Vibrio harveyi JMH597		AI-2	*luxCDABE*	Luciferase, Luminiscence	Luminiscence	[5]

*Major sensibility to this signaling molecule.

Table 2. Biosensor for quorum sensing signaling molecules.

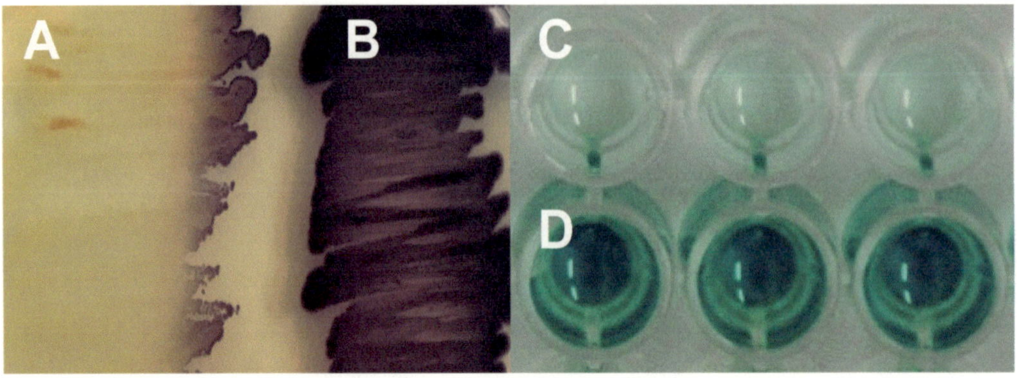

Figure 2. Bacterial biosensors for AHL detection. *Chromobacterium violaceum* CV026 (A) exposed to diffusible AHLs produced by *C. violaceum* wild type (B). *Agrobacterium tumefaciens* NT1 pZLR4 supplemented with X-gal (C) and *A. tumefaciens* NT1 pZLR4 supplemented with X-gal and C6-AHL (D).

produced by *C. violaceum* wild type (B), inducing violacein synthesis in strain CV026 as a positive reaction for the detection of AHL. On the other hand, *A. tumefaciens* NT1 pZLR4 supplemented with X-gal shows no β-galactosidase activity (colorless) in the absence of AHL (A), while bacterial culture shows a chromogenic reaction when it is exposed to AHL due to this enzyme activity.

4. Choosing the appropriate biosensor phenotype for an indoor detection system

4.1. Quorum sensing microbial-based biosensors

Classically, quorum sensing (QS) has been studied to find new strategies to fight bacterial infections [34]; nevertheless, this system has also been proposed as a biomarker system [35]. Due to QS, autoinducers (AIs) are chemically diverse and are biomolecules produced under conditions by specific bacteria, and detection of AI allows an indirect identification of bacterial pathogens [36, 37]. Because AI concentration increases in a cell-density dependent manner, their detection and quantification also permit to determine the state of infection [38]. Several analytical methods have been used to identify these molecules, like ultra-performance liquid chromatography (UPLC), high-performance liquid chromatography (HPLC) and high-resolution mass spectrometry; nevertheless, these chemical analyses require high-tech equipment as well as sample preparation, extraction and purification [39]. Therefore, it has been proposed that QS microbial biosensors are a potent tool for environmental and healthcare monitoring [40]. Unlike biosensors for inorganic bacterial compounds like ATP [41], biosensors based on QS show higher specificity and consist of viable microbial cells.

4.2. Choosing the adequate quorum sensing biosensor

In order to detect airborne bacterial pathogens in indoor spaces in a more efficient manner, whole cell and cell-free biosensors are able to detect QS signaling molecules, which are of great interest. These sensors are suitable for *in vitro* and *in situ* measurements [42]. As described earlier, reporter methods include luminescent, fluorescent and colorimetric signals (**Table 2**), which required widely available equipment for laboratory usage as well as for *in situ* measurements [43]. Additionally, QS biosensors can detect QS signaling molecules at low concentrations, ranging from pM to μM [28]. **Figure 3** shows a biosensor model for autoinducer detection. This biosensor is composed of four essential genetic elements: promoter R1, gene encoding QS transcriptional regulator, promoter R2 and a reporter system. R1 is a promoter region that regulates gene expression of the transcriptional regulator of QS system. This promoter can be designed in order to respond to different stimuli and induce gene expression of the transcriptional regulator. This transcriptional regulator binds the autoinducer and regulates gene expression of the reporter system by binding promoter region R2, which is a QS promoter region.

The main issues regarding detection of airborne pathogens are related to low bacterial concentration in air samples and interference of other particulate materials in the analyses, requiring appropriate sampling methods and equipment. In this context, QS biosensor technology should contain three essential units: (i) air sampler, (ii) cassette containing active bacterial cells used as biosensor and (iii) a signal processing module that allows data analysis and report generation. There are two main strategies to obtain air samples: (1) to use air samples and (2) harvest particulate matter from air conditioning equipment [44]. Air samples can be

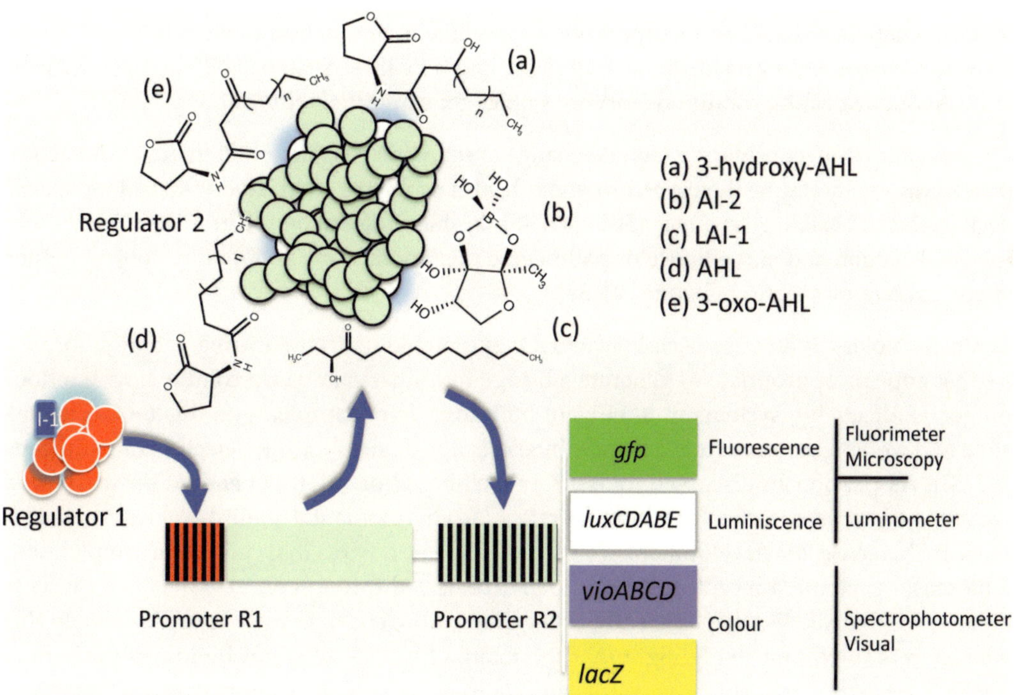

Figure 3. Biosensors for detection of autoinducers (AI) molecules from quorum sensing (QS). Promoter R1 regulates gene expression of the quorum sensing transcriptional regulation (TR) that binds autoinducer (AI) molecules. The TR-AI complex induces gene expression of the reporter system by binding promoter region R2, which is a canonical QS promoter region.

directly coupled to culture medium or inorganic supports containing the biosensor, which will be activated in the presence of QS signaling molecules [45].

The selection of the appropriated biosensor will depend on equipment availability. Colorimetric biosensors do not need a specialized instrument for qualitative analysis due to their visual signal. In case of a quantitative evaluation, a spectrophotometer equipped with specific filters is needed. On the other hand, luminescent and fluorescent biosensors require luminometer and a fluorimeter, respectively, for qualitative and quantitative measurements. Excitation and emission wavelength will depend on the fluorescent protein, which is used as a reporter.

5. A model for future developments: integrating biosensors to global connectivity era and intelligent building to reduce indoor microbiological risks

From a positive and holistic point of view, the vertiginous advances in connectivity, robotics, automation, electronics, computer science, synthetic biology and artificial intelligence allow us to understand that these disciplines will improve our living conditions. In this context, it is easy to imagine the positive impact of automated bioelectronic systems integrated into architecture design and newly build techniques on life quality and health. However, the most revolutionary aspect will be incorporation of intelligent automation devices in cars, houses, hospitals, classrooms or institutional buildings, and how these systems will intelligently generate favorable healthy conditions for the people, cities and their environments [46].

On the other hand, considering climate change and the increase in antibiotic resistance, complex solutions should be developed to avoid health problems associated with indoor spaces such as the *sick building syndrome* (SBS) [47, 48]. In this context, the integration of biosensors for the detection and surveillance of pathogenic microorganisms and quality control indoor spaces is an appropriate challenge [49–52].

Synthetic biology is an interdisciplinary tool based on biology, engineering and bioinformatics that appears appropriate to generate a bridge to connect bio-based solutions with indoor microbial air quality systems in intelligent buildings. For example, with this tool, it is possible to develop genetic circuits and new bioelectronic devices for the detection of pathogens [40, 53]. As previously discussed, biosensors (cell-based or cell-independent sensors) are a suitable tool for the detection of molecules related to environmental quality problems or health risks. In this sense, the development of new bioelectronic devices that consider a sampler unit, a biosensor unit and a receptor unit, remotely connected through online systems represents an advance that allows us to efficiently act against pathogens in indoor environments. In this context, it is important to highlight that the main advantage of smart buildings for human health is related to their ability to couple air quality sensors with automatic control systems.

According to the abovementioned factors, **Figure 4** shows an integrative model of biosensors coupled to an air sampler, equipped with units that allow (i) capturing microorganisms and

http://dx.doi.org/10.5772/intechopen.72390

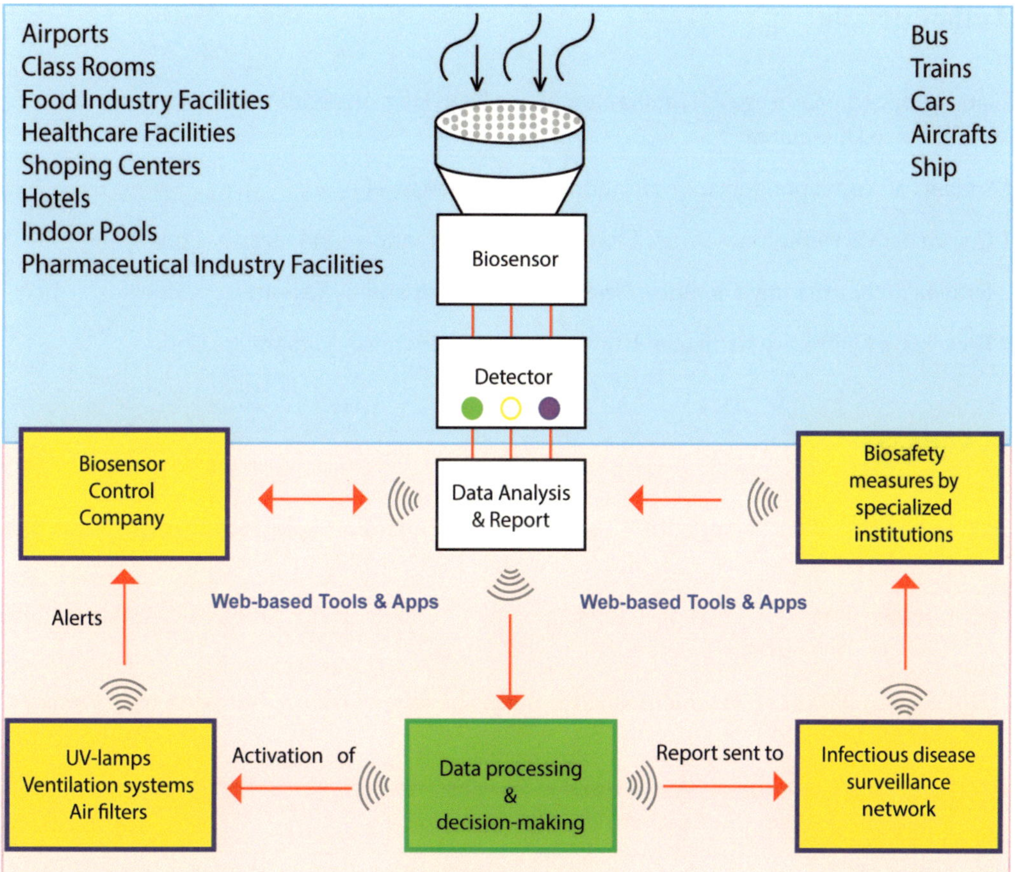

Figure 4. Sensors for detecting and monitoring pathogens in indoor spaces in the era of connectivity, intelligent buildings and automation. Figure shows the integration of a quorum sensing autoinducer biosensor to an intelligent air sampling system, connected to an intelligent control and surveillance system.

their molecules, (ii) exposing them to biosensors, (iii) capturing the signals emitted by the biosensor and (iv) analyzing them and sending a report through web applications to the users. Likewise, the proposed model integrates this technology into intelligent buildings or indoor spaces in general to remotely activate automated systems that reduce the microbial load or informs the health authority in the event of an infectious outbreak occurs.

Acknowledgements

This work was supported by the following grant: CIDI-DIUV 4/2016 from Universidad de Valparaíso and grant: FONDEF VIU140070 from Comisión Nacional de Investigación Científica y Tecnológica (CONICYT).

Author details

Claudia Ibacache-Quiroga[1,2], Natalia Romo[1], Rodrigo Díaz-Viciedo[1,3] and M. Alejandro Dinamarca[1,2*]

*Address all correspondence to: alejandro.dinamarca@uv.cl

1 Centro de Micro-Bioinnovación, Universidad de Valparaíso, Valparaíso, Chile

2 Escuela de Nutrición y Dietética, Universidad de Valparaíso, Valparaíso, Chile

3 Escuela de Química y Farmacia, Universidad de Valparaíso, Valparaíso, Chile

References

[1] Fraser DW et al. Legionnaires' disease: Description of an epidemic of pneumonia. The New England Journal of Medicine. 1977;**297**(22):1189-1197

[2] Gonzalez-Martin C. Airborne infectious microorganisms. In: Reference Module in Life Sciences. Amsterdam, Neetherlands: Elsevier; 2017

[3] Pasquarella C et al. Air microbial sampling: The state of the art. Igiene e Sanità Pubblica. 2008;**64**(1):79-120

[4] Nealson KH, Hastings JW. Bacterial bioluminescence: Its control and ecological significance. Microbiological Reviews. 1979;**43**(4):496-518

[5] Henke JM, Bassler BL. Three parallel quorum-sensing systems regulate gene expression in *Vibrio harveyi*. Journal of Bacteriology. 2004;**186**(20):6902-6914

[6] Papenfort K, Bassler BL. Quorum sensing signal-response systems in Gram-negative bacteria. Nature Reviews. Microbiology. 2016;**14**(9):576-588

[7] Hawver LA, Jung SA, Ng WL. Specificity and complexity in bacterial quorum-sensing systems. FEMS Microbiology Reviews. 2016;**40**(5):738-752

[8] Zhu J et al. Quorum-sensing regulators control virulence gene expression in Vibrio cholerae. Proceedings of the National Academy of Sciences of the United States of America. 2002;**99**(5):3129-3134

[9] Smith RS, Iglewski BH. *P. aeruginosa* quorum-sensing systems and virulence. Current Opinion in Microbiology. 2003;**6**(1):56-60

[10] Burns JL et al. Longitudinal assessment of *Pseudomonas aeruginosa* in young children with cystic fibrosis. The Journal of Infectious Diseases. 2001;**183**(3):444-452

[11] Williams FN et al. The leading causes of death after burn injury in a single pediatric burn center. Critical Care. 2009;**13**(6):R183

[12] Latifi A et al. Multiple homologues of LuxR and LuxI control expression of virulence determinants and secondary metabolites through quorum sensing in *Pseudomonas aeruginosa* PAO1. Molecular Microbiology. 1995;**17**(2):333-343

[13] De Kievit TR et al. Quorum-sensing genes in *Pseudomonas aeruginosa* biofilms: Their role and expression patterns. Applied and Environmental Microbiology. 2001;**67**(4):1865-1873

[14] Pearson JP et al. Structure of the autoinducer required for expression of Pseudomonas Aeruginosa virulence genes. Proceedings of the National Academy of Sciences of the United States of America. 1994;**91**(1):197-201

[15] Pearson JP et al. A second N-acylhomoserine lactone signal produced by *Pseudomonas aeruginosa*. Proceedings of the National Academy of Sciences of the United States of America. 1995;**92**(5):1490-1494

[16] Dou Y et al. *Acinetobacter baumannii* quorum-sensing signalling molecule induces the expression of drug-resistance genes. Molecular Medicine Reports. 2017;**15**(6):4061-4068

[17] Chow JY et al. Disruption of biofilm formation by the human pathogen *Acinetobacter baumannii* using engineered quorum-quenching lactonases. Antimicrobial Agents and Chemotherapy. 2014;**58**(3):1802-1805

[18] Niu C et al. Isolation and characterization of an autoinducer synthase from *Acinetobacter baumannii*. Journal of Bacteriology. 2008;**190**(9):3386-3392

[19] Balestrino D et al. Characterization of type 2 quorum sensing in *Klebsiella pneumoniae* and relationship with biofilm formation. Journal of Bacteriology. 2005;**187**(8):2870-2880

[20] Spirig T et al. The Legionella autoinducer synthase LqsA produces an alpha-hydroxyketone signaling molecule. The Journal of Biological Chemistry. 2008;**283**(26):18113-18123

[21] Hochstrasser R, Hilbi H. Intra-species and inter-kingdom signaling of *Legionella pneumophila*. Frontiers in Microbiology. 2017;**8**:79

[22] Lyon WR et al. Mutation of luxS affects growth and virulence factor expression in *Streptococcus pyogenes*. Molecular Microbiology. 2001;**42**(1):145-157

[23] Rossiter SE, Fletcher MH, Wuest WM. Natural products as platforms to overcome antibiotic resistance. Chemical Reviews. 2017;**117**(19):12415-12474

[24] McNerney MP, Styczynski MP. Small molecule signaling, regulation, and potential applications in cellular therapeutics. Wiley Interdisciplinary Reviews. Systems Biology and Medicine; 2017

[25] Gopinath SC et al. Bacterial detection: From microscope to smartphone. Biosensors & Bioelectronics. 2014;**60**:332-342

[26] Meir D et al. Colorimetric/fluorescent bacterial sensing by agarose-embedded lipid/polydiacetylene films. Journal of Applied Microbiology. 2008;**104**(3):787-795

[27] Scholz RL, Greenberg EP. Positive autoregulation of an acyl-Homoserine lactone quorum-sensing circuit synchronizes the population response. MBio. 2017;**8**(4):e01079-17

[28] Massai F et al. A multitask biosensor for micro-volumetric detection of N-3-oxo-dodecanoyl-homoserine lactone quorum sensing signal. Biosensors & Bioelectronics. 2011; **26**(8):3444-3449

[29] McClean KH et al. Quorum sensing and *Chromobacterium violaceum*: Exploitation of violacein production and inhibition for the detection of N-acylhomoserine lactones. Microbiology. 1997;**143**(Pt 12):3703-3711

[30] Winson MK et al. Construction and analysis of luxCDABE-based plasmid sensors for investigating N-acyl homoserine lactone-mediated quorum sensing. FEMS Microbiology Letters. 1998;**163**(2):185-192

[31] Swift S et al. Quorum sensing in *Aeromonas hydrophila* and *Aeromonas salmonicida*: Identification of the LuxRI homologs AhyRI and AsaRI and their cognate N-acylhomoserine lactone signal molecules. Journal of Bacteriology. 1997;**179**(17):5271-5281

[32] Farrand SK, Qin Y, Oger P. Quorum-sensing system of *Agrobacterium* plasmids: Analysis and utility. Methods in Enzymology. 2002;**358**:452-484

[33] Riedel K et al. N-acylhomoserine-lactone-mediated communication between *Pseudomonas aeruginosa* and *Burkholderia cepacia* in mixed biofilms. Microbiology. 2001;**147**(Pt 12): 3249-3262

[34] Rasmussen TB, Givskov M. Quorum-sensing inhibitors as anti-pathogenic drugs. International Journal of Medical Microbiology. 2006;**296**(2-3):149-161

[35] Struss AK et al. Toward implementation of quorum sensing autoinducers as biomarkers for infectious disease states. Analytical Chemistry. 2013;**85**(6):3355-3362

[36] Singh PK et al. Quorum-sensing signals indicate that cystic fibrosis lungs are infected with bacterial biofilms. Nature. 2000;**407**(6805):762-764

[37] Chambers CE et al. Identification of N-acylhomoserine lactones in mucopurulent respiratory secretions from cystic fibrosis patients. FEMS Microbiology Letters. 2005; **244**(2):297-304

[38] Kumari A, Pasini P, Daunert S. Detection of bacterial quorum sensing N-acyl homoserine lactones in clinical samples. Analytical and Bioanalytical Chemistry. 2008;**391**(5): 1619-1627

[39] Fekete A et al. Identification of bacterial N-acylhomoserine lactones (AHLs) with a combination of ultra-performance liquid chromatography (UPLC), ultra-high-resolution mass spectrometry, and in-situ biosensors. Analytical and Bioanalytical Chemistry. 2007;**387**(2):455-467

[40] Chang HJ et al. Microbially derived biosensors for diagnosis, monitoring and epidemiology. Microbial Biotechnology. 2017;**10**(5):1031-1035

[41] Yao W et al. An aptamer-based electrochemiluminescent biosensor for ATP detection. Biosensors & Bioelectronics. 2009;**24**(11):3269-3274

[42] Struss A et al. Paper strip whole cell biosensors: A portable test for the semiquantitative detection of bacterial quorum signaling molecules. Analytical Chemistry. 2010; **82**(11):4457-4463

[43] Eren H. Electronic Portable Instruments: Design and Applications. Boca Raton, USA: CRC Press; 2003

[44] Napoli C, Marcotrigiano V, Montagna MT. Air sampling procedures to evaluate microbial contamination: A comparison between active and passive methods in operating theatres. BMC Public Health. 2012;**12**:594

[45] Derikvand F et al. Cellulose-based biosensors for esterase detection. Analytical Chemistry. 2016;**88**(6):2989-2993

[46] Podgorny M, et al. Open web services-based indoor climate control system. 2011. Google Patents.

[47] Walls KL, Boulic M, Boddy JW. The built environment-a missing "cause of the causes" of non-communicable diseases. International Journal of Environmental Research and Public Health. 2016;**13**(10):957

[48] Joshi SM. The sick building syndrome. Indian Journal of Occupational and Environmental Medicine. 2008;**12**(2):61-64

[49] Heidari L et al. Integrating health into buildings of the future. Journal of Solar Energy Engineering. 2016;**139**(1):010802-010802-8

[50] Smielowska M, Marc M, Zabiegala B. Indoor air quality in public utility environments – A review. Environmental Science and Pollution Research International. 2017; **24**(12):11166-11176

[51] Salonen H et al. Physical characteristics of the indoor environment that affect health and wellbeing in healthcare facilities: A review. Intelligent Buildings International. 2013;**5**(1):3-25

[52] Salonen H et al. Design approaches for promoting beneficial indoor environments in healthcare facilities: A review. Intelligent Buildings International. 2013;**5**(1):26-50

[53] Slomovic S, Pardee K, Collins JJ. Synthetic biology devices for in vitro and in vivo diagnostics. Proceedings of the National Academy of Sciences. 2015;**112**(47):14429-14435

Chapter 7

Development of a Modular Biosensor System for Rapid Pathogen Detection

René Hanke, Nina Bailly, Philipp Demling,
Florian N. Gohr, Patrick Opdensteinen,
Michael J. Osthege, Markus Joppich,
Suresh Sudarsan, Ulrich Schwaneberg,
Wolfgang Wiechert and Lars M. Blank

Additional information is available at the end of the chapter

http://dx.doi.org/10.5772/intechopen.72457

Abstract

Progress in the field of pathogen detection relies on at least one of the following three qualities: selectivity, speed, and cost-effectiveness. Here, we demonstrate a proof of concept for an optical biosensing system for the detection of the opportunistic human pathogen *Pseudomonas aeruginosa* while addressing the abovementioned traits through a modular design. The biosensor detects pathogen-specific quorum sensing molecules and generates a fluorescence signal via an intracellular amplifier. Using a tailored measurement device built from low-cost components, the image analysis software detected the presence of *P. aeruginosa* in 42 min of incubation. Due to its modular design, individual components can be optimized or modified to specifically detect a variety of different pathogens. This biosensor system represents a successful integration of synthetic biology with software and hardware engineering.

Keywords: quorum sensing, FRET, signal amplification, whole-cell biosensor, customized hardware, online image analysis, point of contact, synthetic biology, iGEM, *Pseudomonas aeruginosa*

1. Introduction

A prerequisite for countermeasures against opportunistic pathogens is their rapid detection [1, 2]. In contrast, conventional diagnostic methods often utilize time-consuming techniques such as microscopy and cultivation in different media [3] and bear the risk of false-positive or false-negative results [4]. Traditionally, microbiological tests have hence been performed by trained personnel in stationary laboratories, because the complex instrumentation hinders transportation [5].

Established methods for detection and identification of pathogenic bacteria most commonly rely on PCR, culture, and counting or immunological techniques such as ELISA. PCR-based methods are extremely sensitive but require purified samples and hours of processing as well as staff trained in molecular biology. Immunological methods are similarly sensitive but often require costly analytes (e.g., labeled antibodies). For detailed information, such as sensitivity, please refer to the "Discussion and outlook" section. Another commercially available technique for pathogen detection is flow cytometry, which offers rapid, quantitative measurements of multiple parameters of individual cells. However, it is expensive and requires stable growth conditions for the organisms to allow reproducible results [6]. Considering these limitations, the need for rapid, specific, and inexpensive point-of-contact tests becomes apparent. Furthermore, these tests should be intuitive to conduct while providing the same or a higher sensitivity than traditional detection methods [1, 7].

Biosensors represent a promising approach for pathogen detection and have the potential to fulfill the aforementioned demands [7]. For example, biosensors offer advantages such as high specificity and sensitivity [6]. Increasing effort has been spent on the development of biosensors that allow for portable microbiological tests since the 1990s [6, 8].

A biosensor can be defined as an analytical device in which a biologically active component (e.g., an enzyme, antibody, whole cell) is immobilized onto the surface of a transducing element (electronic, optic, or optoelectronic), allowing the detection of target analytes in complex mixtures [9]. A typical biosensor comprises three main parts: the bio-recognition component, the interface, and the transducing element [10]. The biological component specifically recognizes the analyte, and the biochemical interaction is then converted into a quantifiable signal via the transducer [9]. The choice of the interface and immobilization technique depends on the selected biological element and transducer [10]. Based on the method utilized for signal transduction, biosensors can be roughly classified into four basic groups, namely, optical, mass, electrochemical, and thermal sensors [6].

Optical biosensors are particularly interesting for detection of pathogens because of their higher sensitivity than electrochemical biosensors. For example, optical biosensors based on surface plasmon resonance (SPR) are already commercially available in a portable format (Spreeta System, Texas Instruments). Drawbacks of this technique are comparably high costs and complexity requiring trained staff for operation [5].

2. The five key elements of the proposed biosensor

The present work provides proof of concept for a novel approach toward a cost-efficient, optical biosensor, which enables safe and simple detection of pathogens and does not require highly trained staff for operation. The detection system was designed for investigation of solid surfaces, for example, to assess cleaning success in a hospital environment, which is receiving increasing interest [10]. This project was performed and has successfully competed in the International Genetically Engineered Machine (iGEM) competition 2014 [11].

The potential of the proposed system lies within the combination of biology and engineering as the development of biosensors is highly interdisciplinary [7]. Five key components, namely, biomolecular detection (I) with intracellular signal amplification (II) embedded into a two-dimensional sensor chip (III), a custom incubation device (IV), and automated image analysis (V), constitute the functional biosensor as displayed in **Figure 1**. In terms of the biological component, the present project comprised the genetic engineering of sensor cells (introduction of the amplifying reporter circuit in *Escherichia coli*) as well as the optimization of the interface and immobilization of the resulting sensor cells. The transduction element (hardware), a customized detection unit, and image analysis software for automated evaluation were developed.

As a model organism for demonstrating the biosensor's functionality, the well-studied opportunistic pathogen *Pseudomonas aeruginosa* [12] was chosen as it has become a major cause of nosocomial infections; about 10% of nosocomial infections in most European Union hospitals are currently caused by *P. aeruginosa* alone [13]. Additionally, this bacterium often acquires multiple drug resistances and is a threat to patients suffering from cystic fibrosis, severe burns, or immunodeficiency [14].

2.1. Quorum sensing in *Pseudomonas aeruginosa*

Bacteria have evolved complex systems to sense their environment. Quorum sensing (QS) networks present a way to synchronize behavior, such as bioluminescence, biofilm formation, sporulation, and the secretion of virulence factors, on a population-wide scale [15].

In QS systems of bacteria, an autoinducer (AI) is produced by one or more synthases and is secreted from the cell. The cell can in turn detect the autoinducers through receptors in the

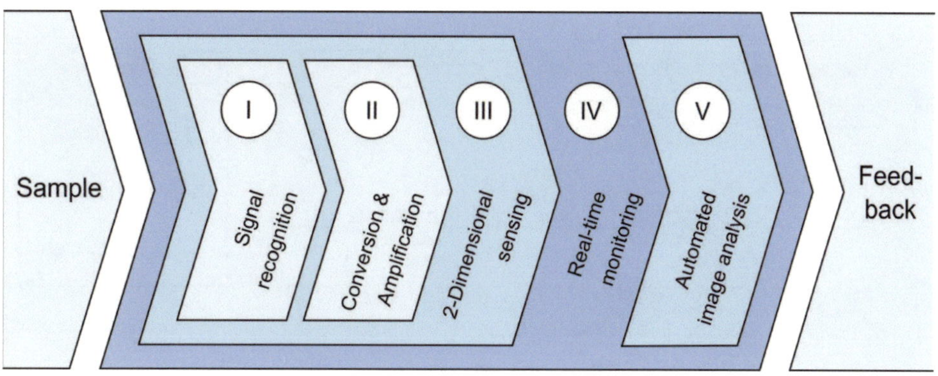

Figure 1. The five key elements of the proposed sensor system. A biomolecular signal originating from pathogens in the sample is recognized (I), converted, and amplified (II) by sensor cells embedded in a two-dimensional sensor chip (III). The chip is incorporated in a detection device capable of real-time monitoring (IV) and equipped with software for an automated image analysis (V). In combination, the setup gives feedback to the user if pathogens were detected.

cytosol (single-step response regulation in Gram-negative bacteria) or in the membrane (two-step response regulation in Gram-positive bacteria). Once a minimal threshold concentration is reached at higher cell densities, the activated AI receptors can induce or repress specific gene expression programs. The induction of the QS regulon leads to the expression of more AI synthase, amplifying the QS signaling [16]. However, most often the QS systems of one bacterial species extend beyond the basic circuit described above. Such configurations can include a multitude of circuits in parallel or series as well as competitive setups and on-off switches [17].

P. aeruginosa is commonly found in soil and is of particular interest due to its role in nosocomial infections. QS is essential for the persistence and disease progression, because it governs cell adhesion, biofilm formation, and virulence factor secretion [14]. The bacterium has three interconnected QS circuits: LasIR and RhlIR, two LuxIR-type circuits, and the *Pseudomonas* quinolone signal (PQS) system. In LasIR, the AI synthase LasI synthesizes the AI 3-oxo-C_{12}-homoserine lactone (3OC_{12}-HSL). LasR is a cytosolic receptor for 3OC_{12}-HSL that acts as an inducer on the *las*I promoter once bound to the AI. LasR is only stable in the complex with its matching AI, in this case 3OC_{12}-HSL. However, LasR not only activates the expression of the Las regulon; it also acts as an inducer for the transcription of *rhlR* and *rhlI*, the receptor and AI synthetase, respectively, in the second LuxIR-type QS system of *P. aeruginosa*. The interaction between the LasIR and RhlIR systems is illustrated in **Figure 2**. The details of *P. aeruginosa* QS have been described in literature [17, 18].

The implementation of the *P. aeruginosa* QS system in *E. coli* is already a well-established example for the use of such components in synthetic biology. Here, the LasIR circuit is used as a reporter system in *E. coli* to detect *P. aeruginosa*. The engineered *E. coli* cells constitutively express the protein LasR. Once 3OC_{12}-HSL is secreted by *P. aeruginosa* cells, it diffuses into the *E. coli* cells and

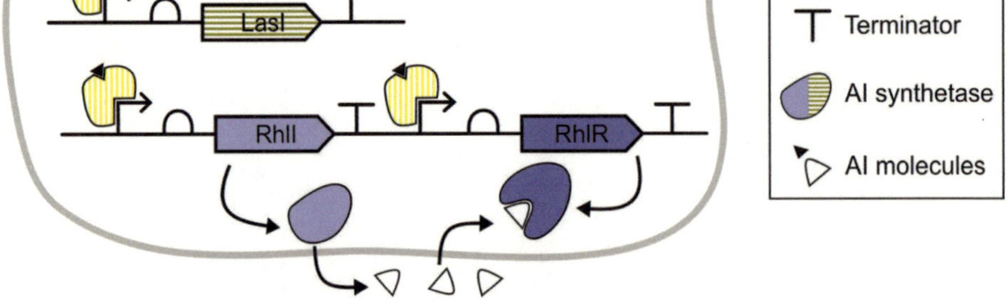

Figure 2. The LuxIR-type QS systems in *P. aeruginosa* and its translation into a biosensor. The AI synthase LasI (horizontal stripes) produces 3OC_{12}-HSL (filled triangles) which bind to the transcription factor LasR (vertical stripes). The LasR-3OC_{12}-HSL complex induces the expression of the Las regulon as well as *rhlI* and *rhlR*. RhlI (light shade) synthesizes the AI C_4-HSL (open triangles) which in turn binds to RhlR (dark shade) and activates the expression of the Rhl regulon as well as the PQS system (not shown). RBS, ribosome binding site; CDS, coding sequence.

binds to LasR. The LasR-3OC$_{12}$-HSL complex then activates the reporter system, resulting in a fluorescent signal that can be read out by the detection device. However, the working principle of the biosensor is not limited to the detection of *P. aeruginosa*. Ultimately, the sensing *E. coli* cells can be engineered to include reporter circuits based on QS systems of other bacteria.

2.2. Molecular signal amplification

The biological component of the proposed biosensor was embodied by genetically modified *E. coli*, which were engineered to generate a fluorescence signal upon the presence of QS molecules specific for *P. aeruginosa* (specifically 3OC$_{12}$-HSL). The core component of the sensor cells is the activation of a pool of quenched fluorophores, which will be discussed in detail later. Desired properties of the sensor cells were a rapid response, specificity, and high sensitivity [10].

The traditional way to report the binding of 3OC$_{12}$-HSL to the constitutively expressed LasR would be the expression of a fluorescent protein, such as GFP, under the control of the *las*I promoter. The presence of the autoinducer would then lead to a detectable fluorescent signal. A rapid generation of the signal, however, would be limited by transcription, translation, folding, posttranslational modification, and maturation of GFP. Therefore, a novel reporter strategy to accelerate the signal generation was chosen. In the proposed system, a quencher-linked GFP fusion protein is constitutively expressed in the cells, but does not exhibit fluorescence as long as the quencher subunit is in close proximity to the GFP subunit. Binding of 3OC$_{12}$-HSL to LasR induces the expression of a tobacco etch virus (TEV) protease, which cleaves the fusion protein. Thereby, GFP is released from the quencher and emits a fluorescence signal. Compared to the conventional approach, the signal is generated faster by maintaining a stock of fusion proteins in the cells, which can be readily cleaved. Additional signal amplification is achieved by the ability of a single TEV protease to cut multiple fusion proteins, while expression of a fluorescent protein upon the presence of 3OC$_{12}$-HSL would only result in a single fluorescent molecule at a time.

2.2.1. Quenching of GFP fluorescence

The quenching of GFP fluorescence in the fusion protein is based on Förster resonance energy transfer (FRET), a process by which the energy of an excited donor fluorophore is transferred to an acceptor molecule whose absorption spectrum overlaps with the emission spectrum of the donor [19]. The energy can then be released, for example, by fluorescence of a longer wavelength or by heat. Yellow fluorescent protein (YFP) represents a suitable FRET acceptor for GFP. Emission resulting from YFP was avoided by using a nonfluorescent mutant of YFP called resonance energy-accepting chromoprotein (REACh [20]). Two REACh variants were generated by introducing the mutation Y145W (REACh1) and the double mutation Y145W/H148 (REACh2) into an enhanced YFP (eYFP) by QuikChange mutagenesis. Ganesan et al. [20] reported a reduction in fluorescence of 82 and 98% for REACh1 and REACh2, respectively.

Both REACh variants were genetically fused to GFP (mut3b [21]) via a linker, which brings both proteins in close proximity, facilitating FRET [22] from GFP to REACh, thus quenching the fluorescence. The linker harbors a cleavage site for the TEV protease (ENLYFQ\S) allowing the separation from the quencher. In the present study, the TEV protease is expressed under control of the *las*I promoter, making it inducible by the QS autoinducer 3OC$_{12}$-HSL. For this purpose, a TEV protease gene with codon optimization for *E. coli* and the anti-self-cleavage mutation S219 V was designed [23]. The GFP-REACh fusion protein is expressed constitutively to ensure continuous supply of protease substrate. **Figure 3** illustrates the interplay between the GFP-REACh fusion protein and the TEV protease. The expression cassette for the GFP-REACh fusion protein was cloned into a pSB3K3 [24] vector backbone, and the TEV protease expression cassette was inserted into a pSB1C3 [25] vector.

2.2.2. *Validation of the reporter system*

For initial validation the developed reporter system was tested via β-D-1-thiogalactopyranoside (IPTG) induction using a well-characterized T7 promoter instead of the *las*I promoter. Two plasmids, one carrying the GFP-REACh fusion protein and one carrying the TEV protease, were introduced into *E. coli* BL21 (DE3). The resulting strain allowed the IPTG-inducible expression of the fusion protein. A growth experiment was conducted in which the fluorescence of the double plasmid strains, containing either variant of the fusion protein and the TEV protease, was compared to cells constitutively expressing GFP as positive control and a nonfluorescent strain as negative control (**Figure 4,** left). For both REACh variants, IPTG-induced as well as IPTG-non-induced cultures were grown in parallel, and all measurements were done in a biological triplicate. The fluorescence was normalized to the observed optical density (OD). The induction with IPTG leads to a rapid increase of the fluorescence signal. At the end point, a signal strength comparable to the positive control was reached, indicating a complete cleavage of the fusion proteins by the TEV protease. The higher base level of fluorescence in the non-induced cells can be attributed to imperfect quenching. This experiment demonstrated the quenching ability of the REACh proteins in our fusion constructs as well as the functionality of the *E. coli*-produced TEV protease.

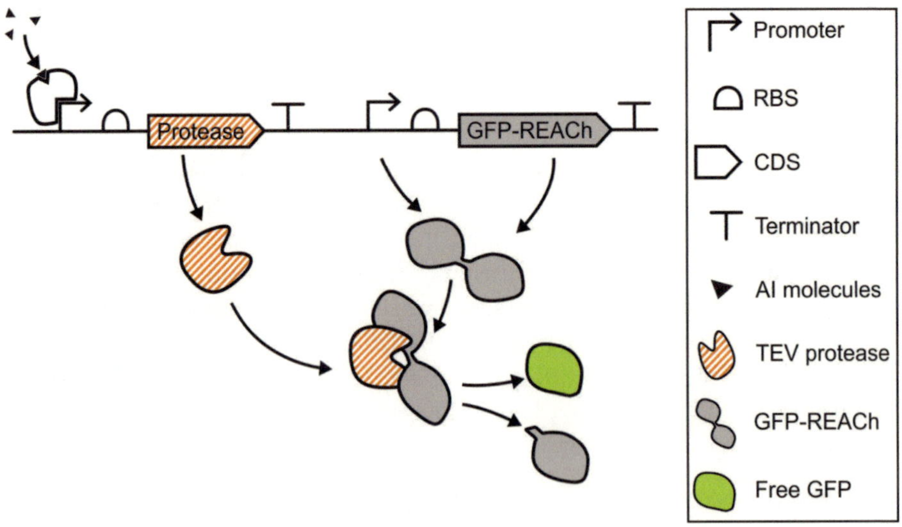

Figure 3. Schematic model of the novel biosensor. Expression of the TEV protease is induced by bacterium-specific HSL bound to its receptor LasR. The protease then activates a pool of readily available fluorophores by cleaving off the quencher (REACh) and releasing fluorescent GFP. RBS, ribosome binding site; CDS, coding sequence.

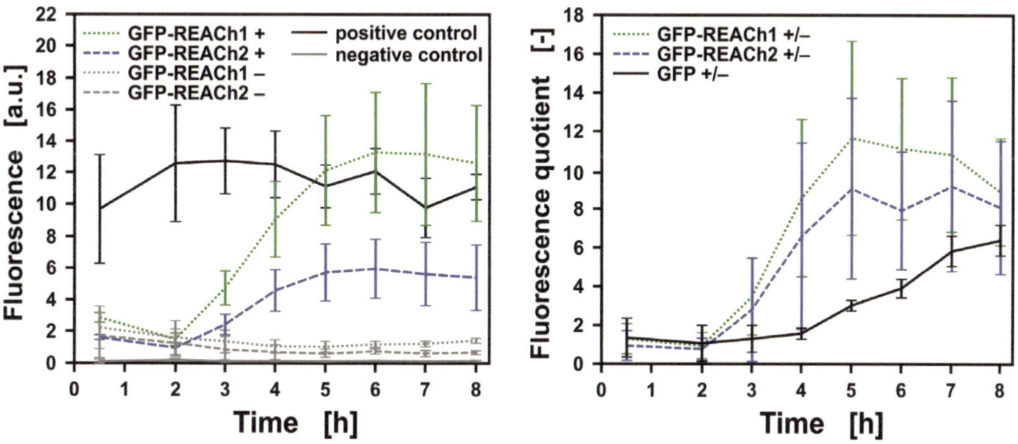

Figure 4. Validation of the reporter system. The production of a fluorescence signal by REACh variants after protease cleavage was compared. Each variant was tested with and without IPTG induction. Constitutive GFP expression and a nonfluorescent strain were used as positive and negative controls, respectively. The fluorescence signal was normalized by the sample OD (left). Comparison of response time of the biosensor setup to conventional GFP expression. The expression of all three systems was under the control of the IPTG-inducible lacI promoter. The fluorescence signal was normalized by the sample OD and based on the signal of a negative control (right). Error bars represent errors as determined by Gaussian error propagation using standard deviations from three biological replicates.

To test the hypothesis that the GFP-REACh fusion proteins in combination with the cleavage amplification results in a faster response than the conventional approach, the kinetics of our reporter strategy were compared to a strain expressing GFP under the control of an IPTG-inducible *lac*I promoter. Using the new reporter strategy, a much stronger and faster increase in fluorescence was observed compared to IPTG-induced expression of GFP (**Figure 4,** right). The high variation for the development of fluorescence by the GFP-REACh systems may have originated from inhomogeneous expression levels of the TEV protease and different sizes of the fluorophore pools. As the signal is amplified by the cleavage of the GFP-REACh fusion protein by the TEV protease, even slight temporal differences in the expression of the TEV protease are expected to cause great shifts in the temporal signal responses, thus resulting in high error bars when different cultures are averaged. The errors were increased even further with the Gaussian error propagation.

2.3. Immobilization of sensor cells

The sensor cells were immobilized in rectangular layers (chips), thus creating an interface between the biological component and the technical component (transducer). Main objectives during the design of the interface were to enable viability and storability of the immobilized sensor cells, reproducibility of the fluorescence response, as well as cost-efficiency. For proof of concept, a simple and robust design was chosen.

A variety of different methods have been used for immobilization of whole cells, which can be divided into six general types: covalent coupling, affinity immobilization, adsorption, confinement in liquid-liquid emulsion, capture behind semipermeable membranes, and entrapment [26]. An established technique for immobilization of living cells is entrapment, which refers to the physical containment of organisms inside a matrix or fibers, thus creating a protective barrier around the cells [27]. Matrices used for entrapment can be synthetic polymers, such as polyester, or natural polymers, such as agar, agarose, or alginate [27]. Entrapment allows to preserve and prolong cell viability, for example, during storage [26, 27], which matched the intentions of this work.

Important prerequisites for the entrapment matrix of the sensor cells were physical rigidity, safety, resistance against biological degradation, transparency, as well as the possibility to conduct matrix synthesis at mild conditions, suitable for living cells. Inorganic polymers such as polyacrylamide were ruled out due to the carcinogenicity of the monomers and rather harsh polymerization conditions [28]. Natural polymers allow for higher diffusion rates than inorganic polymers (tested for small molecules [28]) and are less expensive and less hazardous in production than synthetic polymers. The organic polymer agarose offers several advantages including easy handling, resistance to microbial degradation, and favorable conditions for entrapped cells [27]. Thus, agarose was the polymer of choice for immobilization of cells and formation of chips.

2.3.1. Optimization of chip casting mold and medium

First, a casting mold for rapid and reproducible manufacturing of the 2D sensor chip was developed. A plain surface was a prerequisite for automated image evaluation. Low agarose concentrations (<3.0%) were chosen to reduce consumable costs and to ensure rapid diffusion of the analyte (HSL) to the immobilized sensor cells.

Manufacturing of the agarose gel was conducted based on existing protocols for entrapping living cells in melted polymers. In brief, the temperature of the polymer solution was adjusted to 45°C and was quickly poured into the respective mold after mixing with the sensor cells. Sensor cells were spun down from a liquid culture (50 mL LB, 5 $g \cdot L^{-1}$ NaCl, 10 $g \cdot L^{-1}$ tryptone, 5 $g \cdot L^{-1}$ yeast extract) and resuspended in 1 mL LB medium (21°C) before mixing with the temperature-adjusted agarose solution, resulting in a cell concentration of approximately 5.6×10^9 cells/mL. Before usage, solidified and cutout sensor chips were incubated for 1 h at 37°C.

An open casting mold, which exploited the surface tension of the polymer solution to achieve a plain chip surface, was most successful for the production of sensor chips. After discarding a small gel area in direct contact with the edges of the mold (**Figure 5**, left), bubble-free sensor chips with a plain surface were readily obtained from this approach. The open mold allowed for simple, reproducible, and rapid manufacturing of sensor chips and was hence the method of choice for this work. An agarose concentration of 1.5% was found to be sufficient to cast robust sensor chips. For an accelerated manufacturing process, multiple sensor chips were casted simultaneously using an extended mold (**Figure 5**, left).

Further, to meet the nutritional needs of the sensor cells while minimizing background fluorescence, different complex media (Luria-Bertani or LB medium, Terrific-Broth or TB medium, nutrient agar or NA medium) as well as minimal media (Hartmans minimal or HM medium, M9 minimal medium) were tested with respect to sensor cell growth and the presence of background fluorescence. Background fluorescence was investigated in a commercial gel imaging system (GelDoc™ XR, Biorad, Germany) as well as in the custom-made optical detection device constructed in this work as described in the following section. The results are summarized in **Table 1**, and a comparison of the background fluorescence

http://dx.doi.org/10.5772/intechopen.72457

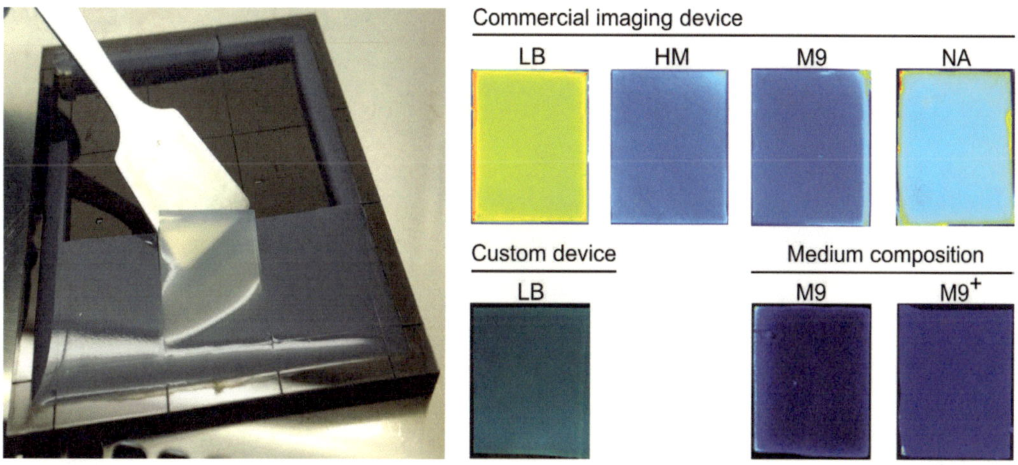

Figure 5. Sensor chip manufacturing and optimization. Sensor chip manufacturing (left) and effect of the medium choice on background fluorescence (right). M9[+] represents supplementation of the M9 minimal medium with Casamino acids. Excitation commercial gel imaging system and in the custom-made optical detection device was conducted at 480 nm. Chips displayed contained 1.5% agarose and no sensor cells.

of sensor chips comprising the respective media is displayed in **Figure 5** (right). Only LB medium allowed for sufficient growth of the sensor cells. Its background fluorescence in the custom-made optical detection device was acceptable, most likely due to the narrow excitation profile compared to the commercial device.

Background fluorescence appeared to be more intense in complex media than in minimal media. To identify a possible cause for this observation, minimal M9 medium was supplemented with 2% Casamino acids (**Figure 5**, right, bottom row). Background fluorescence was stronger in supplemented minimal medium matching reports in literature [29], possibly due to an increased concentration of aromatic amino acids possessing inherent fluorescence.

Activity of the sensor cells after immobilization was investigated in a subsequent experiment by inducing a fluorescent signal with 0.2 μL of a 500 $\mu g \cdot mL^{-1}$ HSL (3-oxo-C_{12}) solution (**Figure 6A**).

	Luria-Bertani medium	Terrific-Broth medium	Nutrient agar medium	M9 minimal medium	Hartmans minimal medium
Growth of sensor cells	+	+	−	−	−
BF, gel imaging system	−	−	+	+	+
BF, custom-made device	+	−	+	+	+

Fluorescence in the commercial gel imaging system and in the custom-made device was measured at λ_{ex} = 480 nm. Growth in the respective media was investigated in liquid culture; background fluorescence was investigated in chips containing 1.5% agarose and no sensor cells. + indicates either growth of the sensor cells or the absence of background fluorescence (BF); − indicates the absence of growth or the presence of background fluorescence.

Table 1. Compatibility of different growth media with the proposed 2D biosensor.

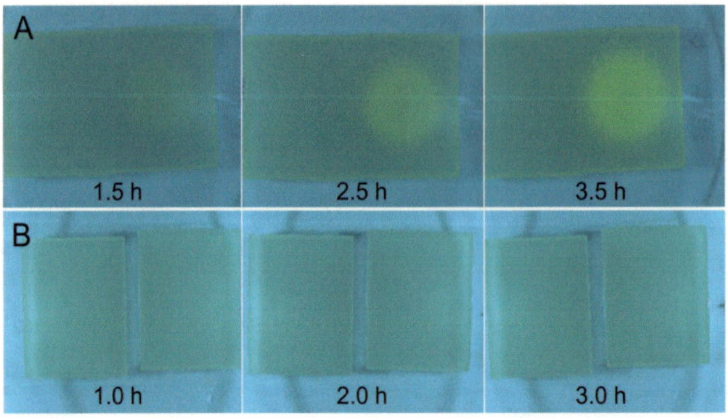

Figure 6. Assessment of the sensor cell viability after immobilization. (A) Fluorescence was induced with 0.2 μL of a 500 μg·mL^{-1} HSL (3-oxo-C_{12}) solution. (B) a non-induced negative control was included to ensure that observed fluorescence only originated from induced sensor cells. Pictures were taken with the custom-made device (λ_{ex} = 480 nm) at different times after induction. Sensor chips were prepared as described in the text section and incubated for 1 h at 37°C before induction.

One and a half hours post induction, a fluorescence signal was visible even to the naked eye, indicating that the sensor cells were in fact still viable after immobilization. No apparent change in fluorescence was observable for the negative control (**Figure 6B**).

For easier handling and experimentation, storability of the sensor chips of several days was desired. Activity of the immobilized sensor cells after storage under different conditions was investigated by induction with HSL. Generation of a fluorescence signal was used as an indicator for cell viability. After storage at −20°C, no fluorescence was observed after thawing and inducing the sensor chips. The addition of glycerol in different concentrations (5–10% v/v) did not improve cell survival at −20°C. The shelf life at 4°C was 5 days, allowing a batch-wise production and storage for later use. Exceeding this storage duration led to an insufficient fluorescence response upon induction.

Additional experiments were carried out to investigate the biosafety of the proposed sensor chips, because a release of the genetically modified sensor cells from the sensor chips represented a possible risk in handling. A simple approach for investigating the biosafety of the sensor chips was replica plating on agar plates containing the respective antibiotic. An average of five colony-forming units (CfU) was found (n = 3), indicating that some cells were in fact able to escape the agarose entrapment. Therefore, measures to achieve a complete entrapment, for example by increasing the agarose concentration, should be evaluated to render the system as safe for the use in non–GMO-certified areas.

2.4. Integrated cultivation and detection device

The two-dimensional approach of sensing pathogens on agarose chips requires a specialized device for detecting and interpreting the fluorescent signals generated by the immobilized sensor strain. Since the results from commercially available plate readers and gel imaging systems did not yield a sufficient spatial resolution, a custom-made device was designed and constructed as pictured in **Figure 7** (left).

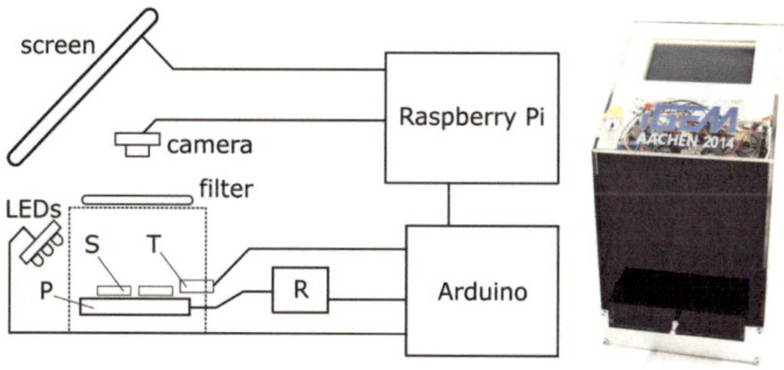

Figure 7. Schematic representation of hardware components and assembled device. Biosensor chips (S) are placed above a Peltier heating element (P) in the incubation chamber (dotted line). An Arduino microcontroller measures the temperature (T) and switches the heating on or off via a relay (R). A Raspberry Pi microcomputer displays the graphical user interface with the analysis software on the touchscreen. Whenever a picture is taken, the two controllers communicate to switch the excitation LEDs on/off. The fully assembled device (right) is sprayed black to avoid interference of ambient light. Stickers of the project logo are visible at the top.

The device consists of two enclosed compartments, separated by laser-cut plates of acrylic glass. The inner compartment serves for cultivation and illumination of the sensor chip. The outer compartment contains a Raspberry Pi microcomputer, an Arduino microcontroller, and a camera for imaging. **Figure 7** (right) schematically shows the individual components of the device and their interaction.

Once the chip is prepared and a sample taken, a petri dish containing the chip is inserted into the inner compartment, which serves as an *in situ* incubation chamber for both pathogens and genetically modified sensor organisms. A UV lamp could be integrated to facilitate built-in inactivation of microorganisms.

During the experiment, the parameters are controlled by an Arduino Uno and a Raspberry Pi. The Arduino has two main functions: first, it is responsible for controlling the incubation temperature in the inner compartment. Based on measurements from the temperature sensor, it sets the power input for the Peltier elements, thus heating or cooling the interior of the device. Second, the Arduino controls the LEDs illuminating the chip. When a control command from the Raspberry Pi is received, the two channels of the connected relay are turned on or off, switching the state of the LEDs, respectively. Thus, the chip is exposed to the specific wavelength emitted by the LEDs, in this case 480 nm for the excitation of the unquenched GFP.

Upon user input, the Raspberry Pi triggers the camera module to take an image of the chip. A filter slide is placed in front of the lens to block the excitation wavelength from the LEDs and to specifically transmit the emission wavelength of the fluorophore. In this configuration, a highly resolved fluorescent signal is obtained. The image is further processed by the Raspberry Pi and displays the analysis results via the graphical user interface (GUI) on a built-in 7-inch display located in the outer casing. The GUI (**Figure 8**, left) runs on either the Raspberry Pi or an externally connected computer; it enables the user to adjust the camera settings, take a single image or start time-lapse imaging, and to monitor the imaging process. Moreover, it allows execution of the analysis software for saved images as described in detail

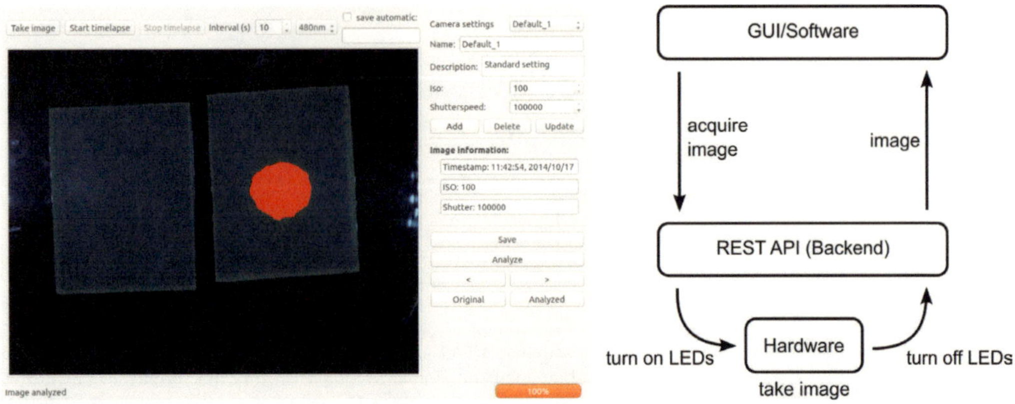

Figure 8. Graphical user interface (GUI) and chain of commands. Using the GUI (left) the user can specify settings for cultivation and imaging. The software instructs the backend via a REST API (right) to execute the imaging command. The acquired image is transferred back to the software which performs an automated analysis.

below. The communication between the GUI and the hardware is ensured by the backend software. It receives the respective commands (e.g., for capturing an image) from the GUI and subsequently forwards them to the according hardware. Therefore, the backend is responsible for image acquisition. An exemplary chain of commands for taking an image is depicted in **Figure 8** (right). The backend runs on the Raspberry Pi.

For the detection of *P. aeruginosa* using the sensor system presented in the previous sections, time-lapse imaging was performed, taking pictures in intervals of 5 min. The agarose chip was incubated at 37°C and excited with four LEDs (Superflux LED blue 3 lm NSPBR70BSS-PU/PV-W, Nichia Corporation) emitting a peak wavelength of 480 nm. The filter "010 Medium Yellow" (LEE Filters) was installed in front of the camera to allow the emission wavelengths of the fluorophore to pass while blocking the peak wavelength of the LEDs.

2.5. Analysis of spatial fluorescence

Automated, fast, and reliable analysis of raw sensor data is critical for a diagnostic device. Since, in the case of the 2D biosensor, the raw sensor measurement is a series of pictures taken by the onboard camera, an image analysis pipeline is required. Here, a novel pipeline is presented involving segmentation through statistical region merging (SRM [30]), thresholding in hue-saturation-value (HSV)-color space, and a final classification step. This leads to segmentation of the fluorescent regions in the biosensor chip, thus identifying chips or chip regions containing pathogens.

2.5.1. Image segmentation

Onboard image analysis on embedded computing hardware is subject to rigorous performance constraints due to the poor availability of existing analysis packages and the limited computing power. This complicates the use of sophisticated analysis pipelines. At the same time, the need for quantification of fluorescent regions on the biosensor mandates the image to be segmented into foreground (fluorescent) and background regions, also called super-pixels. This is necessary because only after a segmentation mask is computed for an input image, the number of

http://dx.doi.org/10.5772/intechopen.72457

independent fluorescent regions in the image, their intensity, and their area can be quantified. Statistical region merging is an image segmentation algorithm which is both light-weight and does not require expensive tuning of algorithm-specific hyperparameters [30]. In contrast to other clustering algorithms, it also produces deterministic results, which increases the reproducibility of the analysis pipeline. The SRM algorithm has one important hyperparameter Q which influences the merging process. A Q-level of 256 resulting in many fine regions was chosen (**Figure 9**, top-left).

The input image (**Figure 10A**) is segmented into super-pixels, and the list of regions is filtered to obtain only candidate regions of fluorescence (**Figure 10B**). Since the color of the fluorescence signal is known, the regions can be thresholded based on their HSV color representation. For selection of GFP-fluorescent regions, super-pixels that have hue (color shade) in the interval [0.462, 0.520], saturation of 0.99, and value (brightness) in the interval [0.25, 0.32] were considered. This thresholding step removes background regions and is performed at low computational cost (**Figure 10C**).

Since false positives can remain after filtering, they are removed from the list of candidate regions by classifying each region into noise or signal. First, the classification applies a smoothing procedure to the region mask. This is achieved by convolving the region mask with a disk filter (**Figure 10D**). Then, for each pixel p' in that smoothed image, the smoothness index [31] is calculated (**Figure 10E**) as the sum of the difference with respect to each of its neighbors N_k (**Eq. (1)**). In the implementation, the neighbors in a radius of i=4px were used. Finally, the matrix of smoothness indices is normalized the interval [0, 1]:

$$S_p = \frac{\sum_{p' \in N_k} \nabla(p')}{\max_p S_p} \quad (1)$$

A subsequent thresholding step selects pixels that fulfill $S_p \geq T_S \wedge I_p \geq 255$ where S_p denotes the smoothness index at pixel p, T_s=0.85 is an empirically determined smoothness threshold, and I_p is the intensity of the pixel in the smoothed mask. The final classification step removes regions with high-edge curvature and selects smooth, blob-like regions (**Figure 10F**). Thereby, artifacts are removed from the analysis, and only fluorescent pixels are quantified.

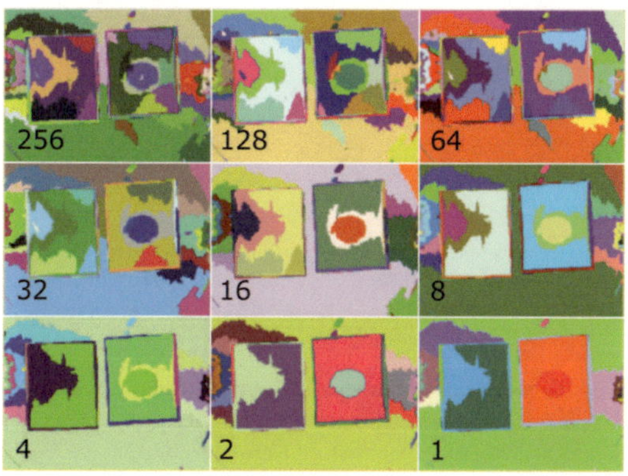

Figure 9. Regions obtained from SRM with different Q-levels. High Q-levels (indicated by numbers) result in many super-pixels (top-left), while low Q-levels correspond to rigorous merging (bottom-right). Segmented regions are randomly colored for better visualization.

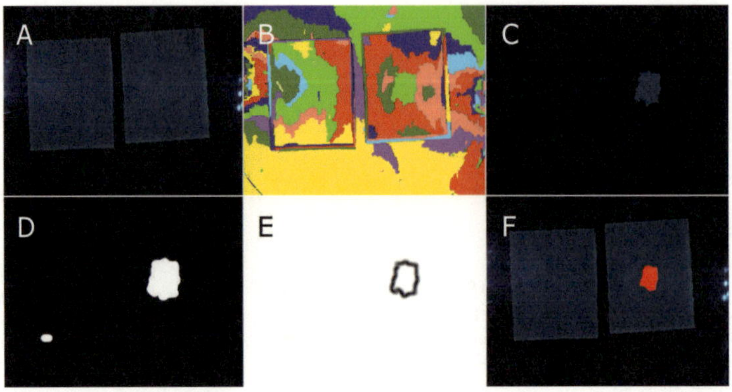

Figure 10. Input, intermediates, and result. The input image (A) is segmented using statistical region merging (B), and superpixels are selected based on the HSV properties (C). The binary region mask is smoothed (D), and smoothness indices are computed (E). Pixels that were classified as foreground in D and smooth (E) are overlaid as red pixels on the input image (F).

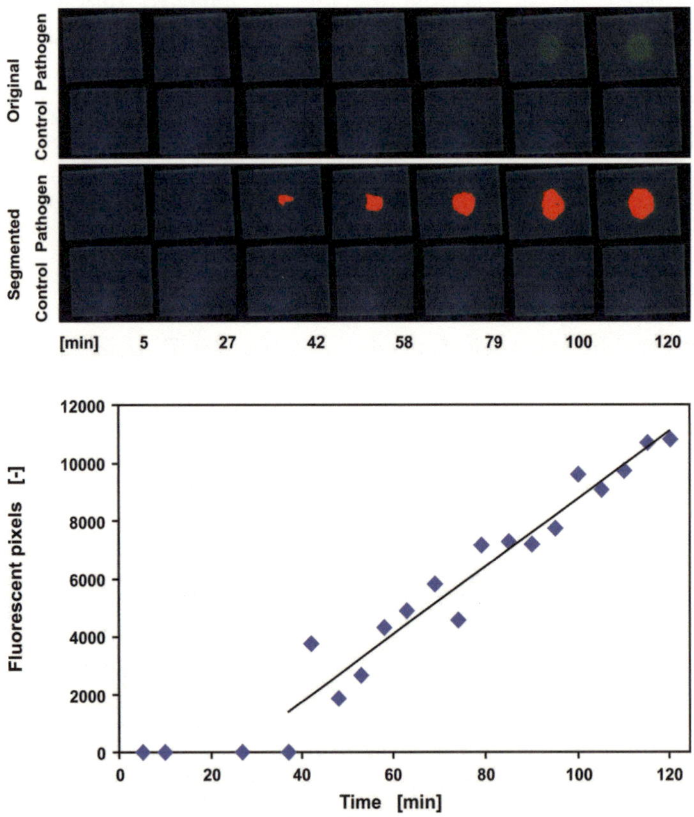

Figure 11. Time series acquired by the measurement device and quantification of fluorescent pixels over time. A volume of 0.2 μL of bacterial culture in LB medium (approximately 6×10^5 CFU) was added onto the center of agarose chips containing the immobilized sensor cells. The negative control culture contained *E. coli* DH5α, the pathogen sample culture *P. aeruginosa* O1. The chips were incubated at 37°C, and pictures were taken approximately every 5 min. The fluorescence signal recognized by the image analysis software is shown as highlighted area. A video sequence of the live pathogen detection can be found at [32] (top). A time series of images taken with the measurement device was analyzed using the outlined image analysis pipeline. Counts of foreground pixels (dots) are plotted against incubation time. Starting after 40 min of incubation, the number of fluorescent pixels linearly increased (117 pixels/min, $R^2 \approx 0.936$; bottom).

2.5.2. *Quantification of the fluorescence signal*

The image analysis pipeline outlined above was implemented in both MATLAB and C++. It allowed the detection of fluorescence with little tuning of hyperparameters (*Q*-level and thresholds). When a time-lapse of images is automatically acquired with the software, the image analysis pipeline can be applied to each frame (**Figure 11**, top). The number of pixels in the resulting foreground regions can be quantified over time. After about 40 min of incubation, a region of pathogen-induced fluorescence was detected, which then grew linearly with respect to its area over time (**Figure 11**, bottom). As a proof of principle, 6×10^5 cells were applied on the chip. However, serial dilution testing is needed to determine the lower detection limit. The expected lower limit of detection is 1 CFU due to cell proliferation during the incubation step.

3. Discussion and outlook

In this work, a modular biosensor for the detection of the opportunistic human pathogen P. aeruginosa was developed. Five key components, (2.1) a selective molecular detection mechanism, (2.2) an integrated amplification step, (2.3) a gentle immobilization technique, (2.4) a low-cost cultivation and optical detection device, and (2.5) a graphical analysis software, were integrated. The resulting modular biosensor demonstrates the power of combining synthetic biology with software and hardware engineering by detecting P. aeruginosa in less than 1 h of analysis time. **Table 2** provides a comparison of the sensor system developed in this study to existing detection methods for P. aeruginosa.

In addition to the detection methods compared in **Table 2**, there are several whole-cell approaches. Most of the previously developed whole-cell biosensors deliver an optical output [39]. In a previous work, Struss et al. developed a whole-cell biosensor detecting AHLs of gram-negative bacteria, particularly *P. aeruginosa* [40]. Similar to the approach presented herein, they used components of the AHL-mediated QS regulatory system to generate an optical signal. A portable format was developed by liquid-drying the sensor cells on filter paper strips. While Struss et al. met many criteria for a successful portable on-site field kit, such as easy handling, inexpensiveness, and simple transportation, it lacks a rapid, integrated analysis and is dependent on the user's subjective evaluation.

Enhancement and optimization of the proposed biosensor system beyond the proof of principle demonstrated in this work can be realized by modifying each of the five key elements as well as their interactions. The individual key elements can be optimized as follows.

The utilization of the pathogen's inherent QS system guarantees a high specificity as the receptor for the AI is unique. However, this poses a challenge if multiple pathogens are desired to be detected simultaneously. First, only QS molecules can be recognized by a molecular sensing system of the presented type. In theory, other secreted compounds can be used for detection, though potentially reducing the specificity. Second, the sensing system should be introduced into a separate sensing organism to completely avoid interaction, especially if a closely related QS system and a signal amplification as presented here are utilized. This may lead to insufficient spatial resolution as many different sensing cells are required to be incorporated in the same sensor chips. An equal distribution of each type of sensing cell needs

Principle of detection	Details	Advantages	Disadvantages
PCR	Targeting *gyrB* gene using real-time PCR, sensitivity: 3.3×10^2 to 2.3×10^3 CFU/PCR [33]	High selectivity and reliability, conclusive and unambiguous results, fast compared to culturing methods	No discrimination between viable and nonviable cells, purification step required
Culture and colony counting	Simple and traditional plating method, sensitivity: 20 CFU/mL [34]	Moderate selectivity, simple, inexpensive, low detection limit	Time-consuming cultivation of several days, detects only viable/culturable organisms, unspecific
Immunology	ELISA applying antibodies to detect cell surface antigens [35], typical sensitivity: 10^6 CFU/mL [6]	High selectivity, faster than PCR-based techniques	Complex and expensive, less sensitive than PCR, regularly requires cultural enrichment
Modular biosensor presented in this study	Transcription factors recognize pathogen-specific quorum sensing molecules; signal is transduced through activation of quenched fluorophores, tested number of cells: 6×10^5 CFU	Inexpensive (no expensive reagents or equipment required), rapid (short cultivation without pretreatment), simple (no highly trained personnel required)	Selectivity and sensitivity dependent on detection system, viable cells required
Nucleic acid biosensor	Reception through (-)ssDNA probe coupled to piezoelectric transduction, sensitivity: 0.1 μg/mL [36]	Detection in under 3 h, high selectivity	Low sensitivity, complex immobilization on hybrid membrane
Molecular imprinting polymer-based biosensor	Recognition of bacterial structure in combination with dielectrophoresis, sensitivity 10^3 CFU/mL [37]	Detection time of 3 min, high sensitivity, no pretreatment necessary	Cross-reactivity with bacteria of similar shape
Droplet-based microfluidic biosensor	Detection of virulence factors via surface-enhanced Raman spectroscopy, sensitivity: 0.5 μM pyocyanin [38]	Low sample volume, low detection limit for pathogen-specific virulence factor pyocyanin	Expensive, trained personnel required, increased technological effort, fluid samples only, extensive interpretation of data needed

Table 2. Conventional methods and biosensor approaches for detection of *P. aeruginosa*.

to be ensured and reciprocal interference avoided. The feasibility hereof has already been proven in previous work [41].

By introducing the REACh quenching system, the fluorescence response was amplified and accelerated compared to conventional GFP expression. Quenched fluorophores are constitutively expressed, and a constant pool of reporter molecules is built up. Upon the presence of inducers and a subsequent expression of the protease, they are unquenched resulting in a fast and strong fluorescent signal. Since the two expression cassettes for the GFP-REACh fusion protein and the TEV protease are currently on two separate plasmids, using a single plasmid would increase the robustness of the detection system, as two plasmid expression systems are considered less stable. As a proof of principle, the system was tested using IPTG-induced expression of the TEV protease. As a next step, the system would be adjusted by exchanging the T7 promoter with the HSL-bound LasR-inducible *las*I promoter to render the expression of the TEV protease inducible by $3OC_{12}$-HSL. Subsequently, extensive testing with different concentrations of $3OC_{12}$-HSL and varying cell numbers of *P. aeruginosa* should be performed to determine detection limits. Based on the results, the expression can be fine-tuned, for example, by improving the promoters. On the protein level, the linker length between GFP and REACh can be optimized with respect to the protein folding, protease accessibility, and quenching efficiency [22].

Engineering of the agarose chips for entrapment of the sensor cells represents a simple yet efficient way for a two-dimensional detection method. The immobilized sensor cells survived and still performed as expected, even after short-term storage at 4°C. A fluorescence signal was generated upon induction, thus proving a sufficient diffusion of the inducer through the chip. As discussed above, adjustment of the agarose concentration used for production of the sensor chips represents a simple way to further optimize the sensor chips. Increasing the agarose concentration could focus the fluorescent response on a smaller area by restricting diffusion of the analyte, however, under the prerequisite that the diffusion is fast enough to reach the sensor cells within a short time. Additionally, adjustment of the agarose concentration affects the biosafety as the ability of the chip to contain the sensor cells is altered. To ensure a sufficient quantity and spread of the cells, an array-based technique for pattering the sensor cells onto a chip surface could be used to enable high-throughput analysis [41]. Several techniques for printing bacteria on surfaces have already been used successfully [42, 43].

The optical detection device represents a simple and cost-effective solution for the rapid visualization and analysis of the 2D fluorescent signal. In situ cultivation with automatic, real-time monitoring of the fluorescence resulted in the detection of *P. aeruginosa* within 42 min, even without using the optimized sensor cells. Compartmentation and the possibility to install a UV sterilization light ensures a high standard of biosafety. The settings described in Section 2.4 are highly specific for the presented two-dimensional biosensor; however, as the device is modular, single components such as the LEDs and the filter sets can be exchanged to adjust the optical settings to different reporter systems. An extension of the device, for example, by using a filter wheel or a monochromator and LEDs emitting different wavelengths bears the potential of simultaneously detecting various pathogens if respective molecular reporter systems can be constructed, thus allowing a high degree of multiplexing. The extensive modularity and the inexpensive parts in comparison to common commercial devices grant an easy access for potential users and researchers customizing the system for other biosensors.

The analysis software pipeline recognized and distinguished fluorescent signals of certain shapes and marked them for an easy interpretation by the user. However, the lack of sufficient amounts of real input data may imply a subjectivity of the analysis. Further testing needs to be done to prove universal applicability. In this regard, the precision vs. recall trade-off of the software is required to be further investigated to determine ratios between false positives and false negatives. Additionally, time-lapse data should be featured not only in the GUI but in the analysis as well. Since the project was conducted, the computational capabilities of embedded hardware have dramatically improved. Future adoptions of this work should therefore utilize state-of-the-art embedded hardware and software packages.

In general, the presented biosensor represents a proof of concept of a modular whole-cell, point-of-contact biosensing system. It enables rapid and inexpensive detection of *P. aeruginosa*, providing intuitive feedback through integrated, real-time analysis. The applicability of this sensor platform in other fields, such as food, water, and environmental safety, offers further innovation potential.

Acknowledgements

The biosensor system presented in this chapter was developed by the 15 members of the "iGEM Team Aachen 2014" [44]. The team was supported by the Institute of Applied Microbiology (iAMB), the Institute of Biotechnology, and the Institute for Molecular Biotechnology, all three at RWTH Aachen University as well as the Institute of Bio- and Geosciences Biotechnology (IBG-1) at Forschungszentrum Jülich GmbH. Financial support originated from numerous organizations, including the aforementioned institutes, the Helmholtz Initiative for Synthetic Biology as well as other institutional and private donors listed on the project website [11].

Contributions

Experiments were performed by the "iGEM Team Aachen 2014" members, namely, Vera Alexandrova, Nina Bailly, Philipp Demling, Florian Gohr, René Hanke, Markus Joppich, Ansgar Niemöller, Patrick Opdensteinen, Michael Osthege, Björn Peeters, Julia Plum, Stefan Reinhold, Anna Schechtel, Eshani Sood, and Arne Zimmermann. The team was advised by Suresh Sudarsan and Ljubica Vojcic and instructed by Lars Blank, Wolfgang Wiechert, and Ulrich Schwaneberg. The chapter was written by (alphabetically) Nina Bailly, Philipp Demling, Florian Gohr, René Hanke, Patrick Opdensteinen, and Michael Osthege. Markus Joppich, Suresh Sudarsan, Ulrich Schwaneberg, Lars Blank, and Wolfgang Wiechert reviewed this chapter.

Author details

René Hanke[1,†*], Nina Bailly[1,†], Philipp Demling[1,†], Florian N. Gohr[1,†], Patrick Opdensteinen[1,†], Michael J. Osthege[1,†], Markus Joppich[1], Suresh Sudarsan[2], Ulrich Schwaneberg[3], Wolfgang Wiechert[4] and Lars M. Blank[2]

*Address all correspondence to: rene.hanke@rwth-aachen.de

1 iGEM Team Aachen 2014, RWTH Aachen University, Aachen, Germany

2 Institute of Applied Microbiology, RWTH Aachen University, Aachen, Germany

3 Institute of Biotechnology, RWTH Aachen University, Aachen, Germany

4 Forschungszentrum Jülich GmbH, Institute of Bio- and Geosciences, IBG-1: Biotechnology, Jülich, Germany

† These authors contributed equally to this work

References

[1] Tallury P, Malhotra A, Byrne LM, Santra S. Nanobioimaging and sensing of infectious diseases. Advanced Drug Delivery Reviews. 2010;**62**(4):424-437. DOI: 10.1016/j.addr.2009.11.014

[2] Byrne B, Stack E, Gilmartin N, O'Kennedy R. Antibody-based sensors: Principles, problems and potential for detection of pathogens and associated toxins. Sensors. 2009;**9**(6):4407-4445. DOI: 10.3390/s90604407

[3] Singh R, Das Mukherjee M, Sumana G, Gupta RK, Sood S, Malhotra BD. Biosensors for pathogen detection: A smart approach towards clinical diagnosis. Sensors and Actuators B: Chemical. 2014;**197**:385-404. DOI: 10.1016/j.snb.2014.03.005

[4] Behzadi P, Behzadi E, Ranjbar R. The application of microarray in medicine. ORL.ro. 2014; **7**:24

[5] Lazcka O, Del Campo FJ, Munoz FX. Pathogen detection: A perspective of traditional methods and biosensors. Biosensors and Bioelectronics. 2007;**22**(7):1205-1217. DOI: 10.1016/j.bios.2006.06.036

[6] Ivnitski D, Abdel-Hamid I, Atanasov P, Wilkins E. Biosensors for detection of pathogenic bacteria. Biosensors and Bioelectronics. 1999;**14**(7):599-624. DOI: 10.1016/S0956-5663(99)00039-1

[7] Rocha-Gaso MI, March-Iborra C, Montoya-Baides A, Arnau-Vives A. Surface generated acoustic wave biosensors for the detection of pathogens: A review. Sensors. 2009;**9**(7):5740-5769. DOI: 10.3390/s90705740

[8] Zourob M. Biosensor using magnetic particles for pathogen detection. US20170038373 A1. 2015. DOI: 10.3390/s17081704

[9] Montoya A, Ocampo A, March C. Fundamentals of piezoelectric immunosensors. In: Vives AA, editor. Piezoelectric Transducers and Applications. 1st ed. Berlin: Springer; 2009. pp. 289-306. DOI: 10.1007/978-3-540-77508-9_12

[10] Eltzov E, Marks RS. Whole-cell aquatic biosensors. Analytical and Bioanalytical Chemistry. 2011;**400**(4):895-913. DOI: 10.1007/s00216-010-4084-y

[11] iGEM Team Aachen Wiki [Internet]. 2014. Available from: http://2014.igem.org/Team:Aachen/ [Accessed: 2017-10-28]

[12] Wu L, Estrada O, Zaborina O, Bains M, Shen L, Kohler JE, et al. Recognition of host immune activation by *Pseudomonas aeruginosa*. Science. 2005;**309**(5735):774-777. DOI: 10.1126/science.1112422

[13] de Bentzmann S, Plésiat P. The *Pseudomonas aeruginosa* opportunistic pathogen and human infections. Environmental Microbiology. 2011;**13**(7):1655-1665. DOI: 10.1111/j.1462-2920.2011.02469.x

[14] Nadal Jimenez P, Koch G, Thompson JA, Xavier KB, Cool RH, Quax WJ. The multiple signaling systems regulating virulence in *Pseudomonas aeruginosa*. Microbiology and Molecular Biology Reviews. 2012;**76**(1):46-65. DOI: 10.1128/MMBR.05007-11

[15] Ng WL, Bassler BL. Bacterial quorum-sensing network architectures. Annual Review of Genetics. 2015;**43**:197-222. DOI: 10.1146/annurev-genet-102108-134304

[16] Li YH, Tian X. Quorum sensing and bacterial social interactions in biofilms. Sensors. 2012;**12**:2519-2538. DOI: 10.3390/s120302519

[17] Waters CM, Bassler BL. Quorum sensing: Cell-to-cell communication in bacteria. Annual Review of Cell and Developmental Biology. 2005;**21**(1):319-346. DOI: 10.1146/annurev.cellbio.21.012704.131001

[18] Latifi A, Foglino M, Tanaka K, Williams P, Lazdunski A. A hierarchical quorum-sensing cascade in *Pseudomonas aeruginosa* links the transcriptional activators LasR and RhlR (VsmR) to expression of the stationary-phase sigma factor RpoS. Molecular Microbiology. 1996;**21**(6):1137-1146. DOI: 10.1046/j.1365-2958.1996.00063.x

[19] Broussard JA, Rappaz B, Webb DJ, Brown CM. Fluorescence resonance energy transfer microscopy as demonstrated by measuring the activation of the serine/threonine kinase Akt. Nature Protocols. 2013;**8**(2):265-281. DOI: 10.1038/nprot.2012.147

[20] Ganesan S, Ameer-beg SM, Ng TTC, Vojnovic B, Wouters FS. A dark yellow fluorescent protein (YFP)-based resonance energy-accepting chromoprotein (REACh) for Förster resonance energy transfer with GFP. Proceedings of the National Academy of Sciences of the United States of America. 2006;**103**(11):4089-4094. DOI: 10.1073/pnas.0509922103

[21] Cormack BP, Valdivia RH, Falkow S. FACS-optimized mutants of the green fluorescent protein (GFP). Gene. 1996;**173**(1):33-38. DOI: 10.1016/0378-1119(95)00685-0

[22] Van Der Meer BW, Coker G, Chen SYS. Resonance Energy Transfer: Theory and Data. 1st ed. Weinheim: Wiley-VCH; 1994

[23] Kapust RB, Tözsér J, Fox JD, Anderson DE, Cherry S, Copeland TD. Tobacco etch virus protease: Mechanism of autolysis and rational design of stable mutants with wild-type catalytic proficiency. Protein Engineering. 2001;**14**(12):993-1000. DOI: 10.1093/protein/14.12.993

[24] Shetty R. pSB3K3 Vector Backbone Specification [Internet]. 2004. Available from: http://parts.igem.org/Part:pSB3K3. [Accessed: 2017-10-28]

[25] Che A. pSB1C3 Vector Backbone Specification [Internet]. 2008. Available from: http://parts.igem.org/Part:pSB1C3. [Accessed: 2017-10-28].

[26] Mallick N. Biotechnological potential of immobilized algae for wastewater N, P and metal removal: A review. Biometals. 2002;**15**(4):377-390. DOI: 10.1023/A:1020238520948

[27] Nilsson K, Birnbaum S, Flygare S, Linse L, Schröder U, Jeppsson U, et al. A general method for the immobilization of cells with preserved viability. Applied Microbiology and Biotechnology. 1983;**17**(6):319-326. DOI: 10.1007/BF00499497

[28] Leenen EJTM, Dos Santos VAP, Grolle KCF, Tramper J, Wijffels R. Characteristics of and selection criteria for support materials for cell immobilization in wastewater treatment. Water Research. 1996;**30**(12):2985-2996. DOI: 10.1016/S0043-1354(96)00209-6

[29] Stricker J, Maddox P, Salmon ED, Erickson HP. Rapid assembly dynamics of the *Escherichia coli* FtsZ-ring demonstrated by fluorescence recovery after photobleaching. Proceedings of the National Academy of Sciences of the United States of America. 2002;**99**(5):3171-3175. DOI: 10.1073/pnas.052595099

[30] Nock R, Nielsen F. Statistical region merging. IEEE Transactions on Pattern Analysis and Machine Intelligence. 2004;**26**(11):1452-1458. DOI: 10.1109/TPAMI.2004.110

[31] Joppich M, Rausch D, Kuhlen T. Adaptive human motion prediction using multiple model approaches. Virtuelle und Erweiterte Realität 10. Work. der Gi-fachgr. VR/AR. 2013; 169-180.

[32] iGEM Team Aachen Wiki [Internet]. 2014. Available from: http://2014.igem.org/Team:Aachen/Project/Measurement_Device#watsonmeasurarty. [Accessed: 2017-10-28]

[33] Lee CS, Wetzel K, Buckley T, Wozniak D, Lee J. Rapid and sensitive detection of *Pseudomonas aeruginosa* in chlorinated water and aerosols targeting gyrB gene using real-time PCR. Journal of Applied Microbiology. 2011;**111**(4):893-903. DOI: 10.1111/j.1365-2672.2011.05107.x

[34] Mohammadi Kouchesfahani M, Alimohammadi M, Nabizadeh Nodehi R, Aslani H, Rezaie S, Asadian S. *Pseudomonas aeruginosa* and heterotrophic bacteria count in bottled waters in Iran. Iranian Journal of Public Health. 2015;**44**(11):1514-1519

[35] Brett MM, Ghoneim AT, Littlewood JM, Losowsky MS. Development of enzyme linked immunosorbent assay (ELISA) to detect antibodies to *Pseudomonas aeruginosa* cell surface antigens in sera of patients with cystic fibrosis. Journal of Clinical Pathology. 1986;**39**(10):1124-1129. DOI: 10.1136/jcp.39.10.1124

[36] He F, Liu S. Detection of *P. aeruginosa* using nano-structured electrode-separated piezoelectric DNA biosensor. Talanta. 2004;**62**(2):271-277. DOI: 10.1016/j.talanta.2003.07.007

[37] Tokonami S, Nakadoi Y, Takahashi M, Ikemizu M, Kadoma T, Saimatsu K, et al. Label-free and selective bacteria detection using a film with transferred bacterial configuration. Analytical Chemistry. 2013;**85**(10):4925-4929. DOI: 10.1021/ac3034618

[38] Žukovskaja O, Jahn IJ, Weber K, Cialla-May D, Popp J. Detection of *Pseudomonas aeruginosa* metabolite pyocyanin in water and saliva by employing the SERS technique. Sensors. 2017;**17**(8):1704. DOI: 10.3390/s17081704

[39] Ahmed A, Rushworth JV, Hirst NA, Millner PA. Biosensors for whole-cell bacterial detection. Clinical Microbiology Reviews. 2014;**27**(3):631-646. DOI: 10.1128/CMR.00120-13

[40] Struss A, Pasini P, Ensor CM, Raut N, Daunert S. Paper strip whole cell biosensors: A portable test for the semiquantitative detection of bacterial quorum signaling molecules. Analytical Chemistry. 2010;**82**(11):4457-4463. DOI: 10.1021/ac100231a

[41] Melamed S, Elad T, Belkin S. Microbial sensor cell arrays. Current Opinion in Biotechnology. 2012;**23**(1):2-8. DOI: 10.1016/j.copbio.2011.11.024

[42] Kim K, Lee BU, Hwang GB, Lee JH, Kim S. Drop-on-demand patterning of bacterial cells using pulsed jet electrospraying. Analytical Chemistry. 2010;**82**(5):2109-2112. DOI: 10.1021/ac9027966

[43] Merrin J, Leibler S, Chuang JS. Printing multistrain bacterial patterns with a piezoelectric inkjet printer. PLoS One. 2007;**2**(7):e663. DOI: 10.1371/journal.pone.0000663

[44] iGEM Team Aachen Wiki [Internet]. 2014. Available from: http://2014.igem.org/Team:Aachen/Attributions. [Accessed: 2017-10-28]

Chapter 8

Detection of Pathogens Using Microfluidics and Biosensors

Natalia Lopez-Barbosa, Ana Lucia Campaña,
Mabel Juliana Noguera, Sergio Leonardo Florez,
Miguel Angel Aroca, Juan C. Cruz and
Johann F. Osma

Additional information is available at the end of the chapter

http://dx.doi.org/10.5772/intechopen.72443

Abstract

Point-of-care devices technology are a promising way towards the recognition of pathogens in early-stage diagnosis, which is critical for the success of inexpensive treatments as opposed to the high costs of managing the disease. The integration of immunoassays with read out circuitry allows the implementation of diagnostic devices for their use by untrained personnel, without compromising reliability. In the following chapter, three different biosensors based on lab-on-a-chip (LoC) and microfluidic technologies were designed, assembled and tested for pathogen diagnosis. The devices allowed the effective detection of the human papilloma virus, *Mycobacterium tuberculosis* and Chagas parasite in shorter times and with smaller sample volumes than those required by current clinical diagnosis techniques. All devices were benchmarked against commercial techniques in terms of cost and time requirement per test.

Keywords: microfluidics, biosensors, electroimmunosensors

1. Introduction

Diagnostic of pathogenic driven diseases has become a global concern due to the rapid growth of infectious diseases around the world [1]. For decades, pathogen detection has been mainly attained through cell culture, nucleic amplification and enzyme-linked immunoassays, which rely on tedious protocols and are generally time consuming [2]. According to the World Health Organization (WHO), novel technologies for pathogen diagnosis urgently need to address issues regarding affordability, sensitivity, specificity, ease of use, robustness, response time and deliverability to end-users [3]. For this reason, lab-on-a-chip (LoC) and microfluidic systems, with the inclusion of biosensors, emerge as an attractive alternative due to their low sample volume requirements, rapid response, and ease of integration [4].

The first generation of electrochemical biosensors emerged from the incorporation of immobilized enzymes on conventional electrodes. They were firstly thought for laboratory instruments, but rapidly penetrated into the medical device industry thanks to diagnostic companies [5]. Enzyme-based biosensors exploit the specificity of enzymes towards a particular substrate for sensing purposes [4]. In such devices, immobilized enzymes serve as mediators, easing electron transport from the active site to the electrode [6] and providing a clear signal for substrate recognition. Due to the rather limited availability of substrates, enzyme-based biosensors were rapidly replaced in the medical industry with immunoassays. Antibody-based biosensors rely on the transduction of signals from immobilized antibodies upon binding of specific analytes. This type of biosensors is well accepted in the medical industry for the detection of proteins specific to a particular disease or condition. Electroimmunosensors are antibody-based biosensors that employ electrochemical transducers to obtain an electrical response [7]. The charge transport capacity of the electrodes employed in electroimmunosensors can be monitored via cyclic voltammetry (CV) or as an electrical impedance change via electrochemical impedance spectroscopy (EIS). These two techniques, in conjunction with microfluidics, allow the fabrication of what is usually known as LoC devices.

In the following chapter, we present the design and fabrication of three different systems for detection of human papilloma virus (HPV), tuberculosis and Chagas. Detection of HPV and tuberculosis is effectively achieved by electroimmunosensor LoC technology, while Chagas relies on a microfluidic device for separation and impedance measurement for sensing. The devices are benchmarked against commercial diagnostic devices in terms of ease of use, time of testing and cost.

2. Case of study: HPV

The human papilloma virus (HPV) is a double DNA chain viral pathogen that is sexually transmitted. HPV has been associated with several diseases, such as cervical lesions, condylomas and cervical cancer [8]. Recent studies estimate that between 50 and 80% of sexually active women around the world have been infected with HPV at least once in their lifetime [9]. There are more than 100 different types of HPV strands, some of which are low risk and are generally associated with genital warts. Some other strands, such as HPV 16, are more virulent and may lead to the development of cervical cancer [10]. It is estimated that every year some 500,000 new cases of HPV are diagnosed with condyloma or cervical cancer, which cause around 240,000 deaths in the U.S. [11].

Currently, the preferred assays for diagnosis of HPV infections are hybrid capture (HC) and polymerase chain reaction (PCR) [12]. HC is based on the hybridization of denatured cells with a RNA probe followed by capturing the hybrids via specific binding to antibodies. Signal is amplified by chemiluminescent compound binding through a specific enzyme. This is attained by the conjugation of a secondary antibody with an enzyme that catalyzes the chemiluminescent reaction. Conversely, in PCR, virus detection is performed by the amplification of target DNA aided by DNA polymerases.

Regardless of the accuracy and standardization of laboratory testing, reducing long times of diagnosis and the requirement of specialized personnel, remain as major challenges.

Miniaturization in LoC devices has been widely explored to attain these issues. For instance, Kim et al. [13] developed a microcantilever-based biosensor for the electrical detection of HPV by its conjugation with specific proteins and magnetic beads. Similarly, Huang et al. [14] implemented electrical impedance spectroscopy (EIS) and differential pulse voltammetry on graphene/gold electrodes to detect specific DNA strands of HPV. Although these biosensors have proved to enhance the sensitivity of the detection, Their manufacturing processes are not cost-effective, limiting their accessibility.

Hereby, an antibody-based biosensor with an electronic readout is presented and compared with HC2 and RT-PCR cobas® 4800. The system consists of almost 100 individual test chambers, and was tested with real samples for the detection of HPV.

2.1. Methodology and results

2.1.1. Fabrication of the biomicrosystem

The biomicrosystem was fabricated by self-assembly technique as described in [15]. Briefly, a gold nanolayer was deposited on a poly(methyl methacrylate) (PMMA) substrate via physical evaporation. A second PMMA slide was patterned by laser engraving with 2 mm wells organized in 7 rows and 14 columns. The slide was adhered to the gold-coated PMMA with methylene chloride. Wells were equipped with square holes for electrical connectors. A total of 98 independent biosensors were embedded as shown in **Figure 1**.

Antibody immobilization was attained by placing 4 μL of 97% 4-aminothiolphenol (ATP) (Sigma-Aldrich, USA) in each well. Excess thiols were removed by further ethanol and deionized water rinses. 4 μL of monoclonal antibody (mAb) 5051 was added to each well for immobilization via covalent coupling to the pendant amine group. The biomicrosystem was incubated for 1 h at 37°C and washed with PBS and deionized water.

2.1.2. HPV detection

HPV detection was achieved by EIS and cyclic voltammetry (CV) measurements, and was compared with PCR technique. Samples were obtained from a specialized clinical laboratory

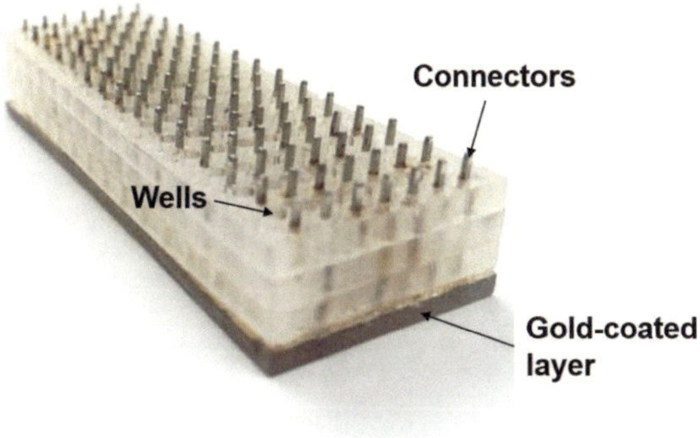

Figure 1. Biomicrosystem for HPV detection.

(PATOLAB, Colombia) from women between 25 and 40 years old. Changes on the impedance were recorded for biomicrosystems with only the gold layer (gold); the gold layer and the thiol (gold-4-ATP); and the gold layer, the thiol and the mAb 5051 (gold-4-ATP-mAb 5051). 10 μL of sample with or without HPV 16 was pipetted in each well and incubated for 1 h at 37°C. Wells were washed with deionized water prior to impedance measurements.

2.1.3. Results

Samples placed in gold-4-ATP-mAb 5051 wells and containing HPV 16 exhibited an impedance change of approximately 40% when compared with initial measurements, while samples without HPV 16 showed an impedance change of less than 5%. Changes in impedance between clean wells and wells of 40 samples with HPV 16 are shown in **Figure 2**.

Impedance changes were significant in wells were the mAb 5051 was immobilized due to its affinity towards HPV 16 proteins.

2.2. Cost analysis

An analytic hierarchy process (AHP) was performed to compare our biomicrosystem with RT-PCR cobas® 4800 and HC2 Test in terms of cost, effectiveness, time required and test analysis. RT-PCR cobas® 4800 allows an automated sample preparation without the need of thawing or mixing, giving results in less than 20 min for up to 94 different samples. HC2 test utilizes *in vitro* nucleic acid hybridization assay with signal amplification towards 13 different HPV specimens.

Cost was considered as the local price of performing one test; effectiveness as the probability of encountering false positives or false negatives; time required as the total time per test; and test analysis as a compounded weigh of the probability of sample contamination, the capacity of

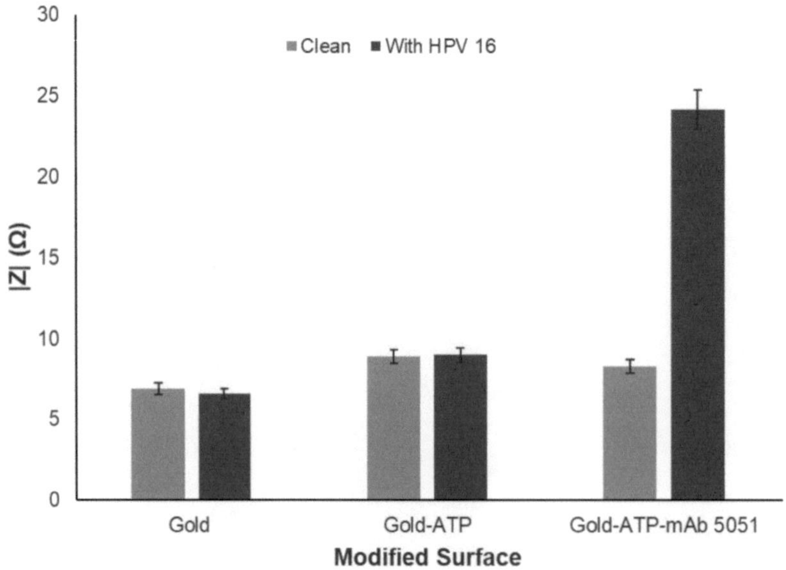

Figure 2. Changes in impedance after exposure to HPV 16 samples.

Test	Cost	Time per test	Contamination probability	Effectiveness with blood in sample	Amount of HPV genotypes per test	Effectivity of the test
Biomicrosystem	Less than commercial tests	2 h	High	High	1	High
RT-PCR cobas 4800	55 USD	2–3 h	None, process is automatized	Medium	14	High
Hybrid Capture 2	63 USD	2–3 h	Low	High	13	High

Table 1. Information used for matrix pairwise comparison.

the test to diagnose with blood in the sample and the number of different HPV genotypes that can be detected per test.

Information for RT-PCR cobra® 4800 and HC2 Test was obtained from three independent specialized laboratories; namely SIPLAS, Quimiolab and Fundacion Santafe de Bogota. Matrix pairwise comparisons based on the scale of Saaty were then conducted on the software Expert Choice 11.5 (ExpertChoice, USA) to evaluate each method [16]. **Table 1** shows the criteria selected and the values for each of the tests.

Global relative weighs of the biomicrosystem, RT-PCR cobas® 4800 and HC2 Test were of 0.343, 0.458 and 0.199, respectively. Our biomicrosystem lags behind the PCR technique due to its inability to detect more than one genotype of HPV. Nonetheless, since the biomicrosystem consists of 98 independent wells, an increase on genotype detection can be achieved by varying the types of antibodies immobilized per well.

3. Case of study: tuberculosis

Tuberculosis (TB) is a disease caused by the pathogenic bacterium *Mycobacterium tuberculosis*. This disease can be effectively controlled by early diagnosis and treatment [17]. Conventional detection technologies include polymerase chain reaction (PCR), enzyme-linked immunosorbent assay (ELISA), and immunochromatographic assay. PCR utilizes oligonucleotides towards a specific gene in *M. tuberculosis* [18]; ELISA is used as a solid phase immunoassay for the detection of an antigen [19]; and immunochromatographic assay is based on the analysis of antigens in a sandwich-based format [20]. These detection technologies exhibit; however, issues regarding long-time of analysis and lack of reliability and sensitivity, which ultimately limit their ability to recognize *M. tuberculosis* [21]. Furthermore, other techniques require various reagents and fluorescent or chemiluminescent labeling for sensing, exhibit low-yields, and may even require further purification steps [22]. Currently, TB is the leading cause of death in people within the most economically productive age-groups and the second deadliest infectious disease in the world [23]. Since diagnosis represents a vital link in the TB control chain, new cost-effective detection platforms are required to achieve quality results in a shorter time span [24].

An alternative route is the use of biosensors, which have attracted significant attention due to their high sensitivity, short analysis time, ease of miniaturization and cost-effectiveness.

Biosensors can be manufactured by the immobilization of biomolecules via self-assembled monolayers (SAMs), which can be generated with the use of thiols, disulfides, silanes, or acids [25]. Among biosensors, immunosensors are devices based on antigen–antibody interaction for the recognition of specific proteins. This interaction is usually transduced into an electrical readable signal [4, 5, 7]. Impedance analysis, a technique based on the measurement of changes in electrical properties of a conductive material [26], is used in this type of biosensors, providing label-free detection and avoiding chemical amplification schemes [27].

In this section, we show the design, manufacturing and testing of biomicrosystems based on printed circuit board (PCB) platforms, with 40 independent electro-immunosensors for the detection of the 6 kDa early secretory antigen target-6 (ESAT-6), which is an immunodominant secreted protein involved in the virulence of *M. tuberculosis* [28]. Sensors were integrated into a microfluidic system that allows the use of a minimum volume of sample per test. Human serum albumin (HSA) was employed as a negative control. Each electro-immunosensor was comprised of a gold nanolayer with an immobilized polyclonal antibody (pAb) attached by a thiol-based SAM. Without the need of intrusive or destructive methods, it was possible to detect probe-target interactions and verify all manufacturing stages of the biomicrosystem via impedance analysis at different frequency ranges [29].

3.1. Materials and methods

3.1.1. PCB design and manufacture

Each biomicrosystem was mounted on a double-layer FR-4 PCB of 142 × 48.7 mm with 2 oz. thickness of copper. Electrodes were patterned on the top layer while interconnection tracks were placed on the bottom layer with CadSoft Eagle Professional 7.4.0. The PCB bottom surface was laminated with antisolder and the top layer was left uncovered for further material deposition. The PCB electrical conductivity was verified through PeakTech 3725 multifunction digital tester (PeakTech, Ahrensburg, Germany).

3.1.2. Lift off and gold deposition

A uniform gold nanolayer was physically evaporated to form the electrodes at the top layer of the board. Briefly, the substrate top surface was laminated with a dry photosensitive film (LAMINAR® E9200) in the RLM 419P (Bungard Elektronik, Windeck, Germany) laminator. The substrate was exposed to UV light to promote free-radical polymerization. The laminated substrate was subjected to a developing process and a uniform gold nanolayer was physically evaporated on the laminated substrate through physical vapor deposition (PVD) with thermal evaporator Edwards Auto 306 (Moorfield Nanotechnology Limited, Cheshire, UK). A 3 A current, vacuum pressure of 4×10^{-5} mbar and an evaporation rate of 0.12 nm/s were used over a tungsten slide for 100 mg gold evaporation. Finally, photoresist sacrificial layer was removed with stripper (Bungard Elektronik, Windeck, Germany), obtaining an 80 nm gold nanolayer on 35 μm copper surfaces. The electrical conductivity of individual electrodes on the board of each biomicrosystem was verified using a PeakTech 3725 multifunction digital tester (PeakTech, Ahrensburg, Germany).

3.1.3. Biomicrosystem development

A 121 × 20.8 mm PMMA slide with 2 mm wells organized in two rows and 20 columns was adhered to the top of the PCB top layer using TESA® 4965 double-sided tape and subsequently fixed with screws (**Figure 3a**), miming a well plate with individual wells for each electrode. Reagents were deposited inside each well for the biosensor fabrication (**Figure 3b**) and electrical connectors were placed between each well for electrical measurements (**Figure 3c**). Three biomicrosystems were fabricated and tested in different batches, each biomicrosystem containing 40 independent electro-immunosensors, which were individually measured for each batch (**Figure 3d**) to assure the reproducibility and repeatability of the manufacturing process. A total of 120 electro-immunosensors were tested.

3.1.4. Reagents immobilization

SAM were produced in each well following the procedure in [15]. Shortly, 10 μL of 20 mM 4-aminothiophenol (4-ATP) solution were added as cross-linkers in each well and left at room temperature for 4 h. To remove excess of thiols, wells were washed with ethanol and deionized water. 10 μL of 100 μg/mL pAb 45073 solution were added into each well. The system was stored at 4°C overnight. PBS and deionized water were used to remove excess biomolecules.

3.1.5. Immobilization tests

Impedance measurements of each well of the electro-immunosensor were according to the diagram shown in **Figure 3d** and using an impedance analyzer (Agilent 4294A) at a frequency

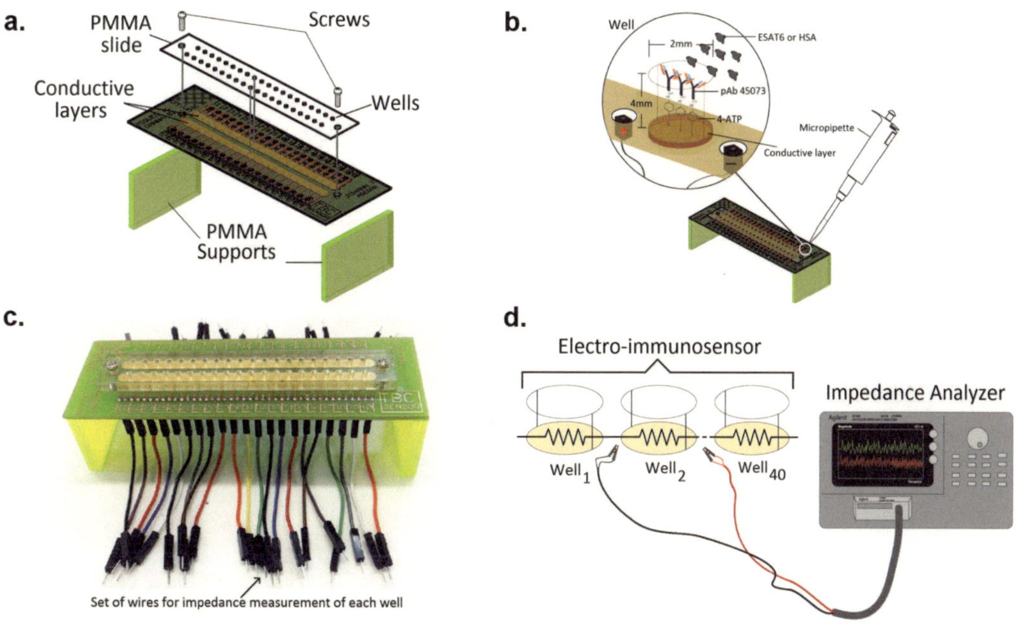

Figure 3. (**a**) Schematic representation of the biomicrosystem, (**b**) illustration of the self-assembly process for each well, (**c**) actual image of the fabricated biomicrosystem, and (**d**) equivalent measurement circuit of the biomicrosystem.

range from 40 to 120 Hz, 120 to 200 Hz and 200 to 280 Hz. Frequencies were selected as reported in [15]. Sensors were manufactured in three main stages, first a gold nanolayer (Au), followed by a gold nanolayer with a SAM of 4-ATP (Au + ATP), and finally a gold nanolayer with a SAM of 4-ATP and pAb 45073 (Au + ATP + pA). Eight replicates of the impedance measurements were collected at each stage for the specific frequencies above. Impedance analysis was also performed for analyte recognition in the presence of both 0.5 μg/mL of ESAT6 (Au + ATP + pA-ESAT6) (positive control) and HSA (Au + ATP + pA-HSA) (negative control). After analyte deposition, wells remained at room temperature and under static conditions for 1 h prior to electrical measurements.

3.2. Results

3.2.1. Immobilization testing by impedance analysis

The average impedance magnitude of the three manufacturing stages of the sensors (Au, Au + ATP, Au + ATP + pA) was determined by its response to an AC current as a function of frequency [30]. To determine the variation of the copper with gold evaporated prior to the immobilization (conductive layer), 40 individual wells of three biomicrosystems were measured by impedance analysis at different frequency ranges. The mean value of the 120 wells was 0.1588 Ω with a standard deviation of 0.0142, 0.1591 Ω with a standard deviation of 0.0142, and 0.1584 Ω with a standard deviation of 0.0102 Ω, for ranges 40–120 Hz, 120–200 Hz and 200–280 Hz, respectively. This suggested small variance and good reproducibility of the manufacturing processes of all wells regardless of the fabrication batch. The largest significant differences within immobilization stages were observed for 40 and 120 Hz (**Figure 4**, **Table 2**).

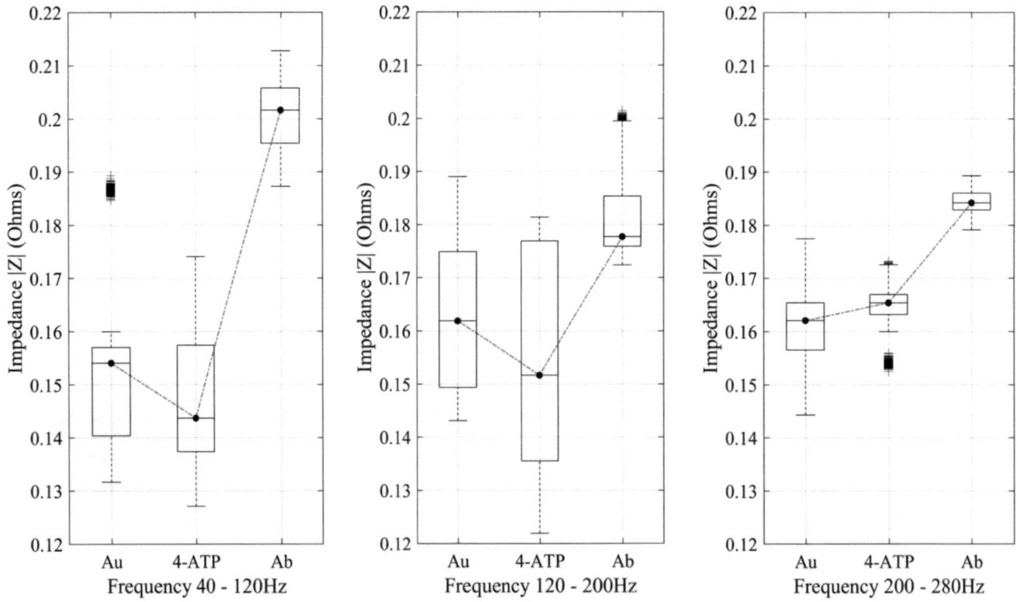

Figure 4. Analysis of impedance variation for the three main manufacturing stages. (**a**) Impedance magnitude at 40–120 Hz, (**b**) impedance magnitude at 120–200 Hz, and (**c**) impedance magnitude at 200–280 Hz.

Frequencies	|Z| Au		|Z| 4-ATP		|Z| Ab	
	Average (μ) Au	Standard Deviation (σ) Au	Average (μ) 4-ATP	Standard Deviation (σ) 4-ATP	Average (μ) Ab	Standard Deviation (σ) Ab
40	0.1526	0.0167	0.1466	0.0145	0.1986	0.0070
50	0.1523	0.0165	0.1482	0.0142	0.1997	0.0067
60	0.1517	0.0169	0.1472	0.0141	0.2004	0.0065
70	0.1523	0.0167	0.1475	0.0144	0.1996	0.0065
80	0.1530	0.0160	0.1473	0.0139	0.2009	0.0068
90	0.1528	0.0159	0.1470	0.0144	0.2018	0.0071
100	0.1530	0.0165	0.1471	0.0142	0.2016	0.0068
110	0.1525	0.0159	0.1470	0.0143	0.2003	0.0070
120	0.1532	0.0166	0.1472	0.0140	0.2009	0.0070
130	0.1629	0.0159	0.1542	0.0220	0.1819	0.0083
140	0.1627	0.0156	0.1540	0.0213	0.1821	0.0084
150	0.1629	0.0158	0.1540	0.0216	0.1814	0.0083
160	0.1624	0.0157	0.1549	0.0219	0.1815	0.0084
170	0.1624	0.0159	0.1534	0.0216	0.1807	0.0081
180	0.1627	0.0155	0.1535	0.0216	0.1812	0.0085
190	0.1624	0.0154	0.1535	0.0218	0.1809	0.0082
200	0.1629	0.0155	0.1537	0.0216	0.1805	0.0084
210	0.1612	0.0088	0.1653	0.0052	0.1846	0.0022
220	0.1614	0.0089	0.1646	0.0052	0.1844	0.0020
230	0.1605	0.0088	0.1655	0.0051	0.1850	0.0021
240	0.1605	0.0089	0.1644	0.0051	0.1839	0.0019
250	0.1619	0.0087	0.1649	0.0051	0.1846	0.0021
260	0.1613	0.0089	0.1646	0.0052	0.1838	0.0023
270	0.1611	0.0090	0.1646	0.0049	0.1845	0.0019
280	0.1610	0.0087	0.1654	0.0047	0.1843	0.0022

Table 2. Impedance magnitude values (mean and standard deviation) of the manufacturing stages at 40–280 Hz.

In this range, there is a non-significant variation of impedance (−3.81%) between the first two manufacturing stages, Au and Au + ATP. Nonetheless, a 31.21% of impedance variation between Au and Au + ATP + pA was measured. Also, impedance measurements between the first two manufacturing stages varied −5.51% and 2.16%, from 120 to 200 Hz and from 200 to 280 Hz, respectively. Similarly, variations of 11.4 and 14.37% between Au and Au + ATP + pA were detected at frequencies ranges of 120 to 200 Hz and 200 to 280 Hz, respectively. Finally, there was a correspondence between the impedance value of the last immobilization step and negative controls, which was 0.20 Ω [29].

3.2.2. *Detection of protein ESAT6*

Impedance analysis was used to verify the detection of ESAT6 as means of *M. tuberculosis* diagnosis. 0.5 μg/mL ESAT-6 were used as a positive control and 0.5 μg/mL HSA as a negative control, and their detection was compared to the dot blot assay. **Figure 5** and **Table 3** show that the frequency range from 40 Hz to 120 Hz has the largest significant variation in impedance among all investigated ranges. **Figure 5c** and **d** shows significant changes in other frequency ranges (120–200 Hz and 200–280 Hz). Between 40 and 120 Hz, the detection of the *M. tuberculosis* protein has an impedance increase of 171% compared to the impedance measured for the negative control (HSA), which showed a negligible impedance variation. No overlapping values between the negative and the positive control were identified. All the results of the negative controls were under 0.20 Ω while impedance values for the positive controls were above 0.54 Ω. This defined an interval where protein detection is not attainable.

3.3. Analytic hierarchy process (AHP) for comparison of the biomicrosystem with traditional detection techniques

AHP was utilized to study the viability of the electro-immunosensor compared with traditional TB diagnostic techniques (Xpert MTB/RIF, culture, and smear test). Expert Choice 11.5® software was used to perform matrix pairwise comparisons in light of the scale of Saaty [16]. **Table 4** summarizes the required parameters for the pairwise comparison matrix. This weighed analysis compared cost, effectiveness, time, and test analysis for each diagnostic platform. This program assigns a weight to each of the alternatives relative to the criteria. The total weight is distributed among the diagnostic alternatives, which were the electro-immunosensor, Xpert MTB/RIF, culture and smear test. **Table 5** shows the results obtained [29].

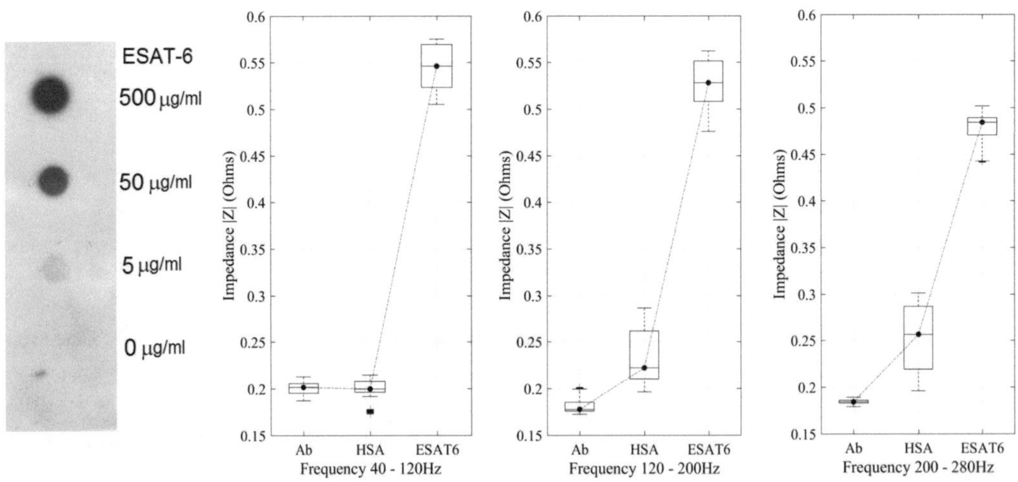

Figure 5. (**a**) Detection limit for the dot blot assay compared to the electro-immunosensor. (**b, c, d**) Analysis of impedance variation for 0.5 μg/mL of analyte. (**b**) Impedance magnitude at 40–120 Hz, (**c**) impedance magnitude at 120–200 Hz, and (**d**) impedance magnitude at 200–280 Hz.

Frequencies	ǀZǀ Ab		ǀZǀ HAS		ǀZǀ ESAT6	
	Average (μ) Ab	Standard Deviation (σ) Ab	Average (μ) HSA	Standard Deviation (σ) HSA	Average (μ) ESAT6	Standard Deviation (σ) ESAT6
40	0.1986	0.0070	0.2016	0.0114	0.5462	0.0264
50	0.1997	0.0067	0.1986	0.0116	0.5440	0.0254
60	0.2004	0.0065	0.1986	0.0118	0.5439	0.0260
70	0.1996	0.0065	0.2000	0.0112	0.5446	0.0260
80	0.2009	0.0068	0.1991	0.0114	0.5443	0.0259
90	0.2018	0.0071	0.1988	0.0109	0.5440	0.0256
100	0.2016	0.0068	0.1988	0.0114	0.5438	0.0260
110	0.2003	0.0070	0.1986	0.0113	0.5437	0.0260
120	0.2009	0.0070	0.1986	0.0114	0.5434	0.0263
130	0.1819	0.0083	0.2340	0.0320	0.5266	0.0292
140	0.1821	0.0084	0.2338	0.0317	0.5267	0.0288
150	0.1814	0.0083	0.2337	0.0318	0.5264	0.0292
160	0.1815	0.0084	0.2338	0.0316	0.5264	0.0294
170	0.1807	0.0081	0.2336	0.0315	0.5262	0.0295
180	0.1812	0.0085	0.2337	0.0319	0.5262	0.0296
190	0.1809	0.0082	0.2340	0.0315	0.5260	0.0294
200	0.1805	0.0084	0.2336	0.0318	0.5266	0.0291
210	0.1846	0.0022	0.2540	0.0373	0.4820	0.0153
220	0.1844	0.0020	0.2537	0.0372	0.4805	0.0156
230	0.1850	0.0021	0.2532	0.0371	0.4798	0.0154
240	0.1839	0.0019	0.2527	0.0372	0.4786	0.0159
250	0.1846	0.0021	0.2522	0.0370	0.4779	0.0163
260	0.1838	0.0023	0.2519	0.0368	0.4784	0.0169
270	0.1845	0.0019	0.2515	0.0371	0.4789	0.0177
280	0.1843	0.0022	0.2513	0.0367	0.4826	0.0144

Table 3. Impedance magnitude values (mean and standard deviation) of different analytes at 40–280 Hz.

The AHP analysis confirmed that the designed electro-immunosensor is a superior alternative for detection compared with traditional TB diagnostic techniques. For instance, it requires a shorter time of analysis per test and allows high throughput screening (a single device handles 40 independent replicas), and even the identification of different *M. tuberculosis* epitopes by varying the bio-recognition probe in each well. Despite these advantages, the electro-immunosensor is not the preferred choice locally mainly due to its prohibitive price (attributed to the cost of required bioreagents) and the untested effectiveness in clinical contexts.

Test	Cost	Time of analysis	Probability of contamination	Difficulty of analysis with blood in sample	Test effectiveness
TBC biosensor	7 USD (without labor and overhead)	1 h	Low: although it is a manual process, there are mechanical barriers to avoid filtration between wells	It is based on antigen-body recognition, so bleeding is not supposed to affect the results	Results confirm that reliable data is obtained with the biosensor
Xpert MTB/RIF	98.10 USD	2 h	None: completely automated	There is no interference after the pretreatment	High sensitivity, specificity and reproducibility. Avoid false positive/negative results
Culture (MGIT)	36.56 USD	1 month	Medium: microbial growth can be affected by accompanying microbiota	Bleeding does not affect the results	Reliability between 70 and 90%
Smear microscopy test	4.07 USD	More than 1 day	None: it is a fast and direct method	There is no interference after the pretreatment	It depends on the sample and technician. Reliability can vary between 22 and 80%

Table 4. Criteria for the establishment of the pairwise comparison matrix for the diagnostic techniques for *M. tuberculosis*.

	Electro-immunosensor (%)	Xpert MTB/RIF (%)	Culture (%)	Smear test (%)
Retail price	31.0	4.3	11.3	53.4
Analysis of tests	35.6	15.8	28.1	20.5
Effectiveness	10.6	14.4	54.3	20.8
Time of test	50.2	29.0	4.1	16.7
Global weights	32.5	16.7	22.5	28.3

Table 5. Local weights for each diagnostic platform.

4. Case of study: Chagas

Development of methods that can facilitate low-cost diagnosis of infectious and particularly neglected tropical diseases has been widely studied in the last few decades. In this section, we outline the design, fabrication and evaluation of a portable system for the detection of Chagas Disease during the Acute phase of the disease, called Chagas Biosense, as an alternative to perform a quick, on-site, and low-cost diagnosis. Furthermore, we describe its potential impact on alleviating the economic burden on the healthcare system by improving rural diagnostics of Chagas in developing and tropical countries.

4.1. Theoretical framework

4.1.1. *Fundamentals of Chagas disease*

The World Health Organization (WHO) classifies 17 major parasitic and bacterial infections as neglected tropical diseases (NTDs) [31]. NTDs are characterized by affecting vulnerable populations (where healthcare systems are generally inefficient), and their survival under tropical and subtropical conditions [32]. American trypanosomiasis, better known as Chagas disease, is one of the most common NTDs in the world, which is caused by the parasite *Trypanosoma cruzi*. Recent estimates indicated that between 6 and 7 million people are infected worldwide [32].

Chagas is a vector-born disease transmitted by triatomine insects. This hematophagous insect of the *Reduviidae* family, transmits the disease while feeding [33]. The infection starts with the movement of the parasite from the insect feces into human blood streams. From this point, the disease will develop in two consecutive phases. First, the Acute phase, characterized for a high number of parasites present in the bloodstream, lasting for about 4 to 8 weeks and showing very mild or non-existent symptoms [34]. Second, the Chronic phase, where the immune system of individuals is compromised and some organs are infested with the *Trypanosoma cruzi* [34]. In fact, when the patient reaches the Chronic phase, the parasite invades the digestive system and the heart tissues, which can cause damages that will be evidenced up to 20 years after the infection [35]. Most commonly, patients will manifest progressive heart damage, which may eventually require a heart transplant [34, 35].

Nowadays, treatments to the disease include benznidazole and Nifurtimox. Both treatments are 100% effective in killing the parasite and treating the disease if they are used at the beginning of the Acute phase. The efficacy of both treatments decreases as the infection progresses [32].

4.1.2. Current diagnosis methods

Diagnosis of Chagas Disease is carried out by observation of the parasite in a blood sample by means of microscopy methods, such as blood cultures, xenodiagnoses and thick drop, among others. However, these methods only work during the Acute phase of the disease, due to the important number of parasites in the bloodstream [9]. Diagnosis in the Chronic phase is determined based on the medical history of the patient, and only if the patient has lived in an endemic area. Thus, diagnosis during this phase relies on laboratory tests based on antibodies specific for the disease, ELISA tests, and quick tests such as Chagas STAT-PAK® [36]. **Table 6** summarizes the main characteristics of most popular diagnosis tests, as well as our system.

4.1.3. Chagas biosense concept

An effective detection method of Chagas Disease relies on the basic understanding of the parasite behavior inside the human circulatory system. The parasite in its infectious stage (*metacyclic trypomastigote*) reaches the circulatory system after the vector (triatomine insect) defecates in a superficial skin wound. Once in the bloodstream, the parasite enters red blood cells (RBCs), white blood cells (WBCs) or platelets, where the next development stage (*amastigote*) begins and the parasite reproduces [37].

After infection, the parasite at the *trypomastigote* stage can be easily differentiated from blood cells. For instance, RBCs have a diameter between 6.2 and 8.2 μm and a thickness between 0.8 and 1 μm [38], while the parasite has a length between 15 and 24 μm [39] and a width of

Name	Test category	Use in laboratory	Detection	State	Sample volume (μL)	Test duration (h.min)	Cost/ test (USD)
Chagas Biosense (BIOTROP)	Rapid assays	No	Direct detection of the parasity Trypanosoma cruzi by microfluidics	Acute	5	0.05	10.83
Chagas STAT-PAK® (Chembio Diagnostic Systems, Inc.)		No	Detection of antibodies for Trypanosoma cruzi by immunochromatographic assay	Chronic	10	0.20	—
HBK 740 IMUNOBLOT LINHAS anti-T. cruzi (Innogenetics, Belgium)	Confirmatory assays	Yes	Indirect immunofluorescence antibody detection		10	1.50	0.19
IMUNOCRUZI® (biolab-Merieux S.A.)		No	Detection of antibodies by immunoblot assay		10	18.00	20
TESA-blot (biolab-Merieux S.A.)		Yes	Detection of antibodies by Western blot		10	4.00	—
CHAGAS HAI IMUNOSERUM (Laboratorio Lemos – Polychaco)	Agglutination	No	Detection of specific antibodies in the sample by hemagglutination		10	1.50	0.33
CHAGAS-ELISA (EBRAM Productos Laboratoriais Ltda)	Enzyme immunoassays	No	Detection of antibodies in the sample by ELISA test		10	1.40	1.02

Table 6. Compared analysis between Chagas biosense and some methods evaluated by the WHO.

approximately 1.09 μm [40]. These differences in size and density suggest the possibility of using a microfluidic device as a separation platform.

Microfluidic devices have already been used in the detection of diseases such as malaria, HIV, and tuberculosis. For example, the detection of HIV is attained by counting the number of CD4 + T-lymphocytes cells in a blood sample, based on the fact that HIV leads to an increase in cell concentration (to levels above 200 cells/mL) [41]. In the case of malaria, the parasite enters RBCs and changes their weight and density, allowing their separation from healthy cells by means of centripetal force [41].

4.2. *In silico* design

4.2.1. *Microfluidics fundamentals*

Fluid mechanics under the confinement of a microsystem differs from that at the macroscale. For instance, parameters like viscosity, diffusion, adhesion forces and density become significant, while gravity loses strength at the microscale [42]. One of the most important parameters in microfluidics is the Reynolds number (Re), which can be estimated by the following equation:

$$Re = \frac{\rho v D_h}{\mu} \quad (1)$$

Where ρ is the density of the fluid, μ is the viscosity of the fluid, v the velocity of the fluid, and D_h is the hydraulic diameter [43]. The Re can be understood as the ratio of inertial forces to viscous forces [43]. In microfluidics, typical values of Re oscillate around 1, which correspond to the laminar flow regime where viscous forces dominate [42, 44]. In addition, microfluidic devices operating at low Re number can be used for particle separation in a predictable manner [44].

When particles are immersed in a fluid flowing in a microchannel, they are subjected to the Lift force (F_L), which drives them towards zones of higher shear stress [44]. The Lift force can be calculated with the following equation:

$$F_L = \rho G^2 C_L a_p^4 \quad (2)$$

where G is the shear rate of the fluid and is given by $G = v/D_h$, C_L is the lift coefficient, which is a function of the particle position in the channel, and a_p is the diameter of the particle [44].

Particles are also subjected to a secondary force known as the Drag force (F_D). This force is generated by the curvature of the geometry leading to particle trajectories perpendicular to the main flow direction [44]. The Drag force can be evaluated from the following equation:

$$F_D = 5.4*10^{-4}\pi\mu De^{1.63}a_p; \;\; De = Re\sqrt{\frac{D_h}{2R}} \quad (3)$$

where De is the Dean number, which describes the effect of curvature in flow nature, and R is the radius of curvature.

As these two forces counterbalance along the microchannel, particle separation is promoted as a strong function of the particle diameter [45]. Thus, the relationship between a_p, F_L and F_D is given by the following set of inequalities, which state that for particles with a large diameter, the dominant force will be F_L. By contrast, if the particle has a small diameter, the dominant force will be F_D.

$$a_{p1} > a_{p2} > a_{p3}; \;\; \frac{F_{L1}}{F_{D1}} > \frac{F_{L2}}{F_{D2}} > \frac{F_{L3}}{F_{D3}} \quad (4)$$

4.2.2. Simulations

Prior to microchannel fabrication, particle separation was evaluated *in silico* with the aid of COMSOL Multiphysics®. This tool allowed us to test different microchannel curvatures, diameters and lengths. To set up the simulations, the Computational Fluid Dynamics (CFD) and particle tracing modules were coupled to study the separation of parasites from RBCs for different microchannel configurations. A non-slip condition was defined at the boundaries. **Figure 6** shows the tested design, which consisted of 5 turns of a 0.5 mm wide microchannel that ended up in 4 outlets.

Proper meshing was determined from a mesh convergence analysis by evaluating the magnitude of flow velocity at different locations within the domain. Convergence was met when there was

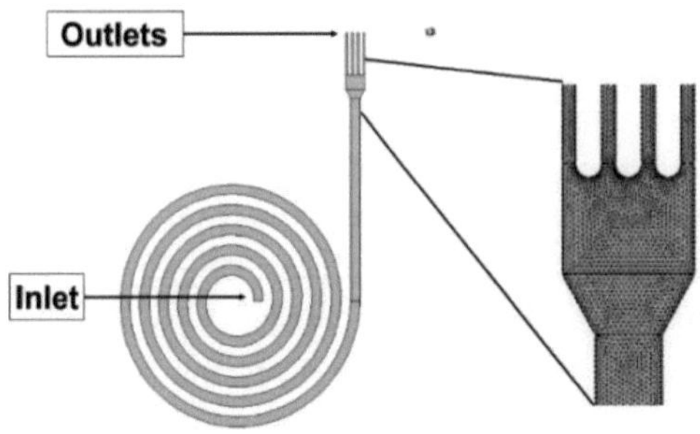

Figure 6. Computational domain and meshing.

less than 2% change on the magnitude of the velocity at each location after duplicating the number of mesh elements in the domain [46]. The parameters for the simulations are listed in **Table 7**:

Fluid density	1030 (Kg/m^3)
Fluid dynamic viscosity	1.5×10^{-3} (Pa s)
Input velocity	0.1 (m/s)
Parasite density	1030 (Kg/m^3)
Parasite diameter	30 (μm)
RBCs density	1030 (Kg/m^3)
RBCs diameter	6 (μm)

Table 7. Simulation parameters.

4.3. Prototypes fabrication

Different manufacturing strategies were used to fabricate the device prototype. These strategies were classified into chemical etching and physical treatments strategies and are described in the following sections.

4.3.1. Chemical etching: photolithography

Chemical etching is a process in which microstructures are generated by the chemical abrasion of a material. Through this process, microstructures can be fabricated on a glass substrate by using hydrofluoric acid (HF) as the etching agent [47]. The protocol for manufacturing the prototype is shown in **Figure 7a**. Briefly, a photoresist layer was spin coated onto a glass slide prior to photolithography (**Figure 7a**). The glass slide was then exposed to HF for 15 seconds to obtain the microchannel. PDMS was adhered to the glass via oxygen plasma irradiation, and served as a sealing layer (**Figure 7a**).

4.3.2. Physical treatment: laser engraving and cutting

Laser engraving and cutting were used as physical techniques for the fabrication of the prototype onto a PMMA substrate. The overall manufacturing process is shown in **Figure 7b**.

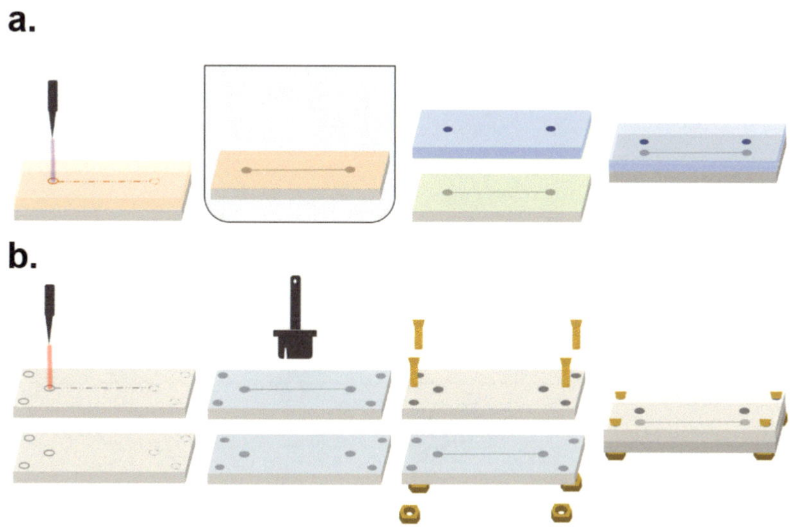

Figure 7. Manufacturing process of biomicrosystems. (**a**) Chemical etching process, and (**b**) laser engraving and cutting.

In brief, the design was engraved into PMMA with a laser cutter (TROTEC® Speedy 100, 60 w). Sealing of the microchannel was attained by application of methyl methacrylate and constant pressure between the layers.

4.4. Results

Currently, the described device is at a design stage. Accordingly, parasite separation has been mainly tested in silico with the aid of the Multiphysics simulation platform COMSOL®. Nonetheless, simulations have given us important insights to be taken into account for preparing more robust prototypes

4.4.1. Simulations

Convergence was attained with 150,000 triangular mesh elements (**Figure 8**). Velocity profiles and particle distributions at the outlets are shown in **Figures 9** and **10**, respectively.

Maximal separation of parasites from RBCs was evidenced in outlets 1 and 3. Nonetheless, there is still a percentage of cross-contamination at the outlets (approximately 25% per outlet). This could be overcome by changing the length of the microchannel or increasing the number of outlets.

4.4.2. Prototypes and proof-of-concept

Functionality and proper sealing of prototypes was tested with water as flowing fluid. Syringes were connected at the inlets through MEDEX® fr 6 urethral nelaton catheters. A Touch Screen (Cole-Parmer®, USA) syringe pump was used to control water flow. Laser engraved prototypes showed leaks when subjected to pressure. In addition, their microchannels dimensions doubled those expected since the manufacturing technique had a low precision in micrometric scales. Furthermore, in the chemical etched prototype, fluid flow was restricted

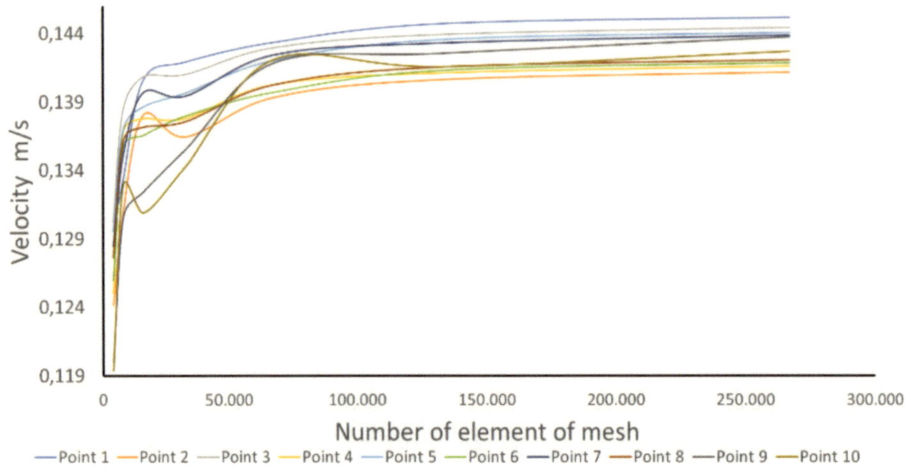

Figure 8. Mesh convergence analysis.

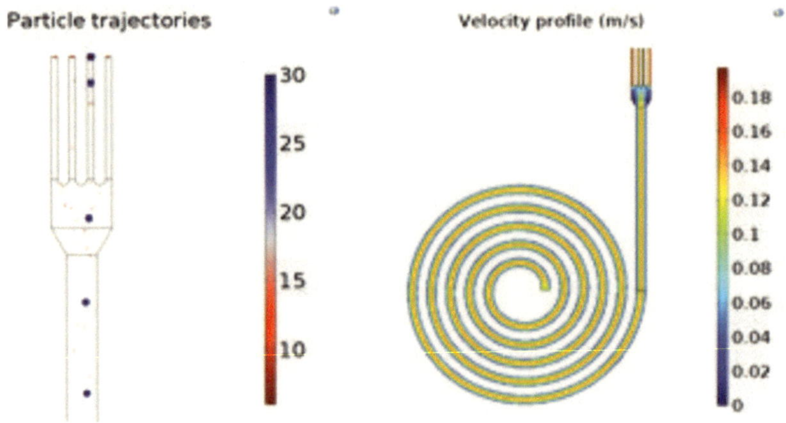

Figure 9. Particle distribution and velocity profile obtained in COMSOL Multiphysics®.

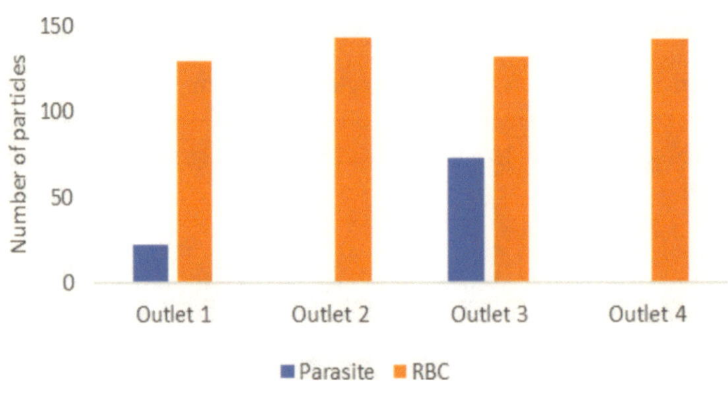

Figure 10. Particle distribution per outlet when simulating 600 particles (100 parasite particles and 500 RBCs particles).

due to the high hydraulic resistance inside the microsystem. To overcome these issues, several strategies can be implemented including a push-in fitting at the inlets to minimize leakages; improved adhesion processes at the interfaces and etched channels with larger dimensions.

4.5. Cost analysis

4.5.1. Disease cost and impact of the device

According to Lee et al. [48], the worldwide expenditure on Chagas Disease is estimated to lay between $186′282,994 and $1638′807,623 USD. 78.35% of which correspond to Latin-America while 18.6% are from the United States and Canada. These costs are principally derived from the treatment of cardiac and digestive complications associated with the disease during the Chronic phase. This roughly represents expenditures of $5900 USD per patient. By contrast, the costs during the Acute phase represent only a single expenditure of $200 USD per patient, which makes diagnosis for the Acute phase the best strategy to reduce the economic burden of treatments on the health care system [49].

The proposed microfluidic system serves as a portable diagnostic device that eliminates the need to attend to specialized laboratories to obtain a diagnosis. This allows rural populations at endemic areas to have a prompt knowledge of their state of health regarding the presence of the Chagas parasite. Also, being able to obtain a diagnosis during the Acute phase will help government agencies to assess the real number of Chagas disease cases, which will result in better awareness and additional research funding.

The expenditure per test of diagnosis varies depending on the stage of the disease. As depicted in **Table 5**, most of the procedures for Chronic phase diagnosis have an approximate cost of $1 USD per test. However, some of the commercially available tests such as the HBK 740 IMUNOBLOT LINHAS anti-T cruzi could have a cost as high as $20 USD per individual test [37]. By contrast, blood testing for Acute phase diagnosis has an approximate cost of $17 USD per patient (Tauramena local Hospital, Colombia).

The Acute phase diagnostic device proposed in this section has an approximate cost of $8 and $4 USD if manufactured via chemical or physical processes, respectively. These costs correspond to expenditures on materials and equipment. In addition to low manufacturing costs, this device does not require specialized laboratory equipment for the diagnosis, allowing its use at remote rural areas, which are usually endemic areas as well.

4.5.2. Future perspectives

Although geometries were verified by simulation processes, there is still a gap between simulated geometries and manufactured prototypes. Sealing techniques must be improved to avoid leaks and increase the life of the device. Also, the microfluidic separation device needs to be coupled with sensing techniques to unequivocally identify the parasite. This could be achieved by including specific antibodies towards *Trypanosoma cruzi* or by placing electrodes at the outlets to determine effective separation by electrical measurements such as electrochemical impedance spectroscopy (EIS).

5. Concluding remarks and future perspectives

Point-of-care devices are ideal for providing reliable information in a fast, user-friendly, accurate, and low-cost manner. Electro-immunosensors offer an attractive option for pathogen detection with high sensitivity and affinity, which can ultimately respond to the challenge of bringing electrochemical sensing techniques to patients. Also, microfluidic separators provide an avenue for isolating and rapidly estimating the relative abundance of pathogens in biological fluids. Rapid diagnosis devices such as those introduced here facilitate clinical decision making and effective treatment thereby leading to greater patient survival rates. The presented case studies show examples in which LoC technology is exploited for pathogen detection. Although the devices show promising results towards early diagnosis of HPV, Tuberculosis and Chagas disease, further work is still needed to bring the developments to commercial success. For instance, the possibility of effectively handling information by end users should be included in the proposed technologies as well as their integration with internet of things (IoT) and cloud computing technology. Also, manufacturing methods that involve drilling can be easily substituted with injection technology, which may reduce costs and time of production. Point-of-care devices constitute the ideal direction towards providing a reliable diagnosis in remote areas without the need of a specialized laboratories or clinical facilities.

Author details

Natalia Lopez-Barbosa[1,2], Ana Lucia Campaña[1,2], Mabel Juliana Noguera[2], Sergio Leonardo Florez[2], Miguel Angel Aroca[1], Juan C. Cruz[2] and Johann F. Osma[1*]

*Address all correspondence to: jf.osma43@uniandes.edu.co

1 CMUA, Department of Electrical and Electronics Engineering, Universidad de los Andes, Bogota, Colombia

2 Department of Biomedical Engineering, Universidad de los Andes, Bogota, Colombia

References

[1] Hay SI, Battle KE, Pigott DM, Smith DL, Moyes CL, Bhatt S, Brownstein JS, Collier N, Myers MF, George DB, Gething PW. Global mapping of infectious disease. Philosophical Transactions of the Royal Society B. 2013;**368**:1-11

[2] Su W, Gao X, Jiang L, Qin J. Microfluidic platform towards point-of-care diagnostics in infectious diseases. Journal of Chromatography. A. 2015;**1377**:13-26. DOI: 10.1016/j.chroma.2014.12.041

[3] Urdea M, Penny LA, Olmsted SS, Giovanni MY, Kaspar P, Shepherd A, Wilson P, Dahl CA, Buchsbaum S, Moeller G, Hay Burgess DC. Requirements for high impact diagnostics in the developing world. Nature. 2006;**444**:73-79

[4] Lopez-Barbosa N, Gamarra JD, Osma JF. The future point-of-care detection of disease and its data capture and handling. Analytical and Bioanalytical Chemistry; 2016. DOI: 10.1007/s00216-015-9249-2

[5] Lopez-Barbosa N, Osma JF. Biosensors: Migrating from clinical to environmental industries. Biosensors Journal. 2016;**5**:1

[6] Wang J. Electrochemical glucose biosensors. Chemical Reviews. 2008;**108**:814-825. DOI: 10.1021/cr068123a

[7] Lopez-Barbosa N, Segura C, Osma JF. Electro-immuno sensors: Current developments and future trends. International Journal Biosensors and Bioelectronics. 2017;**2**:1-6. DOI: 10.15406/ijbsbe.2017.02.00010

[8] Dunne EF, Park IU. HPV and HPV-associated diseases. Infectious Disease Clinics. 2013;**27**: 765-778

[9] Jemal A, Clegg LX, Ward E, Ries LAG, Wu X, Jamison PM, Wingo PA, Howe HL, Anderson RN, Edwards BK. Annual report to the nation on the status of cancer, 1975–2001, with a special feature regarding survival. Cancer. 2004;**101**:3-27

[10] Stanley M. Pathology and epidemiology of HPV infection in females. Gynecologic Oncology. 2010;**117**:S5-S10

[11] Ferlay J, Shin H, Bray F, Forman D, Mathers C, Parkin DM. Estimates of worldwide burden of cancer in 2008: GLOBOCAN 2008. International Journal of Cancer. 2010;**127**:2893-2917

[12] Kornya L, Cseh I, Deak J, Bak M, Fulop V. The diagnostics and prevalence of genital human papillomavirus (HPV) infection in Hungary. European Journal of Obstetrics, Gynecology, and Reproductive Biology. 2002;**100**:231-236

[13] Kim HH, Jeon HJ, Cho HK, Cheong JH, Moon HS, Go JS. Highly sensitive microcantilever biosensors with enhanced sensitivity for detection of human papilloma virus infection. Sensors and Actuators B: Chemical. 2015;**221**:1372-1383

[14] Huang H, Bai W, Dong C, Guo R, Liu Z. An ultrasensitive electrochemical DNA biosensor based on graphene/Au nanorod/polythionine for human papillomavirus DNA detection. Biosensors & Bioelectronics. 2015;**68**:442-446

[15] Urrego LF, Lopez DI, Ramirez KA, Ramirez C, Osma JF. Biomicrosystem design and fabrication for the human papilloma virus 16 detection. Sensors and Actuators B: Chemical. 2015;**207**:97-104. DOI: 10.1016/j.snb.2014.10.036

[16] Saaty TL. Decision making with the analytic hierarchy process. International Journal of Service Science. 2008;**1**:83-98

[17] He F, Xiong Y, Liu J, Tong F, Yan D. Construction of Au-IDE/CFP10-ESAT6 aptamer/DNA-AuNPs MSPQC for rapid detection of *Mycobacterium tuberculosis*. Biosensors & Bioelectronics. 2016;**77**:799-804. DOI: 10.1016/j.bios.2015.10.054

[18] Abe C, Hirano K, Wada M, Kazumi Y, Takahashi M, Fukasawa Y, Yoshimura T, Miyagi C, Goto S. Detection of *Mycobacterium tuberculosis* in clinical specimens by polymerase

chain reaction and gen-probe amplified mycobacterium tuberculosis direct test. Journal of Clinical Microbiology. 1993;**31**:3270-3274

[19] Nassau E, Parsons ER, Johnson GD. The detection of antibodies to *Mycobacterium tuberculosis* by microplate enzyme-linked immunosorbent assay (ELISA). Tubercle. 1976;**57**: 67-70. DOI: 10.1016/0041-3879(76)90019-2

[20] Pottumarthy S, Wells VC, Morris AJ. A comparison of seven tests for serological diagnosis of tuberculosis. Journal of Clinical Microbiology. 2000;**38**:2227-2231

[21] World Health Organization. The End TB Strategy: Global Strategy and Targets for Tuberculosis Prevention, Care and Control After 2015; 2014

[22] Zhang QD, March G, Noel V, Piro B, Reisberg S, Tran LD, Hai LV, Abadia E, Nielsen PE, Sola C, Pham MC. Label-free and reagentless electrochemical detection of PCR fragments using self-assembled quinone derivative monolayer: Application to *Mycobacterium tuberculosis*. Biosensors & Bioelectronics. 2012;**32**:163-168. DOI: 10.1016/j.bios.2011. 11.048

[23] Cheon SA, Cho HH, Kim J, Lee J, Kim HJ, Park TJ. Recent tuberculosis diagnosis toward the end TB strategy. Journal of Microbiological Methods. 2016;**123**:51-61. DOI: 10.1016/j.mimet.2016.02.007

[24] Kim J, Lee K-S, Kim EB, Paik S, Chang CL, Park TJ, Kim H-J, Lee J. Early detection of the growth of *Mycobacterium tuberculosis* using magnetophoretic immunoassay in liquid culture. Biosensors & Bioelectronics. 2017;**96**:68-76. DOI: 10.1016/j.bios.2017.04.025

[25] Costa MP, Andrade CAS, Montenegro RA, Melo FL, Oliveira MDL. Self-assembled monolayers of mercaptobenzoic acid and magnetite nanoparticles as an efficient support for development of tuberculosis genosensor. Journal of Colloid and Interface Science. 2014;**433**:141-148. DOI: http://dx.doi.org/10.1016/j.jcis.2014.07.014

[26] Singh A, Pasha SK, Manickam P, Bhansali S. Single-domain antibody based thermally stable electrochemical immunosensor. Biosensors & Bioelectronics. 2016;**83**:162-168. DOI: 10.1016/j.bios.2016.04.054

[27] Daniels JS, Pourmand N. Label-free impedance biosensors: Opportunities and challenges. Electroanalysis. 2007;**19**:1239-1257. DOI: 10.1002/elan.200603855

[28] Sreejit G, Ahmed A, Parveen N, Jha V, Valluri VL, Ghosh S, Mukhopadhyay S. The ESAT-6 protein of *Mycobacterium tuberculosis* interacts with beta-2-microglobulin (β2M) affecting antigen presentation function of macrophage. PLoS Pathogens. 2014;**10**:e1004446. DOI: 10.1371/journal.ppat.1004446

[29] Sepulveda D, Aroca MA, Varela A, Del Portillo P, Osma JF. Bioelectrochemical detection of *Mycobacterium tuberculosis* ESAT-6 in an antibody-based biomicrosystem. Sensors. 2017;**17**:2178

[30] Technologies A. Agilent 4294A precision impedance analyzer: Operation manual. TEST. 2003;**7**:30-42, 64-78, 130-138

[31] Hotez PJ, Pecoul B, Rijal S, Boehme C, Aksoy S, Malecela M, Tapia-Conyer R, Reeder JC. Eliminating the neglected tropical diseases: Translational science and new technologies. PLoS Neglected Tropical Diseases. 2016;**10**:e0003895

[32] WHO Chagas disease (American trypanosomiasis). http://www.who.int/mediacentre/factsheets/fs340/en/. [Accessed: 12 Sep 2017]; 2017

[33] Capinera JL. Encyclopedia of Entomology. Heidelberg, Germany: Springer Science & Business Media; 2008

[34] Social M de la protección. Protocolo para la vigilancia en salud pública de chagas. Bogotá; 2004

[35] WHO Control of Chagas disease: second report of the WHO expert committee

[36] Abcam Anti-Chagas IgG ELISA Kit (ab178637). http://www.abcam.com/chagas-igg-elisa-kit-ab178637.html. [Accessed 12 Sep 2017]; 2017

[37] Prevention C for DC and DPDx - Laboratory Identification of Parasitic Diseases of Public Health Concern. https://www.cdc.gov/dpdx/. [Accessed 12 Sep 2017]; 2017

[38] Turgeon ML. Clinical Hematology: Theory and Procedures. Philadelphia, USA: Lippincott Williams & Wilkins; 2005

[39] Parasitology TAS for Trypanosoma. http://parasite.org.au/para-site/text/cruzi-text.html. [Accessed 12 Sep 2017]; 2010

[40] Navarro MC, De Lima AR, Askue J, Contreras VT. Morphological comparison of axenic amastigogenesis of trypomastigotes and metacyclic forms of Trypanosoma cruzi. Memórias do Instituto Oswaldo Cruz. 2003;**98**:83-91

[41] Lee WG, Kim Y-G, Chung BG, Demirci U, Khademhosseini A. Nano/microfluidics for diagnosis of infectious diseases in developing countries. Advanced Drug Delivery Reviews. 2010;**62**:449-457

[42] Dimaki M, Okkels F. Design and simulation of lab-on-a-chip devices. In: Lab-on-a-Chip Devices Micro-Total Anal. Syst. Springer International Publishing. Cham, Switzerland; 2015. pp. 27-51

[43] Roselli RJ, Diller KR. Shell balance approach for one-dimensional biofluid transport. In: Biotransport Princ. New York, NY: Appl. Springer New York; 2011. pp. 319-388

[44] Martel JM, Toner M. Inertial focusing in microfluidics. Annual Review of Biomedical Engineering. 2014;**16**:371-396. DOI: 10.1146/annurev-bioeng-121813-120704

[45] Kuntaegowdanahalli SS, Bhagat AAS, Kumar G, Papautsky I, Quake SR, Scrivens WA, Kim KS. Inertial microfluidics for continuous particle separation in spiral microchannels. Lab on a Chip. 2009;**9**:2973. DOI: 10.1039/b908271a

[46] Datta A, Rakesh V. An Introduction to Modeling of Transport Processes: Applications to Biomedical Systems. Cambridge, UK: Cambridge University Press; 2010

[47] Madelung O. Numerical data and functional relationships in science and technology. Landolt Bornstein, New Series, Group III. 1982;**22**:117

[48] Lee BY, Bacon KM, Bottazzi ME, Hotez PJ. Global economic burden of Chagas disease: A computational simulation model. The Lancet Infectious Diseases. 2013;**13**:342-348

[49] Ramsey JM, Elizondo-Cano M, Sanchez-González G, Peña-Nieves A, Figueroa-Lara A. Opportunity cost for early treatment of Chagas disease in Mexico. PLoS Neglected Tropical Diseases. 2014;**8**:e2776

Chapter 9

Dielectrophoresis-Assisted Pathogen Detection on Vertically Aligned Carbon Nanofibers Arrays in a Microfluidic Device

Foram Ranjeet Madiyar, Omer Farooq and Jun Li

Additional information is available at the end of the chapter

http://dx.doi.org/10.5772/intechopen.72626

Abstract

In this chapter, we focus on utilizing nanoelectrode arrays fabricated with vertically carbon nanofibers (VACNFs) for pathogen detection based on a "point-and-lid" dielectrophoretic device in a microfluidic channel. This technique is utilized to concentrate particles from the bulk flow and detect pathogens based on fluorescence, surface-enhanced Raman spectroscopy (SERS) and impedance measurements. The advantage of VACNFs is their ultrasmall diameter (~100 nm) and the high aspect ratio (50:1). When coupled with a macroscopic indium tin oxide (ITO) electrode, it produces a large electric field gradient ($\nabla E^2 = \sim 10^{19} - 10^{20}\ V^2\ m^{-3}$) which is harnessed for pathogen detection based on dielectrophoresis. Several noninfectious pathogens including bacteria *Escherichia coli* DHα5, inactivated vaccinia virus (species: *Copenhagen strain*, *VC-2*), and *Bacteriophage* T4r were utilized as model species to study the size effect and kinetics of dielectrophoretic capture in this study. The comparable size of the nanoelectrode produced strong interaction with virus particles, generating striking lightning capture patterns and high detection sensitivity. The dielectrophoretic capture at the nanoelectrode arrays is successfully integrated with a portable Raman probe as a microfluidic chip for ultrasensitive detection of bacteria *E. coli* DHα5 using SERS-tagged gold nanoparticles co-functionalized with specific antibodies.

Keywords: dielectrophoresis, pathogen detection, vertically aligned carbon nanofibers (VACNFs), nanoelectrode array (NEA), indium tin oxide (ITO), microfluidic device, electroporation, plaque-forming units (pfu), bacteria *E. coli* Dhα5, *Bacteriophage* T4r, vaccinia virus, iron-oxide gold nanoovals (IO-Au NOVs), surface-enhanced Raman spectroscopy (SERS), impedance, fluorescence

1. Introduction

The need for rapid and reliable pathogen monitoring and detection is imperative in the food industry, biodefense, drug discovery, animal healthcare, clinical diagnosis, water, and environmental quality control. Among these, the food industry is the area where most attention has been focused on due to public health implications. In 2015, the World Health Organization (WHO) estimated that 77 million people every year fall victim to contaminated food and about 9000 deaths annually. The WHO has identified 31 agents of foodborne diseases including bacteria, virus, parasites, toxins, and chemicals, among which 95% are caused by *Norovirus*, *Campylobacter*, *Escherichia coli*, and non-typhoidal *Salmonella* [1]. In recent years, there have been considerable efforts to develop devices and methods for capturing pathogens in fluids such as blood, food matrices, soil, bodily fluids, and water for rapid detection.

The conventional pathogen identification methods are standard microbiological techniques and involve necessary steps such as preenrichment, selective enrichment, biochemical screening, and serological confirmation [2]. The traditional methods take up to 72 h to obtain confirmed results which are based on the morphological evaluation, culture growth in various media under various conditions, and enumerating colonies of the bacteria [3, 4]. However, the development of polymerase chain reaction (PCR)-based molecular analysis techniques [5–7], the conventional biochemical methods such as enzyme-linked immunosorbent assays (ELISAs), and blot assays have led scientists to target genes, proteins, and carbohydrate moieties instead of the whole microorganisms [8] to obtain molecular fingerprints of the pathogens. These techniques despite being highly sensitive and selective require experienced personnel, expensive equipment, reagents, and long readout time, thus making the process costly and difficult for on-site applications and causing a delay in the pathogen detection, preventing immediate medical action toward infected patients. There is a keen interest in developing new rapid point-of-care biosensing systems for early detection of pathogens with high sensitivity and specificity.

Recent developments in micro- and nanotechnology offer many technological advances in fabricating devices that incorporate nanoscale features to enhance sensitivity, reduce detection time, and enable multiplexing capability [9–12]. Most important, the properties of nanomaterials can be tailored by changing the size, shape, and composition, modifying the nanomaterial surface with appropriate functionalization, and conjugation with affinity ligands, antibodies, epitopes, and aptamers [13, 14]. Representative nanomaterials utilized for pathogen detection include metal nanoparticles [15–17], nanotubes and nanofibers [18], quantum dots [19], and magnetic nanoparticles [20]. These nanomaterials are used in conjugation with signal transduction techniques [21] such as fluorescence [22], bioluminescence [23], flow cytometry [24], colorimetry [25], electrochemistry [26–29], piezoelectrics [30], surface plasmon resonance (SPR) [31], quartz crystal microbalance [32], chemiluminescence [33], optical waveguides [34], and surface-enhanced Raman spectroscopy (SERS) [17, 25, 35–39].

In this chapter, we summarize an innovative pathogen capture and detection system based on dielectrophoresis (DEP). The device is a unique assembly of nanoelectrode arrays (NEAs) fabricated with vertically aligned carbon nanofibers (VACNFs) and a transparent macroscopic indium tin oxide (ITO) glass electrode in a "point-and-lid" geometry in which pathogens are introduced using microfluidic channels. The study of capture kinetics was accomplished using fluorescence, SERS, and impedance measurement techniques. The test pathogens utilized in this study were bacteria such as *E. coli* DHα5 (nonpathogenic) and viruses such as bacteriophage and inactivated vaccinia virus. There have been several reports on using microscale DEP devices for manipulation of mammalian cells (tens of microns) to bacterial cells (~1.0 micron) [40]. The DEP force is proportional to the volume of the target particles [41] and decreases rapidly when the particle size is reduced to only ~100 nm. Therefore it becomes essential to fabricate nanostructured DEP electrodes to capture virus particles due to their small sizes (ranging from 10s nm to 300 nm). We illustrate in this chapter the method to use VACNFs for fabricating stable nanoscale DEP devices. The capture of virus *Bacteriophage* T4r and T1 using fluorescence and impedance sensing of vaccinia virus accompanied by electroporation has been accomplished due to the high electric field focused on the tips on VACNFs. Last, we have demonstrated the specific detection of bacterial cells using SERS reporter QSY21 that is co-functionalized with polyclonal antibodies on a special type of plasmonic nanoparticles, i.e., anisotropic oval-shaped iron-oxide-gold (IO-Au) core-shell nanoparticles. This dielectrophoretic device is integrated with a portable Raman system for rapid pathogen detection in field applications. Such integrated microfluidic systems provide simultaneous concentration and identification of specific microbes in dilute samples.

2. Principles, design, and fabrication

The phenomenon of dielectrophoresis (DEP) is renowned as a particle manipulation technique based on the uneven electrical force on the opposite sides of polarized particles in an electric field with a high gradient produced by the electrodes. The larger the electric field gradient, the stronger the DEP force acts on the particle. This phenomenon was first described by Pohl in 1951 [42] and has been widely used in biological science to separate live and dead bacteria [43, 44], viruses [45–47], cells [48–52], yeast cells [53, 54], and DNA [55–57]. When we consider radius of the particle r, the permittivity of the suspending medium ε_m, the gradient of the square of the applied electric field strength ∇E^2 and the real component of the complex Clausius-Mossotti (CM) factor $Re[K(\omega)]$, the time average DEP force (F_{DEP}) acting on the spherical particles by the nonuniform electric field, and the $Re[K(\omega)]$ are provided by the following equations:

$$\langle F_{DEP} \rangle = 2\pi r^3 \varepsilon_m \mathrm{Re}[K(\omega)] \nabla E^2, \quad (1)$$

where:

$$K(\omega) = \frac{\varepsilon_p^* - \varepsilon_m^*}{\varepsilon_p^* + 2\varepsilon_m^*}, \quad \text{where} \quad \varepsilon^* = \varepsilon - j\frac{\sigma}{\omega} \quad (2)$$

The use of physical fields for the separation of cells takes advantage of the heterogeneity of physical parameters for Eq. (2), such as ε^*, representing the complex permittivity and the indices p and m referring to the particle and medium, respectively; parameter σ is the conductivity; ω is the angular frequency ($\omega = 2\pi f$) of the applied electric field; and $j = \sqrt{-1}$. The direction of the force, either toward the field gradient as in positive DEP or away from it as in negative

DEP, is given by the difference in complex permittivity conductivity between the particle of interest and the suspending media. In this study, the proper medium (280 mM mannitol solution) is chosen to give $Re[K(\omega)] > 0$ so the particles experience a positive DEP (pDEP) force, directing toward higher electric field strength, which is desirable for capture bacteria and viruses at the exposed VACNF tips by selecting a proper frequency.

In the microfluidic device, a particle experiences two forces orthogonal to each other, i.e., DEP force ($\boldsymbol{F}_{DEP}$) forcing the particles to capture on the tips and hydrodynamic force to carry the particles with the flow (i.e., Stokes drag force $\boldsymbol{F}_{Drag}$) (as shown in **Figure 1d**). $\boldsymbol{F}_{DEP}$ is proportional to the volume or cube of the radius (r^3) of the particle. $\boldsymbol{F}_{Drag}$ is directly proportional to the radius of the particle by

$$\boldsymbol{F}_{Drag} = 6\eta\pi rkv \tag{3}$$

where η is the dynamic viscosity, k is a small factor accounting for the wall effects, and v is the linear flow rate (flow velocity). Sedimentation force and Brownian force are negligible for bacteria but not for submicron particles. The advantage of nanostructured DEP devices is that the magnitude of ∇E^2 can be enhanced by orders of magnitude so even small viral particles can be captured.

3. DEP device fabrication and setup for pathogenic particles

Figure 1a is the image of the device produced in the lab at Kansas State University. The detailed procedure of device fabrication is given in reference [58]. **Figure 1a** shows that the size of the devices is comparable to a US penny and illustrates the "points-and-lid" design. **Figure 1b** shows that the NEA comprises randomly distributed VACNFs (diameter ~100–120 nm, the density of ~2×10^7 exposed CNFs/cm^2) embedded in silicon dioxide (SiO_2) matrix (tip exposed) with an average spacing of ~1–2 μ. The active area exposed on NEA is 200 × 200 μm^2, and the rest is covered with a 2-μm-thick photoresist film to shield the effect of the rest of exposed tips. The ITO glass slide containing a photolithographically fabricated 500-μm-wide microfluidic channel in an 18-μm-thick photoresist film is permanently vacuum bonded.

In the experimental setup, DEP device was placed under an upright fluorescence optical microscope (Axioskop II, Carl Zeiss) using 50 X objective lens. The microorganisms such as *Bacteriophage* T4r (labeled with SYBR green I dye) and *E. coli* DHα5 (Alexa 555) fluorescence detection filter sets were configured to an excitation wavelength of 540–552 nm and an emission wavelength of 567–647 nm (filter set 20HE, Carl Zeiss). For vaccinia virus detection, filter sets were configured to 465–505 nm excitation wavelength and an emission wavelength of 515–565 nm (filter set 17, Carl Zeiss) for 3,3′-Dioctadecyloxacarbocyanine (DiO) dye and an excitation wavelength of 620–640 nm and an emission wavelength of 640–740 nm (filter set 60, Carl Zeiss) for propidium iodide (PI) dye. The videos were recorded using Axio Cam MRm digital camera to record fluorescence videos at varying exposure times depending on the pathogen species using multidimensional acquisition mode in the Axio-vision 4.7.1 release software (Carl Zeiss MicroImaging, Inc.). To prevent biofouling, the microfluidic channel was

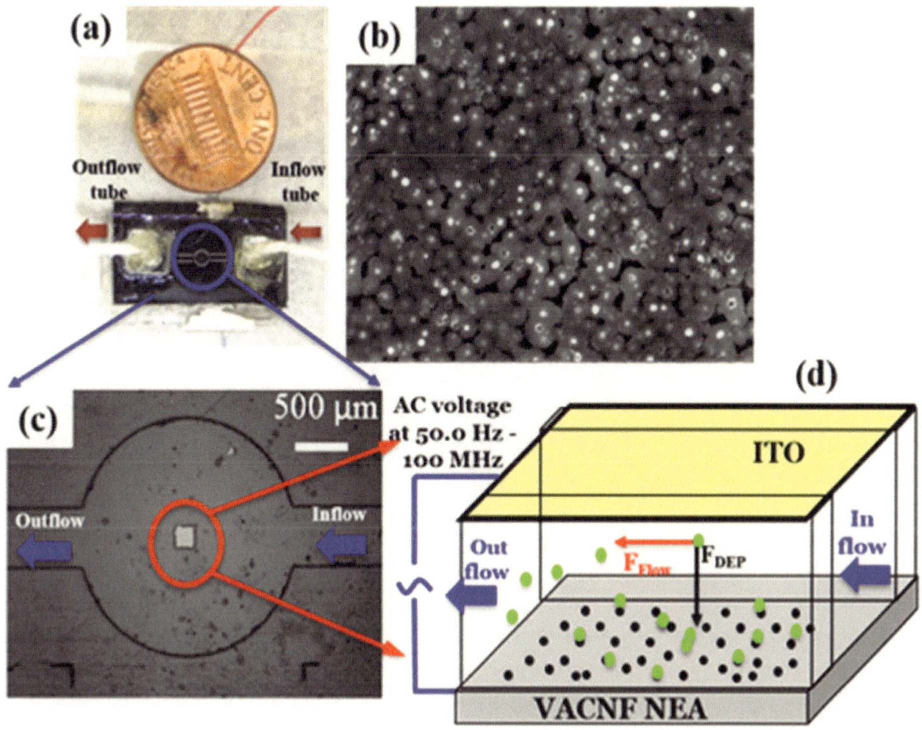

Figure 1. The embedded vertically aligned carbon nanofiber (VACNF) and indium tin oxide (ITO) DEP devices. (a) An example microfluidic device fabricated using indium tin oxide-coated glass and a nanoelectrode array chip covered exposing a 200 × 200 µm² area, glass fluidic connectors, and microbore tubes. (b) Scanning electron microscope (SEM) image of exposed tips (bright spots) of the VACNFs embedded in a silicon oxide layer. (c) A low-magnification optical microscope image showing the 200 × 200 µm² capture area. (d) Schematic diagram of microbial particles in the active nano-DEP area, which is subjected to the hydrodynamic drag force (F_{Drag}) along the flow direction and the dielectrophoretic force (F_{DEP}) perpendicular to the NEA surface. (Reprinted with permission from Madiyar et al. [59]; Foram Ranjeet et al. [61]).

injected with 1.0 mL bovine serum albumin (BSA) solution (2.0 gm in 100 mL of water) at a flow rate of 0.2 µl/min before performing DEP experiments. The channel was then rinsed with 2.0 mL DI water at a flow rate of 5.0 µl/min. **Figure 1c** shows the microfluidic design in which the particles entered from the narrow straight channel (500 µm in width) are distributed into the larger circular microchamber (2.0 mm in diameter), and only a fraction of the particles are passed over 200 × 200 µm active NEA area. Using this setup, bacteria *E. coli* DHα5 counting was accomplished using Axio software. In contrast, when detecting viral particles, it became difficult to distinguish the single viral particles. Hence for virus capture experiments, the integrated fluorescence intensity over the 200 × 200 µm active NEA area was recorded. For this, the initial fluorescence background (F_0) immediately before the V_{pp} was applied was subtracted from the final fluorescence signal (F_F) at the end of the capture period, giving the fluorescence intensity increase (ΔF) to represent the quantity of captured virus. The counts of isolated bright spots of single viral particles were observed at much lower virus concentration and were used in some later experiments to quantify the capture efficiency during the kinetic DEP process [59].

4. Detection of viruses: Bacteriophages and vaccinia virus using fluorescence and impedance method

4.1. DEP capture and kinetics of *Bacteriophage* T4r using fluorescence method

Bacteriophage T4r (Carolina Biological Supply Company, Burlington, NC) and T1 (ATCC, Manassas, VA) were utilized as probes to show the capability of the capture of nano-sized particles on VACNF tips. The culture of the *Bacteriophage* T4r using *E. coli B* is described in the previous report [59]. To label the virus particles, the virus solution was filtered through 0.2 μm filter (Fisher, PA) to remove the live bacteria or bacterial debris. To label the viruses, a 500 X working solution of SYBR® Green I Nucleic Acid Gel Stain (Lonza, Rockland, ME) in TE buffer (100 mM Tris [pH 7.6], 50 mM EDTA) was used, and the washing steps were accomplished using Amicon® Ultra 0.5 centrifugal filter devices (Millipore, Billerica, MA). The counting of viruses was carried out using double-layer agar technique after filtering the virus solution. The final wash was accomplished using 280 mM mannitol solution to enhance the efficiency of pDEP capture by manipulating the CM factor of viruses. The final concentration of the phages was ~5×10^9 pfu/mL except in some concentration-dependent experiments [59].

Figure 2 depicts the increase in an integrated fluorescence intensity to a saturation level in less than 10.0 s as a 10 V_{pp} AC bias when applied to the DEP device while flowing 5×10^9 pfu/mL *Bacteriophage* T4r solution through the channel at the flow velocity varying from 0.085 to 3.06 mm/s while changing the frequency from 100 Hz to 1.0 MHz. **Figure 2a** shows the maximum capture frequency to be 10 kHz. **Figure 2b**, a plot of the integrated fluorescence intensity of captured viruses vs. the flow velocity, showed a maximum at 0.73 mm/s. At $v \leq 0.73$ mm/s, isolated bright spots were seen (**Figure 2c**). At $v \geq 0.73$ mm/s, viruses depicted fractal-like lightening patterns (**Figure 2d**). These patterns are called *Lichtenberg figures*, which occur when the high electric field is produced at a sharp electrode surrounded by a relatively high concentration of polarizable particles. Previously such pattern was observed using *E. coli* cells between interdigitated microelectrodes called as "pearl-chain-like" Suehiro et al. [59, 62] This is first time that such pattern was observed with virus particles with the electric field produced at the nanoelectrode tips [59].

The DEP kinetics dramatically changed with concentration (**Figure 2e**) when two diluted concentrations, i.e., 5.5×10^8 and 2.5×10^7 pfu/ml, were used. The viruses could be individually counted (40 out of 67 particles) at an extremely low concentration of *Bacteriophage* T1 (8.7×10^4 pfu/mL) when passed through the nano-DEP device as the capture was limited by mass transport giving a capture efficiency ~60% [59].

4.2. DEP capture and electroporation of vaccinia virus coupled with real-time impedance detection

Electrochemical sensors based on impedimetric measurements have emerged as an attractive low-cost portable technique for the rapid detection of pathogenic microbes and other microorganisms. In this capture study, vaccinia virus was a probe to study the impedance kinetics and electroporation of the viruses due to high electrical field gradient generated at VACNFs tips.

http://dx.doi.org/10.5772/intechopen.72626

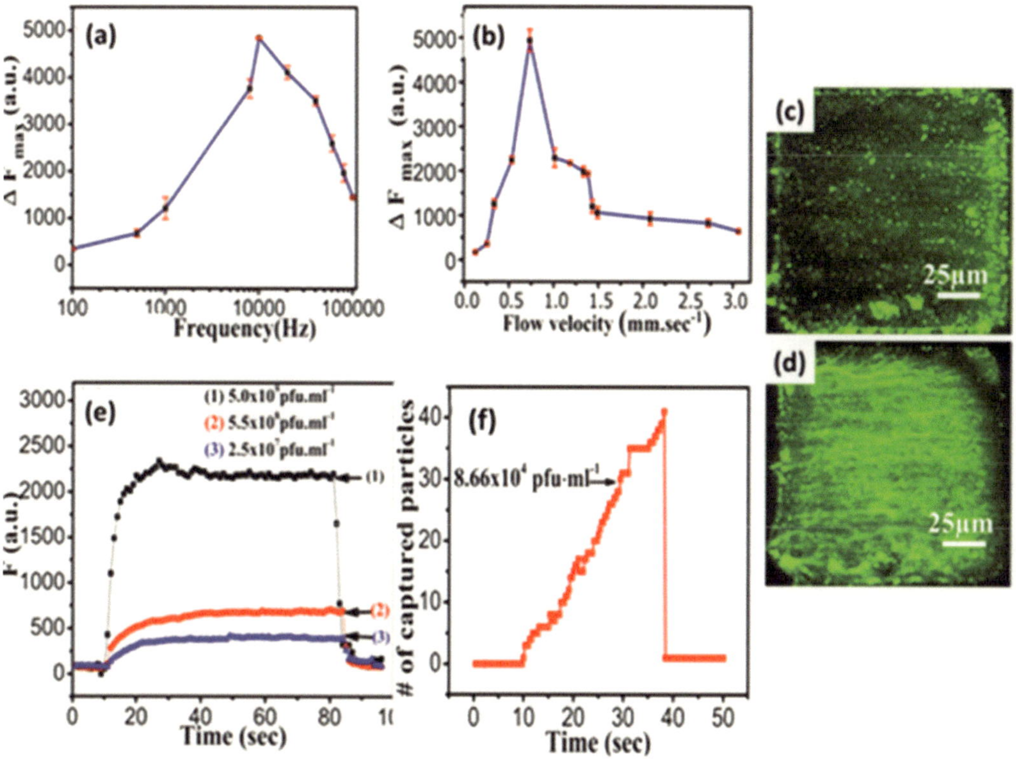

Figure 2. DEP capture of virus particles (*Bacteriophage* T4r) on VACNF in a microfluidic device. (a) The frequency dependence of DEP capture of 5×10^9 pfu/m *Bacteriophage* T4r at a flow velocity of 0.73 mm/s with the AC bias fixed at 10 V_{pp}. The optimum capture was obtained with ~10 kHz AC voltage by measuring integrated fluorescence intensity (ΔF_{max}). (b) The flow rate-dependent DEP capture peaked at 0.73 mm/s. (c) and (d) are the representative snapshots from the videos just before the AC voltage was turned off at a flow velocity of 0.33 and 0.73 mm/s, respectively. (e) The kinetic DEP capture curves at the standard concentration (5×10^9 pfu/ml) and two diluted concentrations (5.5×10^8 and 2.5×10^7 pfu/ml). (f) A kinetic profile of the *Bacteriophage* T1 capture at a low concentration at the flow velocity of 0.87 mm/s showing capture efficiency of 60%. (Reprinted with permission from Madiyar et al. [59]).

The details of the growth and enumeration by conventional techniques are given in a previous report [60]. Briefly, in-house stocks of vaccinia virus (*Copenhagen strain*, VC-2) were amplified by standard virus growth techniques of infecting HeLa cells knocked-down for an antiviral protein kinase, PKR (HeLa PKR-KD), followed by sucrose gradient centrifuge to achieve an optimal yield of 2.0×10^8 pfu/mL quantified via plaque assay. To move the viruses out of biosafety level 2 (BSL-2) containment, a UV-inactivation process was carried out by placing them 3–8 cm directly below a UV lamp (234 nm), and the plate was manually rocked for 10 min. The vaccinia viruses were dually labeled with 50 μM DiO lipophilic dye (Life Technologies, Carlsbad, CA) that stains the outer envelope of the virus by incubating the viruses at 37°C for 2 h. The washing of vaccinia virus was performed similarly as the bacteriophage virus. The concentration of the virus for the experiment was ~3×10^6 pfu/mL (except specified experiments). The nucleic acid (DNA) of the viruses was labeled with 50 μl 20.0 μM of propidium iodide (PI) aqueous solution. All the solutions were filtered with 0.2 μm filter and sterilized at 121°C for 20 min [61].

The details of the fluorescence experiment setup and videos are described in Section 3.0. The frequency (*f*), flow velocity (v), and concentration kinetic response of vaccinia virus cells were monitored using a fluorescence microscope. The experiments lasted for 85 s, during which no voltage (V_{off}) was applied in the first ~16 s, fixed AC voltage at different frequencies was applied (V_{on}) for ~54 s, and no voltage was applied (V_{off}) in the last ~15 s.

The integrated fluorescence intensity was measured at the end of capture period (54.0 s) and compared to the percentage change of the final impedance signal (Z_F) relative to the initial impedance signal (Z_o), i.e., $\%(Z_F - Z_o)/Z_o$. The optimum flow velocity for vaccinia virus was 0.40 mm/s at the frequency of 50.0 Hz and the voltage of 8.0 V_{pp} as shown in **Figure 3a**. The optical image is shown in **Figure 3c** which indicates the *Lichtenberg figures* (similar to *Bacteriophage* T4r) at the frequency of 50.0 Hz, but no capture was observed at 500 kHz (**Figure 3e**). Due to high biofouling of the vaccinia virus at the frequency 50.0 Hz, the frequency of 1.0 kHz (**Figure 3d**)

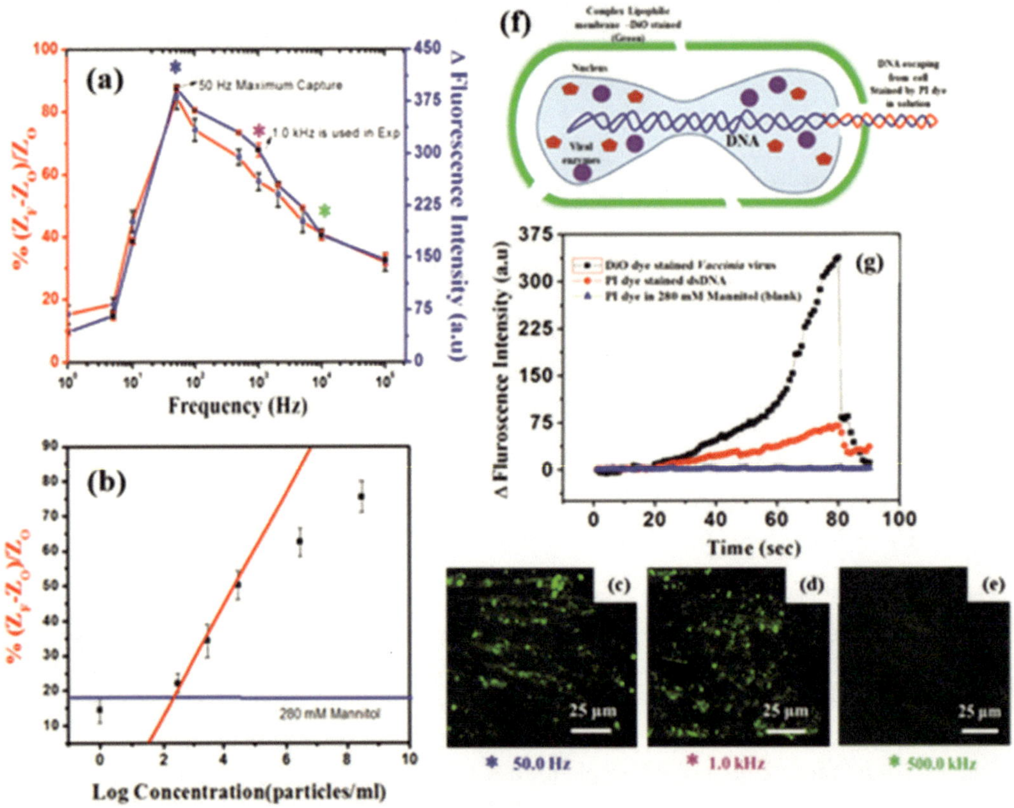

Figure 3. Assessing DEP capture and electroporation of vaccinia virus particles. (a) The frequency dependence of DEP capture ranging from 10.0 Hz to 1.0 MHz at fixed flow velocity (0.40 mm/s) and fixed AC voltage (8.0 V_{PP}) peaking at 50.0 Hz. (b) The calibration curve of the percentage change in the impedance after 54 s DEP versus the logarithm of the virus concentration ranging from 3.0×10^2 to 3.0×10^6 pfu/ml. (c–e) Snapshots from the fluorescence video after 54 s of DEP capture of vaccinia virus at a fixed flow velocity of 0.401 mm/s at various AC frequency of (c) **50.0 Hz,** (d) **1.0 kHz,** and (e) **10 kHz.** (f) The schematic image of electroporation of vaccinia virus particles in which the vaccinia viruses are dually stained using DiO dye for outer lipophilic membrane (green) and propidium iodide (red) for dsDNA (inside or extracted out of the vaccinia virus). (g) The increase in the fluorescence signal of the DiO and PI dye during DEP capture of vaccinia virus and the PI dye mixed in 280 mM mannitol solution as the control experiment. (Reprinted with permission from Madiyar et al. [69]).

was used as the capture frequency (except few experiments). A concentration ~3×10^3 to 3×10^6 pfu/mL was employed to demonstrate concentration-dependent study with the real-time potential and measures the limit of detection of the impedance method. For this experiment, the frequency is fixed at 1.0 kHz, and the 0.5 V_{PP} AC voltage is applied for 16 s to obtain the background impedance value. The AC voltage is then increased to 8.0 V_{PP} for 54 s to capture the virus (indicated by the increase in the impedance signal). The AC voltage is finally reduced back to 0.5 V_{PP}, indicating the release of the virus particles from the VACNF tips. The control experiment is done under the same conditions using blank 280 mM mannitol solution. The calibration curve (**Figure 3b**) shows that the logarithm of virus concentration (C) in the range from ~300 to 30,000 particles/mL is linear with percentage impedance change collected over the 200 × 200 μm active area. Using the calibration curve equation (details in Refs. [61, 66]), the detection limit of vaccinia virus was calculated to be ~ 300 particles/mL [61].

Finally, to investigate the electroporation of lipophilic membrane due to the high electric field on tips of VACNF NEAs, PI dye was added to the mannitol solution containing 3.0×10^6 particles/mL of DiO dye-labeled vaccinia virus and observed in Neubauer chamber. The absence of the red fluorescence indicated there was no structural damage of virus due to UV inactivation [62]. For electroporation experiment in a microfluidic device, the frequency of 50.0 Hz was used. The voltage of 8.0 V_{pp} was turned on for 65 s for maximal DEP capture with the flow velocity set at 0.05 mm/s (for maximum capture and interaction of dye and DNA). **Figure 3f** shows the schematic figure of electroporation of lipophilic membrane of vaccinia virus in the presence of high electric field at the VACNF tips. It is observed that the electroporation made the membrane more permeable and the DNA is likely extracted out of the membrane to interact with PI dye in the mannitol solution which increases the PI dye fluorescence intensity. There is evidence that, after the AC voltage is turned off, some PI-intercalated ds-DNAs are physically adsorbed on the VACNF tip or the NEA chip surface [61, 63].

5. Detection of bacteria: DEP capture and identification of *E. coli* strain DHα5 by surface-enhanced Raman spectroscopy

DEP capture of bacterial cells was demonstrated with nontoxic *E. coli* strain DHα5 (18265-017, Fisher Scientific). The DEP microfluidic device with Raman setup is schematically represented in **Figure 4a**. The procedure for fluorescent labeling and attachment of the bacteria with a unique SERS nanotag consisting of nanooval (NOV)-shaped gold coating on spherical iron-oxide (IO) nanoparticles is reported in Ref. [62]. Gold is coated on the spherical IO nanoparticle cores (~23 nm diameter), forms an outer dimension of ~50 nm with NOVs which demonstrates high SERS enhancement factor due to Raman tag of QSY-21. The NOVs are made biocompatible, and surface active by adding carboxylic acid groups at the surface was accomplished by coating them with carboxyl-polyethylene glycol-thiol (HOOC-PEG-SH, MW 5000) and methoxy-polyethylene glycol-thiol (mPEG-SH, MW 5000). The details of the process are given in Ref. [63, 66]. The carboxylic acid group aids in the formation of amide covalent bonds with secondary IgG antibody conjugated with Alexa 555 making the IO-NOVs fluorescently labeled. These secondary antibodies are complementary to IgG antibody conjugated

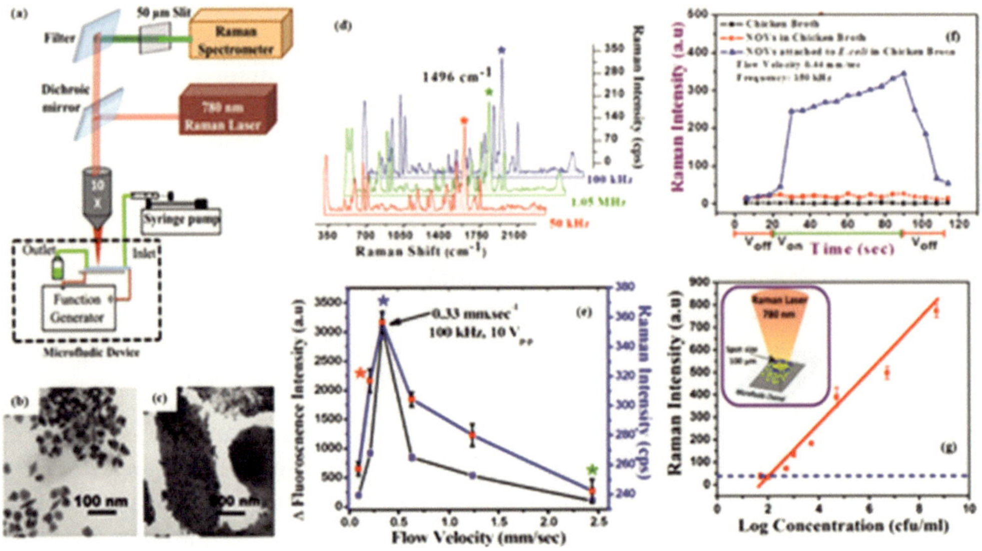

Figure 4. Capture of *E. coli* Dhα5 in NEA microfluidic channel. (a) Schematic of the microfluidic dielectrophoretic device under a Raman microscope for bacteria detection. TEM images of (b) the starting IO-Au NOVs and (c) *E. coli* DHα5 bacterial cells attached with antibody-functionalized IO-Au NOVs. (d) Assessing DEP capture of 5.3×10^5 CFU/mL *E. coli* cells with fluorescence and Raman measurements at varying frequency with the fixed voltage at 10.0 V_{pp} showing 1496 cm^{-1} is the highest peak. (e) The study of *E. coli* cells at varying flow velocity at a fixed frequency (100 kHz) and voltage (10 V_{pp}). (f) The study of DEP capture of *E. coli* cells with Raman measurements in different complex matrices such as chicken broth. The DEP capture kinetics using a chicken solution were performed at 10.0 V_{pp}, 0.44 mm/s flow velocity, and 150 kHz AC frequency. (g) The calibration curve plotted with the concentration varying from 5 CFU/mL to 1.0×10^9 CFU/mL (X-axis) and the Raman intensity after 50 s of DEP capture (Y-axis). The Raman intensity measurements with a ProRaman L portable Raman system (Enwave Optronics) with laser focal spot of 100 µm diameter aligned with active DEP area (inset). (Reprinted with permission from Madiyar [66]).

with FITC primary antibody which was attached to bacteria *E. coli* DHα5. The detailed procedure is given in reference [63, 64]. **Figure 4b** and **c** show TEM images of IO-Au SERS NOVs and those bound to *E. coli*. The typical Raman spectrum of QSY21 has prominent bands at 1333, 1584, and 1641 cm^{-1} which are from the xanthene ring stretching vibrations of the molecule [65]. The intensity of QSY21 marker at the Raman shift of 1496 cm^{-1} is visually separated from the carbon nanofiber signals at 1350 cm^{-1} (D-band) and 1600 cm^{-1} (G-band), respectively [66]. The most reliable characteristic band is seen at 1496 cm^{-1} as seen in **Figure 4d** was used to quantify the SERS signal.

To demonstrate the potential of this method, both confocal (DXR, Thermo Fisher Scientific) and portable systems (ProRaman L, Enwave Optronics. Inc) were used. The similar studies were carried out with the two spectrophotometers at varied flow velocity and frequency. **Figure 4d** shows the full Raman spectrum of QSY21 at different AC frequencies during the capture of bacteria. The highest peak in the full spectra, 1496 cm^{-1}, was used in the further calculation, and the higher capture was seen at the AC frequency of 100.0 kHz. The results between these two Raman systems were very consistent from their fluorescence and Raman intensity plots, with the maximum flow velocity at 0.4 mm/s (0.55 µl/s) (**Figure 4e**).

To analyze the capture in complex samples, one of the representative data is shown in **Figure 4f**, i.e., the capture of *E. coli* in the chicken broth samples. Other samples such as Mott's apple juice and soil samples were also tested, and details are given in Ref. [62]. Complex matrix solution was centrifuged at 14,000 rpm for 10 min, and the supernatant was collected. Complex matrices present different challenges due to inorganic and organic substance interactions, making it difficult to isolate the target to be tested. A concentration of 5×10^5 cells/mL *E. coli* DHα5 was added into the solution of processed chicken broth [66]. The conductivity of bacteria in distilled water (pH 6.8) was 1.22×10^{-4} S/m. The conductivity of commercial chicken broth after sample processing and adding *E. coli* DHα5 cells resulted in conductivity of 1.7×10^{-3} S/m. Due to the change in solution (chicken broth) conductivity, the bacteria in complex matrices have a high Raman intensity at the frequency of 150.0 kHz and for soil solution 100.0 kHz.

Figure 4g summarizes the SERS intensity of the captured NOV-labeled *E. coli* using the portable Raman setup, while the *E. coli* concentration was varied from ~10 to 1×10^9 cells/mL. The probe diameter at the focal point in the portable Raman system is about 100 μm (inset in **Figure 4g**), much larger than the 3.1 μm size in the confocal Raman microscope allowing signals to be collected from many more bacteria, and yields better statistics of the detection limit measurement [66]. The calibration curve for the detection limit measure is shown in **Figure 4g**. The Raman intensity was a linear function of the logarithm of bacteria concentration when the concentration C is above ~100 cells/mL [66]:

$$(\mathrm{RI})_{\mathrm{portable}} = 108.8 \times \log C - 214.7 \quad (4)$$

where RI was the Raman intensity increase after 50 s of DEP capture. For bacteria concentrations below the critical value, C_0 = ~100 cells/mL. There was no measurable signal detected above the background, i.e., $(RI)_{blank}$ = ~36 a.u. Due to the slow mass transport of bacteria to the active area, no captured bacterial cells were detected during the applied DEP period. However, at the time when the high concentration of the bacteria was passed, the Raman intensity increased. The detection limit $\log C_{dl}$ was determined using calibration curve:

$$\log C_{dl} = \log C_0 + 3\, s_{blank}/m, \quad (5)$$

where s_{blank} (~11.7) is the standard deviation of the Raman signal for bacteria concentration below C_0 and $m = 108.8$ is the slope of the calibration curve. The concentration detection limit was determined to be ~210 cells/mL.

6. Discussion and conclusion

The physical phenomenon of DEP was observed on the tips of VACNF NEAs in microfluidic channel design due to high electric field gradient generated by the "point-and-lid" geometry acted as an effective and reversible electronic manipulation technique to rapidly (less than 60 s) concentrate bacteria and viruses into a micro-area from the solution flow. The nanoscale size of the VACNF tips has two critical features: the extremely high electrical field strength at the tip ($E = \sim 10^7$ V m^{-1}) and the large electric field gradient at the tips of nanoelectrode (giving $\nabla E^2 = 10^{19} - 10^{20}$ V^2 m^{-3}) against ITO electrode. The polarizable pathogenic particles in the microfluidic device encounter hydrodynamic drag force along the flow direction and orthogonal (vertical) DEP forces due to the high electric field gradient. Once the pathogens are close to the VACNF tip, the lateral DEP force becomes larger than the hydrodynamic drag force, and the pathogens are captured at the nanoelectrode tip.

According to Eq. (1), the force of DEP highly depends on the volume of the particles (r^3) and the optimal frequency for capture bacteria, *E. coli*, *Bacteriophage* T4r, and vaccinia virus at the NEA tips was found to be 100 kHz, 10.0 kHz, and 50 Hz, respectively. This variation is due to the differences in size, structure, and molecular composition. *Bacteriophage* T4r virus has ~ 80–100 nm icosahedral-shaped protein capsid encapsulating ds-DNAs [67]. Vaccinia virus particles are larger spheres with dimensions of 360 × 270 × 250 nm, which consist of the lipophilic membranes encapsulating ds-DNAs [68]. Bacteria *E. coli* DHα5 is ~1 micron with an elongated shape and more complex internal structures [69, 70].

The second drastic contrast in the capture of viruses is the formation of *Lichtenburg figures* which was absent during capture of the bacteria. This is due to the spatial distribution of the electrical field strength at the nanoelectrode tip. *Bacteriophage* T4r and vaccinia virus are similar in size and are comparable to the diameter of VACNFs, causing the viruses to be polarized to a large extent. The captured virus acts as an extended tip attracting more viruses toward it. For bacteria, the more significant size (~1 μ) and higher internal conductivity may have screened the high electric field at the nanoelectrode tip and reduced the electrical interaction with additional cells [58, 59, 64, 70].

The device successfully captured single virus particles observed at isolated spots in the 200 × 200 μm^2 active NEA surface at an extremely dilute concentration (8.9 × 10^4 pfu/ml) in which facilitated studying the impedance kinetics of real-time DEP capture of vaccinia viral particles, yielding a detection limit of 300 particles/ml. VACNF tips have been found to cause electroporation of the lipophilic membrane of the vaccinia virus due to the large electric field produced on the tips. This electroporation phenomenon has allowed extracting the internal nucleic acid contents to the solution.

Finally, highly sensitive detection of *E. coli* bacteria using the SERS nanotag based on QSY21 on IO-Au NOVs proved to be highly sensitive. This was accomplished using two complementary antibodies, in which the secondary antibody was bonded to nanoovals and other to the bacteria. The attachment of the nanoovals significantly enhanced Raman signals and aided in specific recognition to *E. coli* DHα5 cell. The detection and kinetics of capture were studied using both a confocal Raman microscope and a portable Raman system, and the limit of detection of 210 CFU/mL was calculated by calibration curve using the portable Raman system.

All these studies revealed the exciting interplay between the highly focused electric fields at the nanoelectrode with bioparticles of comparable sizes. The device was successfully integrated with fluorescence, surface-enhanced Raman spectroscopy and electrochemical impedance sensing. All these results are very encouraging and can be further improved by optimizing the DEP design. The combined functions of DEP in concentration, detection, and electroporation make such nano-DEP devices useful to extract intracellular materials, such as DNA or proteins without a lytic agent. It can act as an on-chip portable sample preparation module for potentially capturing pathogenic particles at concentrations approaching 1–10 particles/mL and for future downstream processing and testing of microbial samples.

Author details

Foram Ranjeet Madiyar[1,2]*, Omer Farooq[2] and Jun Li[1]

*Address all correspondence to: madiyarf@erau.edu

1 Department of Chemistry, Kansas State University, Manhattan, KS, United States

2 Department of Physical Sciences, Embry Riddle Aeronautical University, Daytona Beach, FL, United States

References

[1] WHO news release World Health Organization. 2015

[2] Law JW-F, Ab Mutalib N-S, Chan K-G, Lee L-H. Frontiers in Microbiology. 2014;**5**:770

[3] Ivnitski D, Abdel-Hamid I, Atanasov P, Wilkins E. Biosensors and Bioelectronics. 1999; **14**:599-624

[4] Lazcka O, Campo FJD, Muñoz FX. Biosensors & Bioelectronics. 2007;**22**

[5] Espy MJ, Uhl JR, Sloan LM, Buckwalter SP, Jones MF, Vetter EA, Yao JD, Wengenack NL, Rosenblatt JE, Cockerill FR, Smith TF., Clinical Microbiology Reviews. 2006;**19**:165-256

[6] Mackay IM. Clinical Microbiology and Infection. 2004;**10**:190-212

[7] Fung DYC. Food Reviews International. 1994;**10**:357-375

[8] Ahmed A, Rushworth JV, Hirst NA, Millner PA. Clinical Microbiology Reviews. 2014; **27**:631-646

[9] Mairhofer J, Roppert K, Ertl P. Sensors. 2009;**9**:4804

[10] Heo J, Hua SZ. Sensors. 2009;**9**:4483

[11] Khoshmanesh K, Nahavandi S, Baratchi S, Mitchell A, Kalantar-zadeh K. Microfluidics and Nanofluidics. 2011;**26**

[12] Leonard P, Hearty S, Brennan J, Dunne L, Quinn J, Chakraborty T, O'Kennedy R. Enzyme and Microbial Technology. 2003;**32**

[13] Byrne B, Stack E, Gilmartin N, O'Kennedy R. Sensors. 2009;**9**:4407

[14] Sharma S, Byrne H, O'Kennedy RJ, Essays in Biochemistry. 2016;**60**:9-18

[15] Tu S-I, Reed S, Gehring A, He Y, Paoli G. Sensors. 2009;**9**:717

[16] Sun H, Choy TS, Zhu DR, Yam WC, Fung YS. Biosensors & Bioelectronics. 2009;**24**

[17] Wang C, Madiyar F, Yu C, Li J. Journal of Biological Engineering. 2017;**11**:9

[18] Thuy NT, Tam PD, Tuan MA, Le A-T, Tam LT, Van Thu V, Van Hieu N, Chien ND. Current Applied Physics. 2012;**12**:1553-1560

[19] Liandris E, Gazouli M, Andreadou M, Sechi LA, Rosu V, Ikonomopoulos J. PLoS One. 2011; **6**:e20026

[20] Fauss EK, MacCuspie RI, Oyanedel-Craver V, Smith JA, Swami NS. Colloids and Surfaces B: Biointerfaces. 2014;**113**:77-84

[21] Sethi RS. Biosensors and Bioelectronics. 1994;**9**:243-264

[22] Lu Z, Zhang J, Xu L, Li Y, Chen S, Ye Z, Wang J. Sensors (Basel, Switzerland). 2017;**17**:442

[23] Baker JM, Griffiths MW, Collins-Thompson DL. Journal of Food Protection. 1992;**55**:62-70

[24] Rajwa B, Dundar MM, Akova F, Bettasso A, Patsekin V, Hirleman ED, Bhunia AK, Robinson JP. Cytometry. Part A: The journal of the International Society for Analytical Cytology. 2010;**77**:1103-1112

[25] Vidic J, Manzano M, Chang C-M, Jaffrezic-Renault N. Veterinary Research. 2017;**48**:11

[26] Pedrero M, Campuzano S, Pingarrón J. Sensors. 2009;**9**:5503

[27] DeSilva MS, Zhang Y, Hesketh PJ, Maclay GJ, Gendel SM, Stetter JR. Biosensors and Bioelectronics. 1995;**10**:675-682

[28] Ghindilis AL, Atanasov P, Wilkins M, Wilkins E. Biosensors and Bioelectronics. 1998;**13**: 113-131

[29] Ivnitski D, Wolf T, Solomon B, Fleminger G, Rishpon J. Bioelectrochemistry and Bioenergetics. 1998;**45**:27-32

[30] Prusak-Sochaczewski E, Luong JHT, Guilbault GG. Enzyme and Microbial Technology. 1990;**12**:173-177

[31] Liu Y, Liu Q, Chen S, Cheng F, Wang H, Peng W. 2015;**5**:12864

[32] Carter RM, Mekalanos JJ, Jacobs MB, Lubrano GJ, Guilbault GG. Journal of Immunological Methods. 1995;**187**:121-125

[33] Ramanathan S, Shi W, Rosen BP, Daunert S. Analytica Chimica Acta. 1998;**369**:189-195

[34] Mukundan H, Anderson A, Grace WK, Grace K, Hartman N, Martinez J, Swanson B. Sensors. 2009;**9**:5783

[35] Lazcka O, Campo FJD, Muñoz FX. Biosensors and Bioelectronics. 2007;**22**:1205-1217

[36] Singh R, Mukherjee MD, Sumana G, Gupta RK, Sood S, Malhotra BD. Sensors and Actuators B: Chemical. 2014;**197**:385-404

[37] Stöckel S, Kirchhoff J, Neugebauer U, Rösch P, Popp J. Journal of Raman Specroscopy. 2016;**47**

[38] Wu X, Xu C, Tripp RA, Huang Y-w, Zhao Y. Analyst. 2013;**138**

[39] Yang D, Zhou H, Haisch C, Niessner R, Ying Y. Talanta. 2016;**146**

[40] Toner M, Irimia D. Annual Review of Biomedical Engineering. 2005;**7**:77-103

[41] Wood NR, Wolsiefer AI, Cohn RW, Williams SJ. Electrophoresis. 2013;**34**:NA-NA

[42] Pohl HA. Journal of Applied Physics. 1951;**22**:869-871

[43] Lapizco-Encinas BH, Simmons BA, Cummings EB, Fintschenko Y. Analytical Chemistry. 2004;**76**:1571-1579

[44] Fernandez RE, Rohani A, Farmehini V, Swami NS. Analytica Chimica Acta. 2017;**966**:11-33

[45] Masuda T, Maruyama H, Honda A, Arai F. PLoS One. 2014;**9**:e94083

[46] Hughes MP, Morgan H, Rixon FJ, Burt JPH, Pethig R. Biochimica et Biophysica Acta (BBA) - General Subjects. 1998;**1425**:119-126

[47] Ermolina I, Milner J, Morgan H. Electrophoresis. 2006;**27**:3939-3948

[48] Gascoyne PRC, Ying H, Pethig R, Vykoukal J, Becker FF. Measurement Science and Technology. 1992;**3**:439

[49] Markx GH, Pethig R. Biotechnology and Bioengineering. 1995;**45**:337-343

[50] Becker FF, Wang XB, Huang Y, Pethig R, Vykoukal J, Gascoyne PR. Proceedings of the National Academy of Sciences. 1995;**92**:860-864

[51] Pethig R, Menachery A, Pells S, De Sousa P. Journal of Biomedicine and Biotechnology. 2010;**2010**:182581

[52] Voldman J. Annual Review of Biomedical Engineering. 2006;**8**:425-454

[53] Huang Y, Holzel R, Pethig R, Xiao BW. Physics in Medicine & Biology. 1992;**37**:1499

[54] Markx GH, Talary MS, Pethig R. Journal of Biotechnology. 1994;**32**:29-37

[55] Pethig R. Biomicrofluidics. 2010;**4**:022811

[56] Gascoyne PRC, Vykoukal J. Electrophoresis. 2002;**23**:1973-1983

[57] Asbury CL, Diercks AH, van den Engh G. Electrophoresis. 2002;**23**:2658-2666

[58] Syed LU, Liu J, Price A, Li Y-f, Culbertson C, Li J. Electrophoresis. 2011;**32**:2358-2365

[59] Madiyar FR, Syed LU, Culbertson CT, Li J. Electrophoresis. 2013;**34**:1123-1130

[60] In: Jones TB. ed, Electromechanics of Particles. Cambridge: Cambridge University Press; 1995. pp. 139-180

[61] Madiyar FR, Syed LU, Arumugam P, Li J. Advances in applied nanotechnology for agriculture. American Chemical Society. 2013:109-124

[62] Junya S, Ryuichi Y, Ryo H, Masanori H. Journal of Physics D: Applied Physics. 1999; **32**:2814

[63] Bhana S, Rai BK, Mishra SR, Wang Y, Huang X. Nanoscale. 2012;**4**:4939-4942

[64] Arumugam PU, Chen H, Cassell AM, Li J. The Journal of Physical Chemistry A. 2007; **111**:12772-12777

[65] Huang X, Bhana S. Google Patents; 2015

[66] Madiyar FR, Bhana S, Swisher LZ, Culbertson CT, Huang X, Li J. Nanoscale. 2015;**7**:3726-3736

[67] Prasad BVV, Schmid MF. Advances in Experimental Medicine and Biology. 2012;**726**:17-47

[68] Griffiths G, Wepf R, Wendt T, Locker JK, Cyrklaff M, Roos N. Journal of Virology. 2001; **75**:11034-11055

[69] Madiyar FR, Haller SL, Farooq O, Rothenburg S, Culbertson C, Li J. Electrophoresis. 2017; **38**:1515-1525

[70] Li J, Madiyar FR, Swisher L. Carbon Nanomaterials for Biomedical Applications. In: Zhang M, Naik RR, Dai L, editors. Cham: Springer International Publishing 2016. pp. 113-143

Chapter 10

Application of Electrochemical Methods in Biosensing Technologies

Karolina Dziąbowska, Elżbieta Czaczyk and
Dawid Nidzworski

Additional information is available at the end of the chapter

http://dx.doi.org/10.5772/intechopen.72175

Abstract

Introducing biochemical factor to electronic devices have created a new branch of science. Recent development in biosensing technology enabled progress in pathogens detection. Currently, wide range of biomarkers (enzymes, peptides, DNA, microorganisms, etc.) recognize various target analytes, starting from basic metabolism changes to serious infections caused by pathogens. Improved sensitivity, selectivity and response time of sensors have instantly replaced traditional techniques. Easy handling, low production costs and miniaturization have met therapeutics need. Biosensing technologies are very strong point in telemedicine in public healthcare. This chapter will focus on electrochemical techniques for pathogens detection and show trending applications in biosensing technologies.

Keywords: sensor, biosensing technology, bioelectronics, electrochemistry, impedance spectroscopy, cyclic voltammetry, immobilized electrode, nanomaterials, noble metal nanoparticles, recognition element, human pathogen, pathogens detection, virus, bacteria, DNA, markers, diseases, telemedicine, point-of-care, lab-on-chip

1. Introduction

The biosensor era have started in 1962 by invention the first glucose meter by Clark and Lyons [1] and speeded up in uncontrollable pace. Currently, it embraces fields such as bio-telemedicine, biology, environmental monitoring, drug discovery, food safety controlling and others. The term 'biosensor' stands for the electronic analytical device incorporated with biological sensing element and physiochemical transducer [2, 3]. The main biosensors success was achieved by transforming technological sophisticated machines to small handy devices.

Especially, electrochemical biosensors are in main interest. Implementation of biological factors to electronic devices have improved sensitivity, selectivity, limits of detection (LODs) and limits of quantification (LOQs). Also miniaturization, simplification and portability have made them user-friendly and available for large audience of non-specialists and patients.

2. Biosensors classification

Biosensors classification mainly relies on the receptor and transducer type and is represented in **Table 1** [2, 4, 5]. Besides the suitable measurement technique used, the biosensor have to meet the requirements, which are detection limit, linear response range, response time, sensitivity and selectivity, stability and reproducibility. New types of biosensors are being developed, transducer hybrids, like photoelectrochemical [6].

Great sensing development can be observed in electrochemical field. Initially detected analytes were basic chemical compounds like glucose, urea, subsequently macromolecules like proteins, whole cells, viruses, bacteria and other pathogens. Currently, it is possible to follow antigen-antibody interactions, detect tumor markers, DNA materials, etc.

BIOSENSORS			
BIORECEPTORS	TRANSDUCERS		
ENZYME	OPTICAL	ELECTROCHEMICAL	MASS-BASED
ANTIBODY			
DNA	RAMAN FTIR	IMPEDIMETRIC	PIEZOELECTRIC
CELL	SPR	AMPEROMETRIC	MAGNETOELASTIC
BIOMIMETIC	FIBER OPTIC	POTENTIOMETRIC	
	OTHER	CONDUCTOMETRIC	
		VOLTAMETRIC	

Table 1. Biosensors classification based on bioreceptor and transducer types.

3. Electrochemical detection

Electrochemical biosensors are devices containing electrochemical transducer. They provide semiquantitative or quantitative analytical information, thanks to biochemical receptor. Electrical changes due to reduction/oxidation reactions of analyte can be analyzed in different ways. In this case, measured properties are current or potential. The principle is the change of solution properties due to production/consumption of electrons that is measured relatively to always stable reference electrode. The process depends on the species activity, not on the solution concentration, because it is focused on the working electrode surface. There are also electrochemical techniques

http://dx.doi.org/10.5772/intechopen.72175

which do not use direct electron flow and do not focus on the redox reaction. For example, the changes of electrode's surface deriving from surface biofunctionalization and molecular interactions like antigen-antibody, receptor-ligand and others are analyzed. In this case, measured parameters are resistance, capacitance or impedance. The easy way of transforming a biological interaction to simple electrical signal makes it attractive for sensor industry. The strong advantage is a wide range of electrical properties which can be measured and quantified with methods like potentiometry, amperometry, voltammetry, conductometry and impedance (described below). Moreover, multiple electrode materials used as receptors and methods of their immobilization are available [7].

3.1. Electrochemical cell

The conventional electrochemical cell contains three separate electrodes: the working electrode (WE), the counter electrode (CE) and the reference electrode (RE). The WE material must be a chemically stable conductive material, such as carbon, gold, platinum and more. The redox process occurs on the surface, so can be polarized both, cathodic and anodic, depending on analyzed reaction. The electrode material strongly influences the measurement because every material has different parameters, such as potential window, capacity. The WE should have high reproducibility and S/N characteristics. The toxicity and costs are also important. The CE (auxiliary electrode) provides electron flow between WE and CE and closes the current circuit in the cell. The CE surface area must be much larger than WE, to avoid kinetic limit of the process. It can be carbon, platinum wire. The RE produces constant potential in whole cell, balances the WE reaction. Requirements are low impedance and non-polarizability. The most common RE is standard hydrogen electrode (SHE) with a zero half-cell potential or silver wire coated with silver chloride [2, 7].

Except conventional electrochemical cell with three electrodes, there are variations and miniaturized versions. Microfluidic cells concept offers easier sampling and cleaning, enhanced sensitivity and reduced interferences [8]. Obviously fewer reagents are consumed and less waste is generated. For example, the microbial fuel cell (MFC) can convert organic substrates by microbial catabolism to electrical signal [3]. On the lab-on-a-chip devices (LOC), the three electrode system is miniaturized to few centimeters square platform with multiple laboratory functions. It is possible to handle very small fluid volumes (picoliters level) [7]. Screen-printed electrodes (SPEs), three-minielectrodes are deposited or printed onto polymer substrate forming ultrasmall measuring system. They are mass produced with high reproducibility and low costs. This set allows easy modifications of WE surface [2, 9].

3.2. Electrochemical sensor: potentiometric detection

Potentiometric sensors measure the potential change at one electrode referred to another electrode. The electrical potential difference or electromotive force (EMF) is measured at zero current value [4]. For example, the potential is formed when antigen-antibody interaction occurs. The reaction is described by the Nernst equation. Concentration response is logarithmic, allowing very small changes detection [2, 7]. Zelada-Guillén et al. has first applied this technique for *Staphylococcus aureus* detection in real-time. Single-walled carbon nanotubes

(SWCNTs) were used as transducer and functionalized with anti-*S. aureus* aptamers by two approaches. In covalent functionalization, LOD was 8 × 10^2 colony-forming units (CFU)/mL. Non-covalent approach has had higher sensitivity but LOD was 10^7 CFU/mL level [10].

3.3. Electrochemical sensor: conductometric detection

Conductometric transducers measure variation of the ionic strength of a solution, which changes current flow or electrical conductivity. Despite the few advantages like low-priced thin-film applications [4], direct real-time monitoring [7], no reference electrode need and miniaturization possibilities, this technique gives less sensitive responses than others electrochemical methods [2]. Hnaiein et al. have implemented this technique for *Escherichia coli* detection. Authors have used streptavidin-functionalized magnetite nanoparticles which interact with biotinylated antibodies, anti-*E. coli*. Detection on 1 CFU/mL level causes 35 μS conductivity change [11].

3.4. Electrochemical sensor: amperometric detection

Amperometric transducers measure the direct current from redox reaction under a constant potential applied on WE. The activity of recognition element varies before and after interaction with a target molecule [4]. The product must be electroactive and undergoes a redox process [12]. The current is a rate of the electrons transferred and is proportional to the analyte concentration [2, 7]. Singh et al. have invented novel DNA-based amperometric sensor for one of the most common human pathogens—*Streptococcus pyogenes*. Gold nanoparticles were functionalized with cysteine, PAMAM and genomic single-stranded DNA (ssDNA). The amperometric response was measured after DNA hybridization, with sensitivity of 951.34 (μA/cm^2)/ng DNA and LOD with 130 fg/6 μL sample. Sensor was suitable for throat swabs and needed 30 min for pathogen identification [13].

3.5. Electrochemical sensor: voltammetric detection

Voltammetric transducers are the most comprehensive and mostly used by research groups in biosensing analysis. Sensor measures the current-potential relationship. The potential is measured in 'no-current applied' conditions [12]. The potential where the redox peaks appear is specific for the examined species and the current peak size is proportional to the species. It is possible to detect many compounds with different characteristic potentials in one measurement. Voltammetric methods can be further divided into: cyclic voltammetry (CV), differential pulse voltammetry (DPV), stripping voltammetry, AC voltammetry, polarography, linear sweep voltammetry (LSV) etc., however, the most commonly used are CV, DPV and LSV. The difference is in the way of potential application [2]. The simplest is **LSV**, where at WE, the potential applied increases linearly in time. The flowing current consists of the faradaic current (flowing the Faraday laws, means discharging of active compound) and capacitive current (produced due to double electric layer growth between the solution and electrode). Detection limits are at mg/L level. In **CV**, scanning has a triangular shape characteristic. Obtained voltammogram is a closed curve with redox peaks (two if process is reversible, one if process is irreversible). The low sensitivity makes CV inapplicable for quantitative analysis. **DPV** principle is applying periodical constant potential pulse during linear scanning. Measured is the difference between the current before and after the pulse giving one peak-graph. This technique is very sensitive with detections on 10–100 μg/L limit [2].

3.6. Electrochemical sensor: impedimetric detection

Very strongly exploited are impedimetric transducers. The method, called electrochemical impedance spectroscopy (EIS), characterizers the structure and function of electrodes, especially modified with biological material [14]. It can be further classified as Faradaic or non-Faradaic depending on the presence/absence of redox probe in the solution. The second one is more preferred in point-of-care (POC) devices due to no reagents need. During immobilization of electrode surface, the resistance and capacitance of a double-layer are changing, causing change in the impedance. Thus, the biorecognition process and label-free interactions on the sensor surface can be detected [7]. Two most popular results are expressed as Nyquist and Bode plots. EIS sensors are mainly constructed by self-assembled monolayer (SAM) or a conducting polymer base layer method [12]. Detection limits are worse comparing to potentiometric or amperometric methods. False positive results derived from the electrolytes are the main drawback. It can be overcome by blocking the non-specific binding sites of the electrode surface with, for example, BSA protein [4]. The immunoreaction between antigen and antibody directly indicates impedance changes. Nidzworski et al. have presented the universal biosensor for influenza A virus detection. The principle was attaching appropriate antibodies to gold electrode which detect viral M protein. The difference of electron-transfer resistance was observed before and after influenza virus addition and peptide-antibody interaction. Increasing concentration of peptide causes the increase of resistance. The main advantage was no need for sample pretreatment, just swab suspension in buffer solution. Sensitivity was 80–100 virions/μL [15].

4. Importance of sensing materials choice

The wide range of working electrode materials and the variety of electrode surface biofunctionalization methods [7] make the electrochemistry very strong scientific and industry branch. The choice of active material and functionalization mechanism depends on the type of molecular recognition between the receptor and target analyte. Working electrode materials enhance electroactivity and promote electron-transfer reaction, but differ in reactivity, conductivity and stability so interacts diversely with chemical or biological molecules.

Noble metal nanoparticles (NPs) due to great conductivity, biocompatibility, high surface-to-volume ratio and modification possibilities by hybridization, sol-gel, self-assembly monolayer (SAM) and others methods are very popular and available on the market [16]. Currently, nanomaterials are essential in bio-devices due to enhanced sensitivity and detection limits [17]. Well-known are AuNPs, AgNPs, PtNPs, and their alloys Au-Ag, Au-Pt, Ag-Pt [16]. For example, Liu et al. have used AuNPs combined with *Bam*HI endonuclease for Hepatitis C Virus RNA detection by DPV technique with LOD 3.1×10^{-22} M [18]. Li et al. have detected gene fragments from Hepatitis B Virus, also by DPV, but introducing AgNPs and LOD was 1×10^{-18} M level [19].

Next appreciated materials are (nano-)carbon components, such as carbon nanotubes [20] or carbon nanowires with high stability, great mechanical strength and good conductivity, glassy carbon materials or graphene-based sensors [21, 22]. Bhardwaj et al. have fabricated cheap paper-based sensor for detection of foodborne pathogens: *E. coli*, *B. subtilis* and *S. epidermidis*. Authors have used single-walled carbon nanotubes (SWCNTs) conjugated with corresponding antibodies (Ab). Covalent attachment of Ab-SWCNTs has increased the stability of a sensor. Measurement technique was DPV. This fast, label-free method had LOD on 13 CFU/mL level with linear concentration range from 10 to 10^7 CFU/mL [23]. Gong et al. have proposed impedimetric DNA biosensor for HIV-1 gene determination. Glassy carbon electrode was modified with graphene-Nafion composite and ssDNA. The decrease in the resistance was proportional to gene concentration in a range from 1.0×10^{-13} to 1.0×10^{-10} M with LOD at 2.3×10^{-14} M [24].

Silica is willingly used due to no toxicity, biocompatibility, significant electronic, optical and mechanical properties [17, 25]. Nguyen et al. have used magnetic silica nanotubes (MSNTs) for label-free *Salmonella typhimurium* detection. A positively charged surface of silica attracted bacteria adsorption. This complex interacted with antibody-immobilized gold electrode. Impedance sensor showed linear signals for 10^3–10^7 CFU bacterial concentration. In authors opinion, MSNTs material have a better LOD and sensitivity than other nanomaterials in impedimetric immunosensors [26].

5. Technological comparison

The biosensors will be necessary to provide the consumers with sensing devices having short analysis time, low costs, satisfactory LODs and LOQs, portability possibilities, etc., as it was in the case of glucose meters and pregnancy tests. Electrochemical methods will be compared to optical, piezoelectric and others in reference to technology, detection limits, linear range and specificity.

In optic-based biosensors, single molecule detection, such as DNA, can be done [27]. This technology was later improved due to innovations like combination of biological materials. Also, mixing different optical components on one sensor enables forming multisensing device on a single chip and swift analysis. Hybrids of fluorescence and nanomaterials or biomolecules increase application possibilities and sensitivities. However, the main drawbacks are costs and strict instruments requirements [17]. Optical SPR detection is the most evaluated and calibrated technique for real-time and label-free assays [7]. Piezoelectric devices also offer real-time and label-free analysis, but stand out with the flexibility and low costs, compared to optical methods. Thus, it can be ideal for detection methods optimization [28]. However, from all biosensor types (microbial, electromagnetic, optical and electrochemical), only electrochemical are able to detect both, single or multiple, analytes with the real-time analysis and satisfying (but not the highest) sensitivity [17]. Thus, the electrochemical transducers seem to be the most beneficial. They are widely used in POC devices which are on-site diagnostic tests accessible to the physicians and patients, thanks to user-friendly handling and portability [29]. Another positive aspects are sensitivity, specificity with real-time analysis. Cost values are fluctuating, however they are not the highest (comparing to optical devices) and available for many laboratory industries. Currently, the electrochemical instruments are being miniaturized to hand-size. Application does not require laboratory conditions; simple instrumentation enables analysis in physician's offices or patient's houses. They are the smallest from all the sensors and with the strongest future perspectives [2, 17]. Biosensors industry offers hybrid-methods, such as photoelectrochemistry. The principle is to activate the species on electrode surface by the light, and received photocurrent is detected. The assay has advantages deriving from both methods. High sensitivity is gained from separated excitation and detection sources. Comparing to whole-optical methods such as fluorescence, exchanging detection to electrochemical lowers the costs and simplifies the instrumentation. Moreover, implementation of photoelectrochemical active nanomaterials can be very beneficial for hybrid assays [7].

6. Non-invasive, wearable biosensors

In everyday life, the superior analysis is with so-called 'non-invasive' biosensors, where there is no interruption in patient's body, what happens in blood or serum collecting. Non-invasive specimens are saliva, sweat and tears. The basic example can be breathalyzer for blood alcohol content from a breath sample. The main promise of non-invasive techniques, such as polarimetry or impedance, is non-stop monitoring with real-time results for optimal health status maintaining and deterioration warning. These solutions can help reduce health care costs and time spent in hospitals [7]. Glucose, alcohol, illness-causing pathogen like influenza virus and others can be detected from the samples [30, 31].

Tears are rich in proteins, lipids, metabolite and electrolytes and are used for diabetes monitoring. Saliva analysis can show changes in metabolic, hormonal or even emotional human body states [2]. For example, Kim et al. have invented the wearable mouthguard sensor for uric acid detection as end product of purine metabolism in saliva specimens. Abnormalities indicate diseases like hyperuricemia, gout or Lesch-Nyhan syndrome. Enzyme-modified printed electrode shows amperometric response and is connected to the platform sending analysis results to smartphones and laptops [32]. By breath analysis, viruses causing respiratory infections can be detected [33]. Others wearable biosensors are blood pressure sensor, temperature sensor, breathing sensor for respiration monitoring or so-called 'smart socks' used to individual step characterization [34].

7. Applications

Many biosensors have found everyday appliance, not only the laboratory usage. The main goal of biodevices is to be implemented in medical field. It means detect human illnesses, thus mutations, infections at first stages, pathogens, as 'prevention is better than cure'. Pathogens including bacteria, viruses, fungi, protozoa and are one the main human death causes. They have many transmitters like human, animals and plants [35], thus unchecked can cause pandemics. Early diagnosis is one of the strongest prevention method, but still challenging due to high costs, strict sample preparation mechanisms and long-time analysis. Modern technology biosensors can overcome these drawbacks by device miniaturization or rapid data output. Nowadays detection is possible from common illnesses like virus invasions to serious tumors, due to wide range of bioreceptors and measurement techniques mentioned above. Biosensors application, except human health, is in food processing/monitoring, fermentation processes, biodefence in military and many more described in this chapter.

Biological defense sensors are sensitive for organisms posing threat, called biowarfare agents (BWAs), such as bacteria, viruses and toxins. Most used are molecular techniques recognizing BWAs markers, more preferably nucleic acid-based than antibody-based due to higher sensitivity and specificity. An example is detection of genomic DNA of HPV virus by modified surface acoustic wave (SAW) biosensor [36].

Nano-based biosensors are one of the most willingly investigated and applied due to significant properties described in Section 4. For example, nanomaterials are able to detect antibiotics residues in human body which decrease the treatment efficiency [37]. Others specific interactions were carried on porous silicon, for example, for *E. coli* detection [38]. There are also silica-modified materials, by Hg^{2+} ions [39] or Ag/graphene/silica composites [40]. Quantum dots technology can be used for tumor analysis (targeting ligands can be monoclonal antibodies and peptides) and for nano-medicine delivery [17]. Engineered NPs thrive in POC devices. AuNPs combined with magnetic MNPs can detect *mec*A gene which is a biomarker for methicillin-resistant *S. aureus* (MRSA) at concentration 10 pM of targeted DNA. Optical SPR method acts as HBV sensor using AuNPs with LOD 2 fg/mL and 17 min analysis time. Another material, cadmium tellurite QDs conjugated to silica NPs enhanced the signal of Epstein–Barr virus detection. The square wave voltammetry measurements resulted in LOD of 1 pg/mL [29]. For more examples of pathogens nanodiagnostics, view [41], from all nanomaterials, the main interest arouses the gold. Except biosensing application, it is used in drug delivery or photothermal therapy. Gold nanoparticles are the most stable, have activity to biomolecules, significant optical properties depending on environment. In colorimetric methods, it is used for foodborne, waterborne or hospital pathogens detection. The majority of these assays use SPR technique. The peak absorbance of AuNPs highly depends on their shape (nanorods, star-shaped and more) and size. By DNA targeting, it is possible to detect *Salmonella* species, *Bacillus anthracis, Chlamydia trachomatis* bacteria or HIV-1 and H1N1 influenza viruses. Another use is *Leishmania major*, a protozoan parasite, detection by gold nanorods. Gold as signal enhancer can be used as non-functionalized or functionalized with nucleic acids and proteins [35]. Simplification of the detection process is required for bringing nanoparticles to POC field. User-friendly devices can be achieved by phone-based, strip-based solutions which already exist on the market.

Except optical detection, gold is often implemented in **electrochemical** techniques.

Davies et al. have developed amperometric biosensor for *Listeria monocytogenes* in food samples. Authors have modified screen-printed carbon electrode with gold nanoparticles and specific antibodies. AuNPs have increased the reaction surface and conductivity of the material and lowering the LOD to 2 log CFU/mL in blueberry samples [42]. Yang et al. have reported a sensor for *Salmonella* spp. detection where AuNPs acted as self-assembled layer on glassy carbon electrode and increased the sensitivity and selectivity. Pathogen presence was recorded by EIS method with LOD 100 CFU/mL [43]. Gaffar and Nurmalasari have invented DNA biosensor with thiol-modified gold electrode for of *M. tuberculosis* oligonucleotide sequence detection. Complementary ssDNA were immobilized on SAM of thiol and further used for target DNA hybridization. DPV was chosen as measurement technique for guanine oxidation signal monitoring. LOD is 2.7046 μg/mL and LOQ is 9.0155 μg/mL with accuracy of 99.22% and precision of 99.86% [44].

Aptamer-based systems have recently gained big potential in bacterial pathogens recognition. This method is applicable for food and clinical probes and offers excellent sensitivity and less time than traditional methods. Aptamers are called nucleic acid analogues of antibodies and are chosen via traditional SELEX technique. Main advantages are high surface density, thus better binding properties, temperature stability, easy chemical synthesis comparing to monoclonal antibodies. Alizadeh et al. have reviewed aptasensors for microbial pathogens. Authors showed detection of Gram-positive bacteria, *S. aureus* (by tyramine signal amplification (TSA) detection method with LOD of 9 CFU/mL in milk sample), *Salmonella* spp. (by non-covalent self-assembly of SWNTs with LOD of 10^3 CFU/mL in food, clinical and environmental samples), *E. coli* (by flow cytometric method with LOD of 1.1×10^3 CFU/mL in pure culture sample), *M. tuberculosis, S. mutans*, etc. [45].

Microbial biosensors can monitor fermentation processes. For example, isolated bacteria, like *C. tropicalis, G. oxydans* can determine ethanol generated during fermentation. Others, like *L. bulgaricus* or *S. thermophilus* are used for glucose or lactose control [3]. The World Health Organization (WHO) invented a criteria for diagnostic tests development called 'ASSURED' meaning Affordable, Sensitive, Specific, User-friendly, Rapid, Equipment-free, Delivered to those in need. Sensitivity and specificity are required on 85–95% levels [46].

In **viruses**, the main goal is to detect them at very low level, at the beginning of human or animal infection, it allow the doctor for applying appropriate treatment. Currently, viruses are being detected with time consuming methods, like cell culture protocols (2–10 days) or enzyme-linked immunosorbent assay (ELISA) related to viral antigens. Clinical microbiology is limited due long-time process of isolation and detection of microorganisms [46]. Enzyme-linked immunosorbent assay (ELISA) recognizes the antibodies specified to the target antigens with optical response. There are commercially available kits willingly used in clinical laboratories. However, this technique still suffers from long time and multistep analysis, need specialized handling and does not offer satisfying sensitivities. Another technique is polymerase chain reaction (PCR) with nucleic acid amplification for concentration increase of target DNA sequence, thus offering high sensitivities to even single gene copy. Specificity depends on primers design. Interferences from non-targets cause mismatches and non-specific amplifications, but are overcome by newest techniques like real-time PCR, reverse transcription PCR [5, 35]. The sensitivities between known assays are PCR with 5–100 tissue culture infection dose at 50% endpoint ($TCID_{50}$), cell culture with 104 $TCID_{50}$ and ELISA with 105 $TCID_{50}$. For these reasons a rapid, sensitive, cheap device is pivotal [12]. Virus detection receptors are mainly antibodies, peptides, aptamers and nucleic acids. Antibodies are believed as most common, because are produced as immune response in host organism in the presence of foreign species [2]. They can bind with high affinity (K_d 10^6–10^9 M) [12]. Next are peptides, short amino acid monomers chains. They have specific binding properties to viral proteins or antibodies with high stability. Nucleic acids bind specific, complementary viral (also bacterial) RNA and DNA. Viruses can be also detected by electrochemical methods [15]. By CV and DPV techniques, HBV virus can be detected with LOD 1.94×10^{-8} M of target DNA [47]. EIS method is widely used for many pathogens detection, like influenza virus [48], dengue virus [49], HIV [50], rabies virus [51] and others. From optical methods, SPR was the key for many develops in HIV virus issue, like developing new antiviral drugs [52]. SPR has a potential to be portable rapid viral test, however miniaturization is limited. Optical fiber methods were applied for Ebola virus antibodies detection down to 1 ppm or for HCV RNA quantification with LOD at 60 pM [53].

Among all mentioned applications, especially environmental and medical need simple, fast and very sensitive devices, what is available with immobilizers like gold, carbon materials, silica and others. The discovery of electrochemical biosensors became essential in POC [54] and clinical diagnosis [55]. An early disease monitoring is pivotal in adequate treatment.

Lab-on-chip solutions have broad recent scientists' attention, especially fluidic assays due to sample transport improvement, time saving, reduced volumes and dimension of microfluidic channels, making analysis possible in one blood drop. This kind of biosensors includes electrochemical-based, optical-based, micromechanical-based transduction and others. Detection of many pathogens has been reported, like Ebstein-Barr Virus [56], human immunodeficiency virus [57], *Salmonella typhimurium* [58], H5N1 influenza [59] and more. For more examples, please see [60] .

Following the newest researches, we have described the most interesting examples. Ganguli et al. have proposed smartphone-based POC sensor for Zika, chikungunya and dengue viruses detection. Blood sample was collected and applied to pre-processing module, where automated mechanism mixed the sample with lysis buffer and RT-LAMP reagents. The mixture next went to the amplification chip where reaction was incubated. After that, the LED from cellphone was switched on for sample illumination. Real-time fluorescence results were displayed on the screen. If the channel lighted up, the pathogen was presented. LOD for Zika was 10 PFU in 25 μL sample what corresponds to 6250 PFU/mL in blood [54].

A big part of sensing techniques are **smartphone-based** devices as their components are ideal for common analytical readers such as a screen acting as display and controller, a camera as input for signal capturing, a memory for data storing, connectivity modes (Bluetooth, NFC and Wi-Fi) for data transmission. Also, GPS can help track global health in serious cases like pandemic. Wear possibilities and portability makes it powerful branch in biosensing area. The second fact, they are not expensive devices with high accessibility, as there are billions of mobile phone users globally. Smartphone devices are classified as detectors or instrumental interface for controlling the experiment setup, but this solution is less reported in the literature. This classification means to make a device that can be attached to the smartphone or make independent device and connect it with a smartphone via Bluetooth, etc. Adapters are often required for proper distance maintaining between the sample and the camera or for dark chambers making (in fluorescence). Main attention attracts optical methods, however microscopic, magnetoresistive and electrochemical are also available. The next big advantage is costs reduction. Applications are pH measurements [61], heart rate scanning [62] and others. Noteworthy is that phone's microphone can perform spirometry (lung capacity) by blow-sound measurement. Great idea was to introduce phone sensors platforms to drones for reaching difficult places and providing low weight portable laboratories for human in need [63, 64]. For a critical review, more application examples and commercially available biosensors please see [65].

The point-of-care (POC) diagnostics is the next branch with intention of public health revolution. Rapid disease diagnosis is essential for the accurate treatment. In developed countries, most analysis are performed in traditional way-in specialized laboratories with sophisticated equipment and by qualified personnel. Thanks POC testing allows for in vitro diagnostics with results obtained at ambulances, accident sites or physician's offices. Moreover, self-testing will be provided for patients. The strong advantages are small size, portability and automation, like in smartphones. Actually, smartphones can be classified as POC devices. Many products are currently available on the market, like glucose sensors, pregnancy tests, urine screening and more. The microelectromechanical systems (MEMS) technology is strongly introduced to POC assays. The main advantage is separating, mixing, isolating and more sample treatment steps in one device. Main target analytes are proteins, nucleic acids, cells (blood cells), small molecules (metabolites such as glucose and cholesterol). With features as time-efficiency, easy operating and portability, they are ideal for use in poor countries and difficult geographical regions. Many POC devices use microfluidic assays as paper-based microfluidics are disposable, cheap and easy to storage. However, these microfluidic solutions can only show qualitative answers (yes/no for the presence of target analytes). Challenging is the choice of appropriate marker and optimization of accuracy, sensitivity, speed and more parameters. One of the biggest potential in POC devices is detection of circulating tumor cells for cancer progression monitoring by atomic force microscopy technique. Others common label-free assays are filtration, hydrodynamic chromatography and dielectrophoresis [66, 67]. For more point-of-care sensors, authors recommend reading [68].

The novel pathogen detection method was presented by Waller et al. group. Portable detection of *Bacillus anthracis* spores was done by amperometric immunoassay. Magnetic beads and glucose oxidase, both antibodies-conjugated were used as sensing sandwich-like material on gold matrix. Immunomagnetic spores separation and interferences removal from environmental samples was done. For current signal, samples were incubated with glucose, horseradish peroxidase and electron mediator. Target was captured by polyclonal antisera and signal was generated by monoclonal antibodies. Whole analysis took less than an hour. Authors wanted to increase the sensitivity of available lateral-flow devices and decrease analysis time comparing to ELISA and PCR. LOD was 500 spores and linear quantitative range from 5 × 103 to 5 × 106 CFU/mL [69]. Gouma et al. have introduced novel isoprene sensor for influenza virus detection. Infected patients generate more volatile products like nitric oxide (NO) and volatile organic compounds (VOCs) which are biomarkers in the disease detection. The secretion comes from the alveolar and airway epithelium and leukocytes infiltrating the lungs. The device is a portable 3-sensor microsystem with rapid non-invasive screening. Measurement must be done as fast as disease symptoms are observed, for biomarkers changes in time observation. The sensor is able to detect three gases: isoprene, ammonia and NO in temperature control. The measurement relies on resistance changes of h-WO_3 matrix with exposure to NO, NO_2, isoprene and methanol at 350°C [33]. Influenza virus is notably investigated and described in the literature, as it is believed as the mother of all pandemics. Except conventional detection methods, electrochemical techniques attract the scientific and market worlds. Very practical nature of these biosensors makes them applicable for POC [70]. Another electrochemical biosensor was developed for dengue virus. Nascimento et al. have employed gold nanoparticles–polyaniline composite and immobilized with dengue serotype-specific primers. Chosen measurement technique was CV and EIS. Invented system was able to recognize the dengue serotype at picomolar concentration with high specificity and reproducibility [71]. Ishikawa et al. have used In_2O_3 nanowire in their amperometric sensing platforms for SARS virus detection. Authors have used antibody mimic proteins (AMPs), working as antibodies but smaller I size. The biomarker was viral nucleocapsid (N) protein. LOD of 1 nM was achieved in 10 min long analysis [72].

8. Application of biosensing technologies in telemedicine

Telemedicine is a widely used technology branch in patient's healthcare. It exchanges the specialized care information from a distance via electronic communicators, provides health monitoring, increases the access to health services especially in places limited financially, like rural areas, and geographically, enhancing life quality. More specifically it can be video conversation, an email, by smartphone or other device, sometimes wireless tools. Common fields are telepsychiatry, teledermatology and teleradiology. It is definitely safe and effective in adult and pediatric medicine. Telemedicine is no more theory. A big part of implementation attempts succeed. The US survey in 2014 showed 86% of user's satisfaction and 75% of willing attitude to telemedicine formats [73]. Survey form 2011 has reported very high telemedicine application. About 70% of radiology practices in US are in teleradiology form [74]. Treating patients at home seems to be beneficial for the family and the hospital itself. Also the continuous access to patients and physicians is very convenient. Teleconsultations can reduce the costs associated with the transport, waiting time and physical consultation price. Now it is possible to reach more patients with less time with the same or higher consultations satisfactory [75]. Moreover, 'the medicare' is a good marketing and promoting tool for potential new customers wins. Telemedicine cannot act perfectly, obviously. They were many cases of implementation failures, problems connected with operational costs, technology integration lacks, the devices standard quality and safety. The service implementation is affected by factors like financing, technology, society acceptance and more. Necessary are operation trainings, user-friendly simple handlings and the commitment of specialists (physicians, nurses) and patients. There are few types of services such as telemonitoring, teleconsultations, teleeducation, etc. [74, 76] offering home assistance and psychological support. Nowadays, the telemedicine usage reluctance still is observed, however decreases gradually, because these methods meet users need. Patients, especially elderly, use devices more readily and specialists enhance technology confidence. Helpful are program startups like guidelines published by The American Telemedicine Association (ATA) or The Center for Telehealth [74, 76].

As an example of telemedicine application, Shah et al. have proposed high-intensity model of care for illness care, expanding the access to seriously ill patients using real-time and store-and-forward approaches Authors have reduced the emergency department visits to 34% over 1 year comparing to control group [77]. Newest Nature reports show a big interest in telemedicine field, to fill the disease's data-gaps, like in inflammatory bowel disease (IBD) case. Authors debate if IBD should be implemented in e-care or not. IBD is a chronic disease and its treatment is suboptimal, however implementation it to e-health may bring some profits. As it is relapsing and remitting disease, traditional clinical approach can be insufficient and not fast enough. By e-health approach, patients are believed to become active part in decisions-making when the first symptom occurs. Moreover, introducing IBD to telemedicine may be important financial impact, cost-saving due to eliminating outpatient visits. However, validation costs must be considered too. Currently available e-cases are very small in numbers, still insufficient for global implementation. Real-life patient's data are lacking [78].

Telemedicine is a great field to show biosensors potential. As their main goal is to be cheap, portable and user-friendly, they can be applied for everyday-based monitoring and in epidemics seasons, like during Ebola outbreak from 2014 in Africa, SARS in 2003 and pandemic influenza in 2009 or in moments where local medical centers suspect the danger and need reference center consultations. The next great appliance is for quarantine patients restricted to isolation [79] or any place with poor economic background or geographically difficult places to reach. Patients will be allowed to examine themselves by different integrated systems, for example, by electronic device with easy to collect specimen and further send the results through mobile phone with specially designed app. For this case, the main target could be Africa with a spread of malaria, tuberculosis, HIV and Human Papilloma Virus (HPV). Current biomedical sensors for resource-limited countries suffering from these diseases are reported in Ref. [80]. Telemedicine have already found appliance in pathogens area. Beste et al. have described telemedicine support in Hepatitis C treatment in the American Veterans (VA) group. The main problem was not willingly prescribed antivirals by primary care providers due to health insurers or providers preference. The new program ECHO for promoting and improving telecare was launched offering video conferences with specialists. After this adjustment, the rate of prescribed antivirals to reviewed patients by VA-ECHO has increased [81]. Telemedicine services have been implemented also in HIV/AIDS case. In literature reported, there was raising awareness in pharmacy trainees to optimize patient care [82] or in forming new systems like 'VIHrtual Hospital' with user-friendly interface [83].

9. Conclusion

The features for biosensors developments are mainly sensitivity, specificity and cost-effectiveness detection. These parameters are critical for the high-quality sensing technology. The modern era requires combination of technological and biological approaches for more and more satisfactory devices. The next level is developing robust multi-task biosensor for long-term use. It is necessary due to therapeutics need, it means never ending patients and newly discovered pathogens. Unfortunately, hygiene and sanitation improvement did not reduce the mortality of infectious diseases. Current use of aptamers, peptides and other biomarkers is a key for accurate affection diagnosis. Sensing approaches are a strong factor for time-reduced and more effective treatment than before. The next success is molecules used not only for disease definition, but novel therapeutics, drug delivery, food and environmental monitoring. Invention of chemical, especially electrochemical, biosensors have found application in many fields, except everyday analysis, in sport medicine, doping control analysis and more, giving information about metabolism and physiology states. They offer rapid, real-time, very sensitive analysis. The next advantages, especially for electrochemical techniques, are miniaturization possibilities connected with reduces costs. Point-of-care devices and lab-on-chip technology win in the run. Electrochemical, mainly voltammetric and impedimetric, techniques are uncompetitive due to wide range of target analytes detection. This kind of biosensors keeps a promise for developing complete automatic sensing systems, with no need of sample pretreatment, fast analysis and interfaces with telecommunication devices (smartphones and tablets) and further with specialists. Telemedicine can be an answer for every patient suffering from lack of medical check-ups. It will be possible to detect many dysfunctions at first stages and prevent them with higher cure-impact than treatment in far advanced infections. The ubiquitous smartphones distribution and connectivity changes the concept of public health. E-health solution meets the market need offering easy to operate system that fits in every pocket. Independent connectivity via Wi-Fi or Bluetooth will enable 24 h availability and updates depending on patient's requirements.

Author details

Karolina Dziąbowska[1,2*], Elżbieta Czaczyk[1,2] and Dawid Nidzworski[1,2]

*Address all correspondence to: karolina.dziabowska@gmail.com

1 SensDx Ltd, Warsaw, Poland

2 Institute of Biotechnology and Molecular Medicine, Gdansk, Poland

References

[1] Clark Jr C, Lyons C. Electrode systems for continuous monitoring in cardiovascular surgery. Annals New York Academy of Sciences; 1962

[2] Karunakaran C, Bhargava K, Benjamin R, editors. Biosensors and Bioelectronics. Netherlands: Elsevier; 2015. ISBN: 978-0-12-803100-1

[3] Pacheco JG, Barroso MF, Nouws HPA. Biosensors. In: Current Developments in Biotechnology and Bioengineering: Bioprocesses, Bioreactors and Controls. Netherlands: Elsevier; 2017. pp. 627-648. DOI: 10.1016/B978-0-444-63663-8.00021-5

[4] Salek-Maghsoudi A, Vakhshiteh F, Torabi R. Recent advances in biosensor technology in assessment of early diabetes biomarkers. Biosensors and Bioelectronics. 2018;**99**:122-135. DOI: 10.1016/j.bios.2017.07.047

[5] Alahi MdEE, Mukhopadhyay SC. Detection methodologies for pathogen and toxins: A review. Sensors. 2017;**17**:1885. DOI: 10.3390/s17081885

[6] Zhuang J, Han B, Liu W. Liposome-amplified photoelectrochemical immunoassay for highly sensitive monitoring of disease biomarkers based on a split-type strategy. Biosensors and Bioelectronics. 2018;**99**:230-236. DOI: 10.1016/j.bios.2017.07.067

[7] Bettazzi F, Marraza G, Minunii M. Biosensors and related bioanalytical tools. Comprehensive Analytical Chemistry. 2017;**77**:1-33. DOI: 10.1016/bs.coac.2017.05.003

[8] Chand R, Han D, Kim YS. Voltammetric analysis on a disposable microfluidic electrochemical cell. Bulletin of Korean Chemical Society. 2013;**34**(4):1175-1180. DOI: 10.5012/bkcs.2013.34.4.1175

[9] Yamanaka K, Vestergaard MC, Tamiya E. Printable electrochemical biosensors: A focus on screen-printed electrodes and their application. Sensors. 2016;**16**(10):1761. DOI: 10.3390/s16101761

[10] Zelada-Guillén GA, Sebastián-Avila JL, Blondeau P. Label-free detection of *Staphylococcus aureus* in skin using real-time potentiometric biosensors based on carbon nanotubes and aptamers. Biosensors and Bioelectronics. 2012;**31**:226-232. DOI: 10.1016/j.bios.2011.10.021

[11] Hnaiein M, Hassen WM, Abdelghani A. A conductometric immunosensor based on functionalized magnetite nanoparticles for *E. coli* detection. Electrochemistry Communications. 2008;**10**:1152-1154. DOI: 10.1016/j.elecom.2008.04.009

[12] Caygill RL, Blair GE, Millner PA. A review on viral biosensors to detect human pathogens. Analytica Chimica Acta. 2010;**681**:8-15. DOI: 10.1016/j.aca.2010.09.038

[13] Singh S, Kaushal A, Khare S. DNA chip based sensor for amperometric detection of infectious pathogens. International Journal of Biological Macromolecules. 2017;**103**:355-359. DOI: 10.1016/j. ijbiomac.2017.05.041

[14] Yang L, Bashir R. Electrical/electrochemical impedance for rapid detection of foodborne pathogenic bacteria. Biotechnology Advances. 2008;**26**:135-150. DOI: 10.1016/j.biotechadv.2007.10.003

[15] Nidzworski D, Pranszke P, Grudniewska M. Universal biosensor for detection of influenza virus. Biosensors and Bioelectronics. 2014;**59**:239-242. DOI: 10.1016/j.bios.2014.03.050

[16] Wang J. Electrochemical biosensing based on noble metal nanoparticles. Microchimica Acta. 2012;**177**:245-270. DOI: 10.1007/s00604-011-0758-1

[17] Vigneshvar S, Sudhakumari CC, Senthilkumaran B. Recent advances in biosensor technology for potential applications – An overview. Frontiers in Bioengineering and Biotechnology. 2016;**4**:11. DOI: 10.3389/fbioe.2016.00011

[18] Liu S, Wu P, Li W. Ultrasensitive and selective electrochemical identification of hepatitis C virus genotype 1b based on specific endonuclease combined with gold nanoparticles signal amplification. Analytical Chemistry. 2011;**83**:4752-4758. DOI: 10.1021/ac200624f

[19] Li H, Sun Z, Zhong W. Ultrasensitive electrochemical detection For DNA arrays based on silver nanoparticle aggregates. Analytical Chemistry. 2010;**82**:5477-5483. DOI: 0.1021/ac101193e

[20] Guo X. Single-molecule electrical biosensors based on single-walled carbon nanotube. Advanced Materials 2013;**25**(25):3397-3408. DOI: 10.1002/adma.201301219

[21] Wang J, Lin Y. Functionalized carbon nanotubes and nanofibers for biosensing applications. Trends in Analytical Chemistry. 2008;**27**(7):619-626. DOI: 10.1016/j.trac.2008.05.009

[22] Nehra A, Singh KP. Current trends in nanomaterials embedded field effect transistor-based biosensor. Biosensors and Bioelectronics. 2015;**74**:731-743. DOI: 10.1016/j.bios.2015.07.030

[23] Bhardwaj J, Devarakonda S, Kumar S. Development of a paper-based electrochemical Immunosensor using an antibody-single walled carbon nanotubes bio-conjugate modified electrode for label-free detection of foodborne pathogens. Sensors and Actuators B: Chemical. 2017;**253**:115-123. DOI: 10.1016/j.snb.2017.06.108

[24] Gong Q, Wang Y, Yang H. A sensitive impedimetric DNA biosensor for the determination of the HIV gene based on graphene-Nafion composite film. Biosensors and Bioelectronics. 2017;**89**:565-569. DOI: 10.1016/j.bios.2016.02.045i

[25] Peng F, Su Y, Fan C. Silicon Nanomaterials platform for bioimaging, biosensing, and cancer therapy. Accounts of Chemical Research. 2014;**47**(2):612-623. DOI: 10.1021/ar400221g

[26] Nguyen PD, Tran TB, Nguyen DTX. Magnetic silica nanotube-assisted impedimetric immunosensor for the separation and label-free detection of *Salmonella typhimurium*. Sensors and Actuators B. 2014;**197**:314-320. DOI: 10.1016/j.snb.2014.02.089

[27] Kwon SJ, Bard AJ. DNA analysis by application of Pt nanoparticle electrochemical amplifica tion with single label response. Journal of American Chemical Society. 2012;**134**:10777-10779. DOI: 10.1021/ja304074f

[28] Tombelli S. Piezoelectric biosensors for medical applications. In: Higson S, editor. Biosensors for Medical Applications. Cambridge: Woodhead Publishing Limited; 2012. DOI: 10.1533/ 9780857097187.1.41

[29] Thien NTD, Wang H, Sugiarto S. Advances in nanomaterials and their applications in point of care (POC) devices for the diagnosis of infectious diseases. Biotechnology Advances. 2016;**34**(8):275-1288. DOI: 10.1016/j.biotechadv.2016.09.003

[30] Sueki A, Matsuda K, Yamaguchi A. Evaluation of saliva as diagnostic materials for influenza virus infection by PCR-based assays. Clinica Chimica Acta. 2006;**453**:71-74. DOI: 10.1016/j.cca.2015.12.006

[31] Yoon J, Yun SG, Nam J. The use of saliva specimens for detection of influenza A and B viruses by rapid influenza diagnostic tests. Journal of Virological Methods. 2017;**243**:15-19. DOI: 10.1016/j.jviromet.2017.01.013

[32] Kim J, Imani S, Araujo WR. Wearable salivary uric acid mouthguard biosensor with integrated wireless electronics. Biosensors and Bioelectronics. 2015;**74**:1061-1068. DOI: 10.1016/j.bios.2015.07.039

[33] Gouma PI, Wang L, Simon SR. Novel isoprene sensor for a flu virus breath monitor. Sensors. 2017;**17**(1):199. DOI: 10.3390/s17010199

[34] Crean C, McGeough C, O'Kennedy R. Wearable Biosensors for Medical Applications. Cambridge: Woodhead Publishing Limited; 2012. pp. 301-330. ISBN: 978-1-84569-935-2

[35] Verma MS, Rogowski JL, Jones L. Colorimetric biosensing of pathogens using gold nanoparticles. Biotechnology Advances. 2015;**33**(6 Pt 1):666-680. DOI: 10.1016/j.biotechadv.2015.03.003

[36] Mehrotra P. Biosensors and their applications – A review. Journal of Oral Biology and Craniofacial Research. 2016;**6**(2):153-159. DOI: 10.1016/j.jobcr.2015.12.002

[37] Lan L, Yao Y, Ping J. Recent advances in nanomaterial-based biosensors for antibiotics detection. Biosensors and Bioelectronics. 2017;**91**:504-514. DOI: 10.1016/j.bios.2017.01.007

[38] Mathew FP, Alocilja EC. Porous silicon-based biosensor for pathogen detection. Biosensors and Bioelectronics. 2005;**20**:1656-1661. DOI: 10.1016/j.bios.2004.08.006

[39] Wang Y, Jiang L, Chu L. Electrochemical detection of glutathione by using thymine-rich DNA-gated switch functionalized mesoporous silica nanoparticles. Biosensors and Bioelectronics. 2017;**87**:459-465. DOI: 10.1016/j.bios.2016.08.102

[40] Li Y, Han J, Chen R. Label electrochemical immunosensor for prostate-specific antigen based on graphene and silver hybridized mesoporous silica. Analytical Biochemistry. 2015;**469**:76-82. DOI: 10.1016/j.ab.2014.09.022

[41] Shinde SB, Fernandes CB, Patravale VB. Recent trends in in-vitro nanodiagnostics for detection of pathogens. Journal of Controlled Release. 2012;**159**:164-180. DOI: 10.1016/j.jconrel.2011.11.033

[42] Davies D, Guo X, Musavi L. Gold nanoparticle-modified carbon electrode biosensor for the detection of listeria monocytogenes. Industrial Biotechnology. 2013;**9**(1):13-36. DOI: 10.1089/ind.2012.0033

[43] Yang GJ, Huang JL, Menga WJ. A reusable capacitive immunosensor for detection of *Salmonella* spp. based on grafted ethylene diamine and self-assembled gold nanoparticle monolayers. Analytica Chimica Acta. 2009;**647**:159-166. DOI: 10.1016/j.aca.2009.06.008

[44] Gaffar S, Nurmalasari R, Yohan YW. Voltammetric DNA biosensor using gold electrode modified by self assembled monolayer of Thiol for detection of mycobacterium tuberculosis. Procedia Technology. 2017;**27**:74-80. DOI: 10.1016/j.protcy.2017.04.034

[45] Alizadeh N, Memarc MY, Moaddab SR. Aptamer-assisted novel technologies for detecting bacterial pathogens. Biomedicine & Pharmacotherapy. 2017;**93**:737-745. DOI: 10.1016/j.biopha.2017.07.011

[46] Bissonnette L, Bergeron MG. POC tests in microbial diagnostics: Current status. In: Hardwood C, editor. Methods in Microbiology. Vol. 42. Elsevier; 2015. pp. 87-110. DOI: 10.1016/bs.mim.2015.09.003

[47] Ding C, Zhao F, Zhang M. Hybridization biosensor using 2,9-dimethyl-1,10-phenantroline cobalt as electrochemical indicator for detection of hepatitis B virus DNA. Bioelectrochemistry. 2008;**72**:28-33. DOI: 10.1016/j.bioelechem.2007.11.001

[48] Wang R, Wang Y, Lassiter K. Interdigitated array microelectrode based impedance immunosensor for detection of avian influenza virus H5N1. Talanta. 2009;**79**:159-164. DOI: 10.1016/j.talanta.2009.03.017

[49] Fang X, Tan OK, Tse MS. A label-free immunosensor for diagnosis of dengue infection with simple electrical measurements. Biosensors and Bioelectronics. 2010;**25**:1137-1142. DOI: 10.1016/j.bios.2009.09.037

[50] Zhang D, Peng Y, Qi H. Label-free electrochemical DNA biosensor array for simultaneous detection of the HIV-1 and HIV-2 oligonucleotides incorporating different hairpin-DNA probes and redox indicator. Biosensors and Bioelectronics. 2010;**25**:1088-1094. DOI: 10.1016/j.bios.2009.09.032

[51] Hnaien M, Diouani MF, Helali S. Immobilization of specific antibody on SAM functionalized gold electrode for rabies virus detection by electrochemical impedance spectroscopy. Biochemical Engineering Journal. 2008;**39**:443-449. DOI: 10.1016/j.bej.2007.09.018

[52] Rich RL, Myszka DG. Spying on HIV with SPR. TRENDS in Microbiology. 2003;**11**(3): 124-133. DOI: 10.1016/S0966-842X(03)00025-8

[53] Petrosova A, Konry T, Cosnier S. Development of a highly sensitive, field operable biosensor for serological studies of Ebola virus in central Africa. Sensors and Actuators B. 2007;**122**:578-586. DOI: 10.1016/j.snb.2006.07.005

[54] Ganguli A, Ornob A, Hands-free YH. Smartphone-based diagnostics for simultaneous detection of Zika, Chikungunya, and dengue at point-of-care. Biomedical Microdevices. 2017;**19**(4):73. DOI: 10.1007/s10544-017-0209-9

[55] Gruhl FJ, Rapp BE, Länge K. Biosensors for diagnostic applications. Advances in biochemical engineering/biotechnology. 2011;**133**:115-148. DOI: 10.1007/10_2011_130

[56] Horak J, Dincer C, Bakirci H. A disposable dry film photoresist-based microcapillary immunosensor chip for rapid detection of Epstein–Barr virus infection. Sensors and Actuators B. 2014;**191**:813-820. DOI: 10.1016/j.snb.2013.10.019

[57] Damhorst GL, Smith CE, Salm EM. A liposome-based ion release impedance sensor for biological detection. Biomedical Microdevices. 2013;**15**(5):895-905. DOI: 10.1007/s10544-013-9778-4

[58] Dastider SG, Barizuddin S, Yuksek NS. Efficient and rapid detection of salmonella using microfluidic impedance based sensing. Journal of Sensors. 2015;**2015**:8 ID 293461. DOI: 10.1155/2015/293461

[59] Li Y, Wang R. Aptasensors for detection of avian influenza virus H5N1. In: Prickril B, Rasooly A, editors. Biosensors and Biodetection: Methods and Protocols. Vol. 2. Electrochemical, Bioelectronic, Piezoelectric, Cellular and Molecular Biosensors. Berlin: Springer; 2017. pp. 379-402. DOI 10.1007/978-1-4939-6911-1_25

[60] Lafleur JP, Jönsson A, Senkbeil S. Recent advances in lab-on-a-chip for biosensing applications. Biosensors and Bioelectronics. 2016;**76**:213-233. DOI: 10.1016/j.bios.2015.08.003

[61] Oncescu V, O'Dell D, Erickson D. Smartphone based health accessory for colorimetric detection of biomarkers in sweat and saliva. Lab on a Chip. 2013;**13**:3232-3238. DOI: 10.1039/c3lc50431j

[62] AliveCor. Mobilephone-based EKG recorder [Internet]. 2017. Available from: https://www.alivecor.com/ [Accessed: Oct 30, 2017]

[63] Quesada-González D, Merkoçi A. Mobile phone-based biosensing: An emerging "diagnostic and communication" technology. Biosensors and Bioelectronics. 2017;**92**:549-562. DOI: 10.1016/j.bios.2016.10.062

[64] Roda A, Michelini E, Zangheri M. Smartphone-based biosensors: A critical review and perspectives. Trends in Analytical Chemistry. 2016;**79**:317-325. DOI: 10.1016/j.trac.2015.10.019

[65] Roda A, Calabretta MM, Calab D. Smartphone-based biosensors for bioanalytics: A critical review. Comprehensive Analytical Chemistry. 2017;**77**:237-286. DOI: 10.1016/bs.coac.2017.05.007

[66] Choi S. Powering point-of-care diagnostic devices. Biotechnology Advances. 2016;**34**(3):321-330. DOI: 0.1016/j.biotechadv.2015.11.004

[67] Karsten SL, Tarhan MC, Kudo LC. Point-of-care (POC) devices by means of advanced MEMS. Talanta. 2015;**145**:55-59. DOI: 10.1016/j.talanta.2015.04.032i

[68] Zarei M. Portable biosensing devices for point-of-care diagnostics: Recent developments and applications. Trends in Analytical Chemistry. 2017;**91**:26-41. DOI: 10.1016/j.trac.2017.04.001

[69] Waller DF, Hew BE, Holdaway C. Rapid detection of bacillus anthracis spores using immunomagnetic separation and amperometry. Biosensors. 2016;**6**(4):61. DOI: 10.3390/bios6040061

[70] Tepeli Y, Ülkü A. Electrochemical biosensors for influenza virus a detection: The potential of adaptation of these devices to POC systems. Sensors and Actuators B: Chemical. 2018; pp. 377-384. DOI: 10.1016/j.snb.2017.07.126

[71] Nascimento HPO, Oliveira MDL, de Melo CP. An impedimetric biosensor for detection of dengue serotype at picomolar concentration based on gold nanoparticles-polyaniline hybrid composites. Colloids and Surfaces B: Biointerfaces. 2011;**86**:414-419. DOI: 10.1016/j.colsurfb.2011.04.028

[72] Ishikawa FN, Chang HK, Curreli M. Label-free, electrical detection of the SARS virus N-protein with nanowire biosensors utilizing antibody mimics as capture probes. American Chemical Society Nano. 2009;**3**(5):1219-1224. DOI: 10.1021/nn900086c

[73] Mordechai DR, Kari G, Aronson SD. Telemedicine and Pediatric urgent care: A vision into the future. Clinical Pediatric Emergency Medicine. 2017;**18**(1):24-31. DOI: 10.1016/j.cpem.2017.01.003

[74] Doumbouya MB, Kamsu-Foguem B, Kenfack H. Telemedicine using mobile telecommunication: Towards syntactic interoperability in teleexpertise. Telematics and Informatics. 2014;**31**:648-659. DOI: 10.1016/j.tele.2014.01.003

[75] Ataç A, Kurt E, Yurdakul SE. An overview to ethical problems in telemedicine technology. Procedia-Social and Behavioral Sciences. 2013;**103**:116-121. DOI: 10.1016/j.sbspro.2013.10.315

[76] Segato F, Masella C. Department telemedicine services: How to make them last over time. Health Policy and Technology. 2017;**6**(3):268-278. DOI: 10.1016/j.hlpt.2017.07.003

[77] Shah MN, Wasserman EB, Gillespie SM. High-intensity telemedicine decreases emergency department use for ambulatory care sensitive conditions by older adult senior living community residents. Journal of the American Medical Directors Association. 2015;**16**(12):1077-1081. DOI: 10.1016/j.jamda.2015.07.009

[78] Bossuyt P, Pouillon L, Peyrin-Biroulet L. Primetime for e-health in IBD? Nature Reviews. 2017;**14**:133-134. DOI: 10.1038/nrgastro.2017.11

[79] Ohannessian R. Telemedicine: Potential applications in epidemic situations. European Research in Telemedicine. 2015;**4**:95-98. DOI: 10.1016/j.eurtel.2015.08.002

[80] Ozoemena KI, Carrara S. Biomedical electrochemical sensors for resource-limited countries. Current Opinion in Electrochemistry. 2017;**3**(1):51-56. DOI: 10.1016/j.coelec.2017.06.002

[81] Beste LA, Glorioso TJ, Ho PM. Telemedicine specialty support promotes hepatitis c treatment by primary care providers in the Department of Veterans Affairs. The American Journal of Medicine. 2017;**130**(4):432-438. DOI: 10.1016/j.amjmed.2016.11.019

[82] Badowski ME, Nyberg CR, Chaiyaperm V. Perceptions of pharmacy trainees completing a clinical experience in an HIV telemedicine clinic at an urban academic medical center. Currents in Pharmacy Teaching and Learning. 2016;**8**(6):840-845. DOI: 10.1016/j.cptl.2016.08.019

[83] Caceres C, Gomez EJ, Garcia F. An integral care telemedicine system for HIV/AIDS patients. International Journal of Medical Informatics. 2006;**75**:638-642. DOI: 10.1016/j.ijmedinf.2006.04.010

Chapter 11

Development of HRPzyme-Integrated PCR Platform for Colorimetric Detection of Foodborne Pathogens

Bhagwan S. Batule, Seong U. Kim, Hyoyoung Mun,
Won-Bo Shim and Min-Gon Kim

Additional information is available at the end of the chapter

http://dx.doi.org/10.5772/intechopen.72649

Abstract

In recent years, foodborne illnesses have become the most significant public health issue in both developed and developing countries. The World Health Organization (WHO) reported that in 2010, around 1.8 million people died due to foodborne illness. Therefore, the development of a cost-effective, sensitive, and selective detection method for identifying and monitoring foodborne pathogens is necessary for improved public health. Here, we describe a simple and ultrasensitive colorimetric method for the detection of foodborne pathogens based on HRPzyme-integrated PCR using PC-based ImageJ software. We present insights into different aspects of this method such as the importance of 16S rRNA detection, the modification of traditional PCR primers with a unique functional sequence for generating a color signal, and the application of ImageJ in colorimetric image data acquisition. The performance of the proposed strategy in detecting various foodborne pathogens is comparable to that of the commercial UV-Vis spectrophotometer Tecan Infinite 200 Pro. This detection platform exhibits linearity over wide range, high sensitivity, and high selectivity. The diagnostic capability of this colorimetric system to detect foodborne pathogens was demonstrated with spiked fruit and vegetable samples. This low-cost and effective colorimetric method can be conveniently employed for the analysis of DNA sequences arising from pathogenic bacteria.

Keywords: foodborne pathogens, 16S rRNA, PCR, primer, HRPzyme, colorimetric detection

1. Introduction

1.1. The importance of pathogenic foodborne pathogens

Food safety is critically important to consumer and public health and to the economic sustainability of the agro-food sector. Due to food poisoning incidents, consumers desire food safety assurances before they purchase food items. Foodborne illnesses, mainly caused by pathogens derived from contaminated water or contaminated and uncooked foods, cause many cases of death due to severe infection [1, 2]. The most widely recognized foodborne diseases are caused by pathogens such as *Escherichia coli* O157:H7, *Bacillus cereus, Listeria monocytogenes,* and *Vibrio parahaemolyticus*. Hence, it is important to detect the presence of pathogenic bacteria in food and water before they enter the body and cause serious outbreaks [2–4]. The standard microbiological methods for the detection of food pathogens are bacterial culture and biochemical staining, but the application of these is limited due to the time-consuming nature of analysis (up to 7 days) and their nonspecific results [5]. Therefore, there is a need for sensitive, selective, and point-of-care platforms that allow for both genotypic and phenotypic studies of foodborne pathogens. While the detection of foodborne pathogens has been significantly improved due to recent advances in molecular diagnostics, many of these methods require skilled persons and costly instruments. Therefore, point-of-need diagnostic methods are urgently needed to control the spread of food pathogen infections.

1.2. General overview of the importance and limitations of recent detection methods for foodborne pathogens

In recent years, a variety of diagnostic approaches, for example immunological methods, such as enzyme-linked immunosorbent assays (ELISAs) with detection limit of 10^3 cfu mL^{-1} [6–8] and molecular biological methods such as polymerase chain reaction (PCR) with detection limit of 10^2 cfu mL^{-1} [9–11] have been employed for the identification of foodborne pathogens. These methods vary in their sensitivity, specificity, cost, and efficacy. Owing to the recent availability of genomic information, molecular-based approaches have garnered considerable attention in terms of the development of molecular diagnostic techniques to detect and characterize pathogens [5, 12]. In the last decade, PCR, which can amplify a small amount of DNA through an amplification process, has been employed as a gold standard method for the molecular diagnosis of nucleic acids. Agarose gel electrophoresis [13] and real-time measurements [14] with DNA-binding dyes, such as the SYBR green and EvaGreen dyes, have been employed to detect amplified PCR products. Still, these strategies are expensive, time-consuming, and not user-friendly. Considering these limitations, there is a need to develop advanced methods that can overcome the aforementioned limitations. Thus, several research groups have reported new detection platforms based on molecular beacons [12] and nanoparticle-tagged probes [15, 16]. However, these advanced methods additionally require fluorescence conjugation or probe thiolation procedures [17–20], which are also costly and time-consuming. Therefore, a simple, fast, cost-effective, and user-friendly detection platform remains in high demand.

1.3. The introduction of HRPzyme-integrated PCR and its importance

Recently, novel detection platforms have been developed to detect genomic DNA as a target analyte based on colorimetric reactions generated by biocatalysts, such as horseradish peroxidase-mimicking DNAzymes (HRPzymes). HRPzymes consist of a folded structure of a G-quadruplex nucleotide sequence, and they exhibit peroxidase-like activity by folding with a hemin molecule [21, 22]. Importantly, the hemin-HRPzyme folded structure catalyzes the oxidation of 3,3′,5,5′-tetramethylbenzidine (TMB) or 2,2-azinobis(3-ethylbenzothiozoline)-6-sulfonic acid (ABTS) in the presence of H_2O_2 and produces a colored oxidized product [23, 24]. Based on this remarkable property, HRPzyme-based strategies have significantly improved the detection of proteins [25], small molecules [26], and heavy metal ions [27].

Recently, several researchers have reported the use of colorimetric HRPzyme-integrated PCR for the simple and rapid detection of bacteria [28–31]. This PCR platform can be employed for the simultaneous synthesis of a peroxidase-like DNAzyme using a primer including a complementary DNAzyme sequence. To overcome the need for primer labeling and expensive instrumentation, Cheglakov et al. [31] developed the HRPzyme-integrated PCR for the visual detection of bacteria. Similarly, Cheng et al. [28] reported the HRPzyme-based colorimetric PCR for the simple and cost-effective detection of *V. parahaemolyticus*. Bhadra et al. [29] reported a G-quadruplex-generating PCR for the naked-eye colorimetric analysis of SNPs associated with *Mycobacterium tuberculosis* drug resistance alleles. Finally, Seok et al. [30] devised a colorimetric signal generated by an amplified HRPzyme following the PCR amplification of the 16S rDNA of *Salmonella enterica* Typhimurium.

In the aforementioned studies, researchers utilized a combination of the HRPzyme sequence and a primer to amplify a target gene via PCR amplification. The HRPzyme sequences were generated through PCR amplification of the primer, which is integrated with an anti-HRPzyme sequence. After PCR amplification, in the presence of hemin, the unamplified HRPzyme sequence containing primers forms a catalytic hemin-G-quadruplex structure, which mimics peroxidase activity and produces a colorimetric signal via the oxidation of a peroxidase substrate such as TMB or ABTS. The HRPzyme sequence generated during PCR amplification thus produces an optical signal that can be identified by eyes or with a spectrophotometer. These developed colorimetric protocols have been adopted for the rapid and easy detection of various pathogens by integrating a unique functional sequence with the traditional primer set for the generation of the colorimetric signal. These studies thus demonstrated the broad applicability of a fast, simple, ultrasensitive, and selective detection method for DNA as a target analyte.

1.4. HRPzyme-integrated PCR-based detection of foodborne pathogens using PC-based ImageJ software

We have developed a PCR-based detection platform, termed G-quadruplex-blocking PCR, because the amplification of a specific target blocks the folding of the HRPzyme sequence, inhibiting the peroxidase activity of the HRPzyme. In contrast, in the presence of hemin and the absence of target-specific amplification, the G-quadruplex/hemin complex generates an oxidized substrate by oxidizing ABTS in the presence of hydrogen peroxide (H_2O_2) [32, 33].

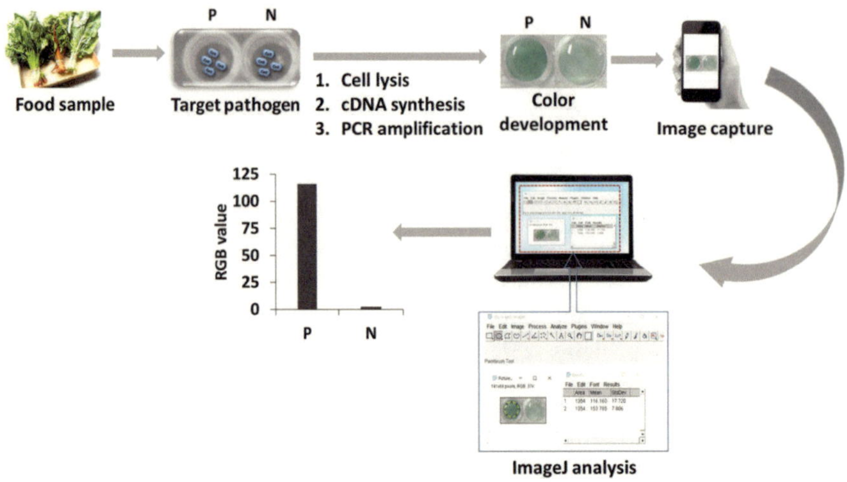

Figure 1. Schematic representation of HRPzyme-integrated PCR-based colorimetric detection of a foodborne pathogen. P: With target pathogen; N: Without target pathogen.

G-quadruplex/hemin complexes can also oxidize different peroxidase substrates such as fluorogenic (e.g., Amplex UltraRed (AUR) and QuantaBlu), electrochemical (e.g., 3-Indoxyl Phosphate and p-aminophenol (PAP)), and luminescent (e.g., luminol), allowing for the combination of the proposed method with fluorometric, electrochemical, and chemiluminescent detection platforms. The developed HRPzyme-integrated colorimetric detection platform allows for color development and provides a simple data analysis tool capable of the detection of specific common foodborne pathogens. Specifically, we used available ribosomal RNA (rRNA) sequence information from microorganisms to design the HRPzyme-integrated PCR assay. The proposed colorimetric detection platform allows the visual detection of food pathogens (even a single cfu per milliliter). In this chapter, we employed sequences of the 16S rRNA, a component of the 30S small subunit of the bacterial ribosome, as a target because several copies of 16S rRNA are present in each bacterium (1×10^3 to 1×10^5 copies) [34]. Further, we demonstrate the integration of this colorimetric HRPzyme-integrated PCR platform with a digital camera and desktop NIH ImageJ software, a simple data analysis tool that is able to measure the gray intensity (32-bit grayscale) of the colored images and further transmit the metadata to a centralized off-site laboratory (**Figure 1**).

2. Material and methods

2.1. Experimental material

DNA polymerase (*Thermus thermophilus* (Tth)) used for PCR reaction was obtained from Epicenter Technologies (Madison, WI, USA), and a DNA Ladder was obtained from Takara Bio (Seoul, South Korea) [35]. The oligonucleotides were obtained from Genotech (Daejeon, South Korea) and dissolved in sterile water and stored at −20°C [35]. Hemin and ABTS were purchased from Sigma-Aldrich (St. Louis, MO, USA). 10X TBE (Tris-borate-ethylene-diamine tetracetic acid) buffer (for gel electrophoresis) was purchased from LPS Solution (Daejeon, South Korea). Phosphate buffered saline-1X (PBS; 137 mM NaCl, 2.7 mM KCl, 4.3 mM Na_2HPO_4, 1.4 mM KH_2PO_4, pH 7.2) was purchased from Bioseasang (Seongnam, Korea). The citrate buffer (0.1 M, pH -7) was prepared by mixing 59 mL of citric acid monohydrate (0.1 M) and 41 mL of trisodium citrate dihydrate (0.1 M). Agarose was purchased from Roche (Seoul, Korea). All reagents and solvents utilized in this study were of analytical grade and utilized without further purification. Target 16S rRNA sequences and primer sets designed for various foodborne pathogens are listed in **Table 1**.

2.2. Microorganism and culture conditions

Foodborne pathogens, including *E. coli* O157:H7 (ATCC 25922), *B. cereus* (KCTC 1092), *L. monocytogenes* (ATCC 19112), *V. parahaemolyticus* (ATCC 27969), *S. enterica* Typhimurium (ATCC 13311), and *C. sakazakii* (KTCT 2949), were grown in tryptic soy broth (Difco Laboratories, Franklin Lakes, NJ, USA) at 37°C. Concentrations of pathogenic bacteria were determined by cell counting on solid culture plates. Samples were collected with sterile plastic inoculating loops from solid culture plates, and culture solutions were prepared by serial dilution into 1× phosphate-buffered saline (PBS) to obtain 10^0–10^6 colony forming units per microliter (cfu mL^{-1}) and were stored at 4°C.

2.3. PCR amplification of 16S rRNA sequences specific to foodborne pathogens without genomic DNA isolation

Various concentrations of bacterial cultures were directly employed as template DNA for amplification with gene-specific primer sets (**Table 1**). Based on our previous report [35], PCR was performed in a total volume of 50 μL containing 5 μL bacterial culture at various concentrations (0–10^6 cfu mL^{-1}), 10× PCR buffer (2.5 μL), 25 mM $MgCl_2$ (6 μL), 2.5 mM dNTPs (deoxynucleotides) mix (8 μL), 10× PCR enhancer (5 μL), 25 mM $MnSO_4$ (1 μL), 20 μM forward primer (1 μL), 20 μM reverse primer (1 μL), and Tth DNA polymerase (0.5 μL). The PCR amplifications were performed under the following conditions: initial denaturation at 95°C for 5 min and 60°C for 20 min, then 35 cycles of 10 s at 94°C, 25 s at 60°C, and 10 s for 72°C adding last one cycle of 1 min for 72°C [35]. The PCR amplification was confirmed using 1.5% agarose gel electrophoresis. Then, to get colorimetric signal, PCR product (10 μL) was mixed with 300 μM hemin (5.5 μL), 5.5 mM ABTS (100 μL), 35% H_2O_2 (0.7 μL), and citrate buffer (1000 μL) with pH 4. After 10 min at room temperature (RT), the absorbance was measured at 410 nm with UV-Vis spectrophotometer (Infinite M2000pro, Männedorf, Switzerland) [35]. All images were taken using a digital camera (Samsung, Seoul, South Korea).

2.4. Spiked sample analysis

Fruit and vegetable samples such as apple, chicory, water dropwort, and white radish samples were purchased from the supermarket, washed with sterile water, and immersed in a plastic bag containing 20% ethanol and 1% lactic acid solution for 10 min. Then, sterilized food samples were cut to specific sizes and inoculated with different concentrations of bacteria, including *E. coli* O157:H7, *B. cereus*, *L. monocytogenes*, and *V. parahaemolyticus*, and kept in Petri dishes at 4°C overnight. Next, 0.1 mL of sterilized PBS was added to the inoculation site,

Pathogens	Target (GenBank number)	Primers (5′→3′) (H-F: Forward primer; H-R: Reverse primer)	Product size (bp)
Escherichia coli	16S rRNA	*H-F: AAAAAAAAAA***GGGTAGGGCGGGTTGGGT**AAAAAAAGCCTGATGCAGCCATGC	166
	(AWXM02000001.1)	*H-R: AAAAAAAAAA***GGGTAGGGCGGGTTGGGT**AAAAAAACAATGAGTAAAGGTATTAACTTTACTC	
Bacillus cereus	16S rRNA	*H-F: AAAAAAAAAA***GGGTAGGGCGGGTTGGGT**AAAAAAACTAGTTGAATAAGCTGGCACCT	164
	(D16266.1)	*H-R: AAAAAAAAAA***GGGTAGGGCGGGTTGGGT**AAAAAAAGATAACGCTTGCCACCTACG	
Listeria monocytogenes	16S rRNA	*H-F: AAAAAAAAAA***GGGTAGGGCGGGTTGGGT**AAAAAAACAAGGATAAGAGTAACTGCTTGT	162
	(JF967621.1)	*H-R: AAAAAAAAAA***GGGTAGGGCGGGTTGGGT**AAAAAAACTTGCCACCTACGTATTACCG	
Vibrio parahaemolyticus	16S rRNA	*H-F: AAAAAAAAAA***GGGTAGGGCGGGTTGGGT**AAAAAAACCTTCGGGGAACGATAACG	162
	(AE006468.1)	*H-R: AAAAAAAAAA***GGGTAGGGCGGGTTGGGT**AAAAAAAGCCATCGTTTCCAATGGTTATC	
Salmonella enterica Typhimurium	16S rRNA	*H-F: AAAAAAAAAA***GGGTAGGGCGGGTTGGGT**AAAAAAAGTTGTGGTTAATAACCGCAGCA	166
	(NR_114632.1)	*H-R: AAAAAAAAAA***GGGTAGGGCGGGTTGGGT**AAAAAAAATTAACGCTTGCACCCTCCG	
Cronobacter sakazakii	16S rRNA	*H-F: AAAAAAAAAA***GGGTAGGGCGGGTTGGGT**AAAAAAAATCCTGCAGAGATGCGGGA	160
	(AE006468.1)	*H-R: AAAAAAAAAA***GGGTAGGGCGGGTTGGGT**AAAAAAACGGGACTTAACCCAACATTTC	

Italic-protector sequence; Bold-HRPzyme sequence; Underline-spacer sequence

Table 1. Oligonucleotide primers used in this work.

and the solution was recovered by pipetting and directly employed in PCR assay following the same experimental conditions mentioned in Section 2.3.

2.5. Data acquisition through ImageJ software

ImageJ is a simple, practical, and freely available downloadable program that can be used on any computer with Java 5 or on a virtual machine [36]. Recently, many researchers have employed the ImageJ software to quantify data [37, 38]. The green color intensities produced during the HRPzyme-TMB-H_2O_2 assay were captured using a digital camera (Samsung, Seoul, South Korea) equipped with a standard 18–55-mm objective lens. Color intensities were measured, quantified, and averaged from three experiments by using the digital camera and ImageJ (Wayne Rasband, National Institutes of Health, Rockville, MD, USA; http://rsb.info.nih.gov/ij). The Δ gray intensity value was obtained by subtracting the average gray intensity of the negative samples from the average gray intensity of the positive samples.

3. Results and discussion

3.1. Principle of HRPzyme-integrated PCR

In this chapter, we established a method for the colorimetric detection of a PCR product generated by HRPzyme-integrated primers, as shown in **Figure 1**. We modified the forward and reverse primers that contain four regions: a protector sequence, HRPzyme sequence, spacer sequence, and sequence complementary to the 16S rRNA sequence from one of several pathogens. The 16S rRNA sequence was employed as a target for the specific detection of food pathogens. During PCR amplification, cells were first lysed by heating PCR samples containing pathogenic bacteria. Then, Tth DNA polymerase was used to successfully transcribe 16S rRNA into complementary DNA (cDNA), which was further employed as a cDNA template for PCR amplification. The thermostable Tth DNA polymerase is obtained from *T. thermophiles* and exhibits optimal activity between 70 and 74°C; therefore, it is suitable for high-temperature PCR. Tth DNA polymerase has intrinsic 5′ → 3′ exonuclease activity but lacks 3′ → 5′ (proofreading) nuclease activity. Tth polymerase is also very effective at reverse transcription in the presence of Mn metal ions, facilitating cDNA synthesis and PCR amplification in a one-step process. Further, as PCR proceeds, the HRPzyme sequence present in the primer is blocked by the formation of double-stranded DNA. Following PCR, the double-stranded HRPzyme sequence prevents the folding of the HRPzyme sequence in the presence of hemin. In contrast, primers that are unincorporated during PCR amplification fold into the G-quadruplex structure in the presence of hemin, oxidizing ABTS and generating a colored product in the presence of H_2O_2. Thus, images of the green PCR products generated from different food pathogens can be captured, and their color intensities were measured using the ImageJ software.

3.2. Feasibility study of the designed strategy

In order to demonstrate the feasibility of this concept, we employed 16S rRNA sequences from various foodborne pathogens as target analytes. According to our previous report [30], this strategy requires two steps for the successful detection of target pathogens: the amplification of target sequences and the subsequent colorimetric signal development. For this reason, we designed 16S rRNA sequence-specific forward and reverse primers containing HRPzyme, protector, and spacer sequences. Under optimized conditions, we confirmed the amplification of 16S rRNA products from *E. coli*. In the agarose gel electrophoresis image, lanes 1 and 2 correspond to samples with and without *E. coli*, respectively (**Figure 2a**). Further, the PCR product could be detected by the generation of a colorimetric signal (**Figure 2b**) as well as the corresponding absorption data (**Figure 2c**). PCR of the negative control (containing no bacteria) did not result in a specific band for the target gene and showed a dark blue color reflecting the presence of unamplified primers.

3.3. Sensitivity and selectivity of proposed study

Based on the optimized conditions, we utilized the proposed detection strategy for the analysis of different foodborne pathogens with HRPzyme-integrated primer sets specific to the 16S rRNA sequences of various bacteria, as shown in **Table 1**. A detailed explanation of the ImageJ-based semiquantitative analysis is illustrated in **Figure 3**. First, a digital image of the green solution is captured using a digital camera. Then, captured images are converted into 32-bit grayscale utilizing the PC-based ImageJ software, and images are inverted (**Figure 3a**). Next, spot areas are individually selected, and their gray intensities are measured (**Figure 3b**). As shown in **Figure 3b**, the performance of the proposed system in the detection of *E. coli* was compared with that of a commercial UV-Vis spectrophotometer, the Tecan Infinite 200 Pro [39]. The results obtained from both systems showed the same linear range from 10^0 to 10^6 cfu mL^{-1} and negligible change in the R^2 value, indicating the applicability of the ImageJ-derived quantitative data for detecting foodborne pathogens.

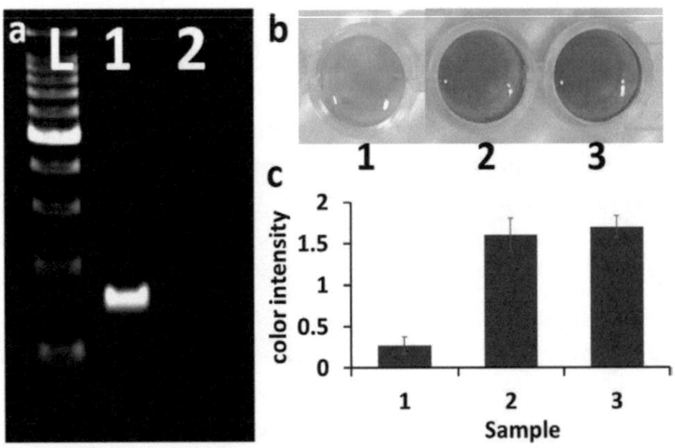

Figure 2. Feasibility study of the colorimetric method involving HRPzyme-blocked PCR for the specific detection of the foodborne pathogen *E. coli* as a model target. (a) Results of agarose gel electrophoresis of diluted PCR products generated using the HRPzyme-integrated primer set. L: DNA marker (100 bp); lane 1: *E. coli* As model target; lane 2: No target bacteria (negative control). (b) Photographs of HRPzyme-integrated PCR colorimetric product. Sample 1: *E. coli*; Sample 2: Negative control; Sample 3: HRPzyme-integrated primer set only. (c) Quantitative results of (b). Error bars represent the standard deviations from three representative experiments (n = 3).

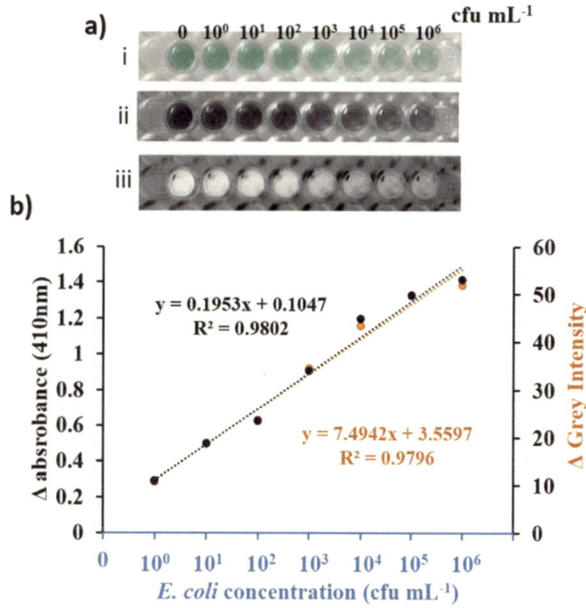

Figure 3. (a) Procedure for ImageJ analysis. (i) a digital image of the colored solution is generated using a digital camera. (ii) the image is converted to 32-bit grayscale utilizing ImageJ. (iii) the image is then inverted. (b) the performance of the proposed system in the detection of *E. coli* was compared with that of a commercial UV-vis spectrophotometer, the tecan infinite 200 pro. Δ absorbance at 410 nm = A0 (without target) – A (with target); Δ gray intensity = blank gray intensity (without target pathogen) – Sample gray intensity (with target pathogen).

Next, we employed this proposed strategy to the detection of different food pathogens. First, we diluted bacteria to different concentrations in the range 0 to 1.0 × 10^6 cfu mL^{-1} in 1× PBS buffer. We then directly employed these diluted samples in PCR amplification without first extracting genomic DNA. After PCR amplification, PCR products of different pathogens were used for colorimetric signal generation. As shown in **Figure 4a**, the electrophoresis gel data reveal the amplification of target gene bands with different concentrations of bacteria. In addition, the results depicted in **Figure 4b** (grayscale images) show that the color intensity signal decreased with increasing concentrations (number of cfu mL^{-1}) of bacteria. The color intensity data show a linear relationship with the concentration of the target pathogens (**Figure 4c**). The standardization curve of Δ gray intensity versus the bacterial concentration (cfu mL^{-1}) exhibited good linearity in the range from 1.0 to 1.0 × 10^6 cfu mL^{-1} (**Figure 4c**). We observed clear differences between negative control samples and those containing various concentrations of bacteria. This strategy showed a 10-fold better performance than the gel electrophoresis-based assay. The proposed method could therefore be used in the diagnosis of pathogenic bacteria without needing to first isolate bacterial genomic DNA.

3.4. Detection specificity

In practical application, the specificity of the detection platform is critical. In order to assess the specificity of the proposed detection strategy, we performed a specificity test using

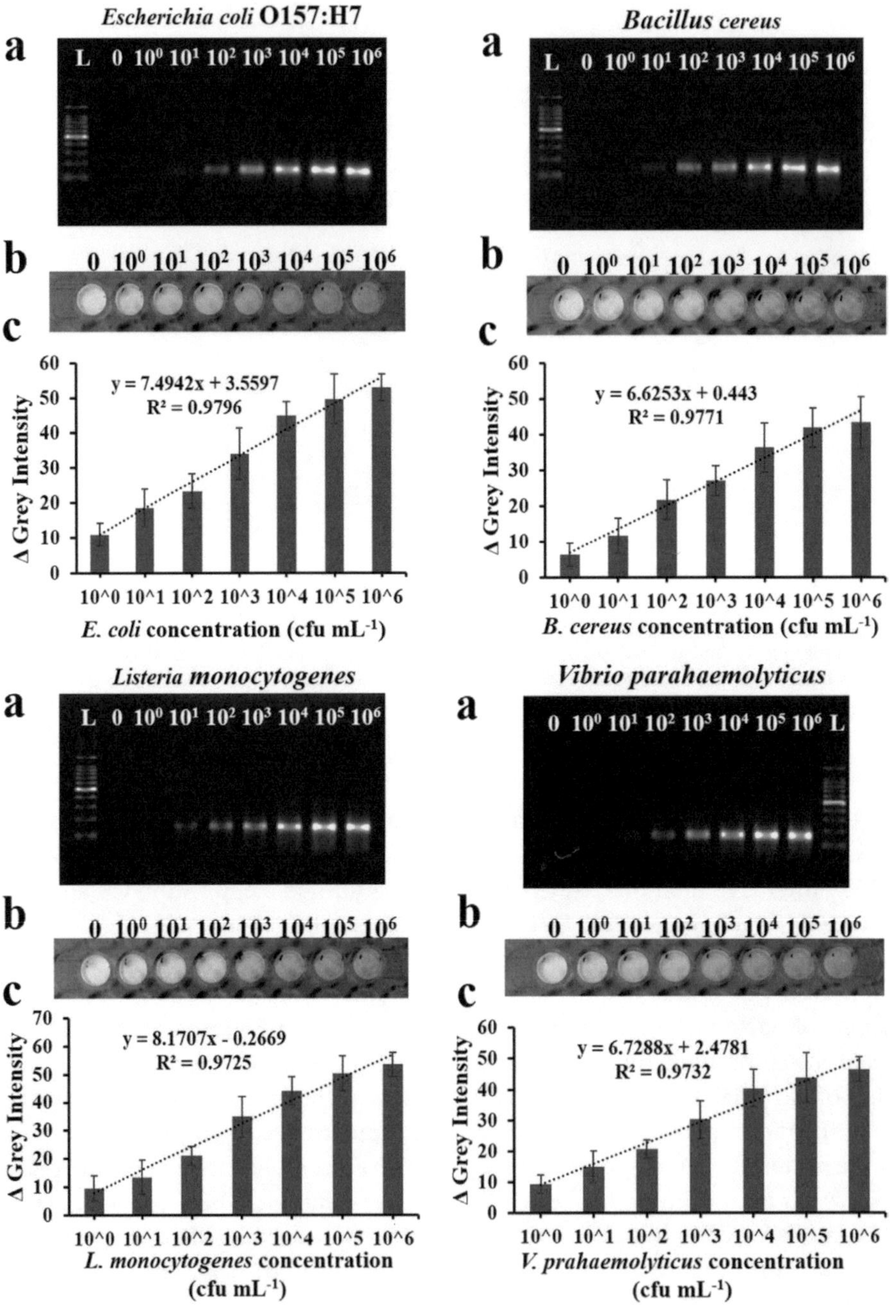

Figure 4. Sensitivity study of HRPzyme-integrated PCR performance in PBS containing different food pathogens (*E. coli* O157:H7, *B. cereus*, *L. monocytogenes*, and *V. parahaemolyticus*). (a) Agarose gel (1.5%) electrophoresis-based analysis. (b) Grayscale images showing different concentrations of bacteria, derived from ImageJ analysis. (c) Δ gray intensities of samples with different concentrations of bacteria, derived from ImageJ analysis. Δ gray intensity = blank gray intensity – Sample gray intensity.

different food pathogens. We successfully demonstrated the selectivity of the method for the detection of several bacteria, including *E. coli* O157:H7, *B. cereus*, *L. monocytogenes*, and *V. parahaemolyticus*, which contain highly homologous 16S rRNA sequences [40, 41]. Selectivity tests including these four pathogens were carried out using the same reaction procedures with the concentration of all pathogens set at 10^4 cfu mL^{-1}. The results are shown in **Figure 5**. We observed specific bands for the target pathogens following 1.5% gel electrophoresis (**Figure 5a**), and the change in color intensity was negligible for nontarget pathogens (**Figure 5b**). This indicates that the PCR products generated during the gene-specific

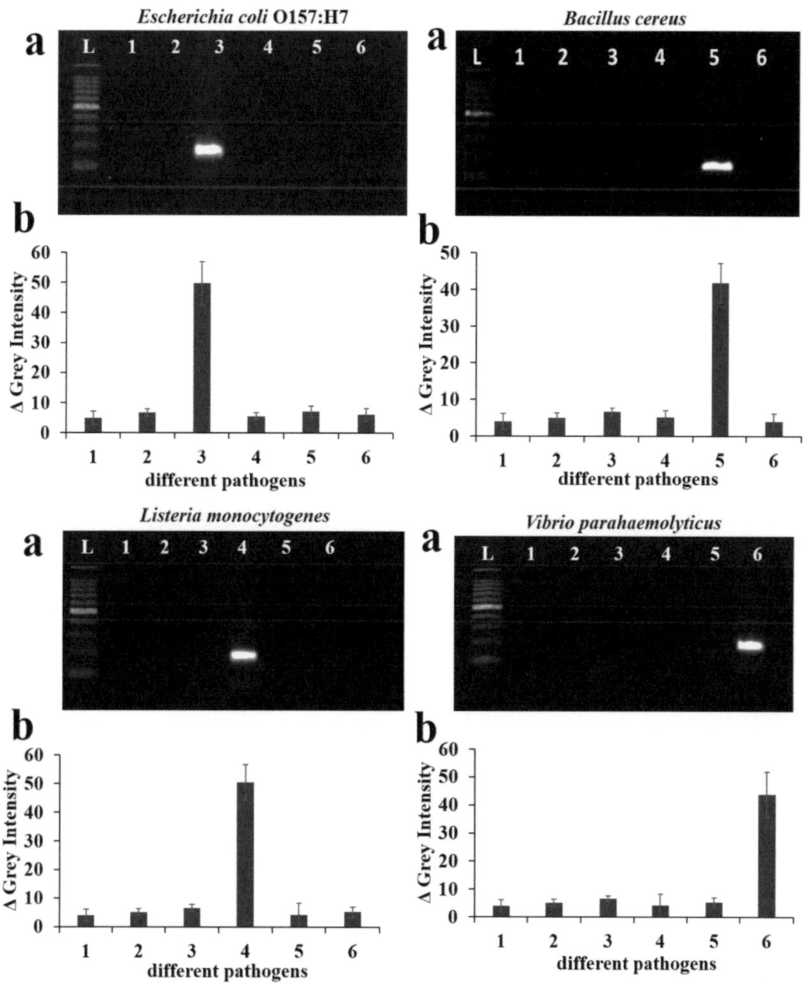

Figure 5. Specificity study of HRPzyme-integrated PCR performed in PBS containing different food pathogens (*E. coli* O157:H7, *B. cereus*, *L. monocytogenes*, and *V. parahaemolyticus*). (a) Agarose gel (1.5%) electrophoresis-based analysis. (b) Δ gray intensities derived from ImageJ analysis. The different pathogens used in this study were *S. enterica* Typhimurium (1), *C. sakazakii* (2), *E. coli* O157:H7 (3), *L. monocytogenes* (4), *B. cereus* (5), and *V. parahaemolyticus* (6).

PCR amplification process successfully blocked the folding of the HRPzyme sequence. In this assay procedure, color generation is dependent upon the application of gene-specific primers integrated with the HRPzyme sequence for the detection of the 16S rRNA sequence, enabling the differentiation of foodborne pathogens. The results in **Figure 5b** show that the presence of the target pathogen results in an intense color intensity signal, while the presence of other food pathogens at the same concentration generates only weak signal. This confirms the high selectivity of the proposed HRPzyme-integrated PCR-based colorimetric strategy for food pathogen detection. Further, in **Table 2**, we have compared our proposed methods with previously reported methods.

3.5. Detection of pathogens from different spiked food samples

A variety of agricultural products have been linked to human illness worldwide. Some agricultural commodities such as fruits and vegetables are more vulnerable to pathogenic bacterial contamination [51]. Therefore, the ability of detection methods to detect pathogens from fresh fruits and vegetables is critical. In this study, we demonstrated the ability of the proposed strategy to detect pathogens among spiked food samples such as apple, chicory, water dropwort, and white radish samples purchased from the local market. Such fruit and vegetable samples contain various biological components [52] such as proteins, phenols, and polysaccharides that may reduce the reliability of the method. **Figure 6** shows the analysis of various food samples spiked with *E. coli*. Based on these results, our method showed good linearity across various concentrations of *E. coli*, indicating the high reliability of the proposed method.

Detection methods	Detection limit (cfu mL^{-1})	Detection range (cfu mL^{-1})	Detection time	Reference
Real-time PCR assay based on immunomagnetic separation	1.0×10^1–1.0×10^4	10	1.2 hrs	[42]
Immunosensors	1.0×10^4–1.0×10^8	1.0×10^5	1.5 hrs	[43]
Antibody-aptamer Sandwich ELISA	1.0×10^3–1.0×10^8	1.0×10^3	<3 hrs	[44]
Selective filtration technique combined with antibody–magnetic nanoparticle nanocomposites	2.0×10^1–2.0×10^4	20	45 min	[45]
Aptasensor, gold-nanoparticles aggregation	1.0×10^2–1.0×10^7	56	1 hr	[46]
Immuno-PCR	1.0×10^3–1.0×10^5	1.0×10^3	4 hrs	[47]
Antibody-conjugated magnetic nanoparticles (MNPs)	1.0×10^2–1.0×10^8	100	1 hr	[48]
Aptasensor, peroxidase mimics magnetic nanoparticles	Not given	7.5×10^5	1 hr	[49]
Aptasensor, gold-nanoparticles aggregation	1.0×10^1–1.0×10^6	10	4 hrs	[50]
HRPzyme-Integrated Polymerase Chain Reaction	1.0×10^0–1.0×10^6	1	~1.2 hrs	This study

Table 2. Comparative study of the proposed method with previously reported methods of foodborne pathogen detection.

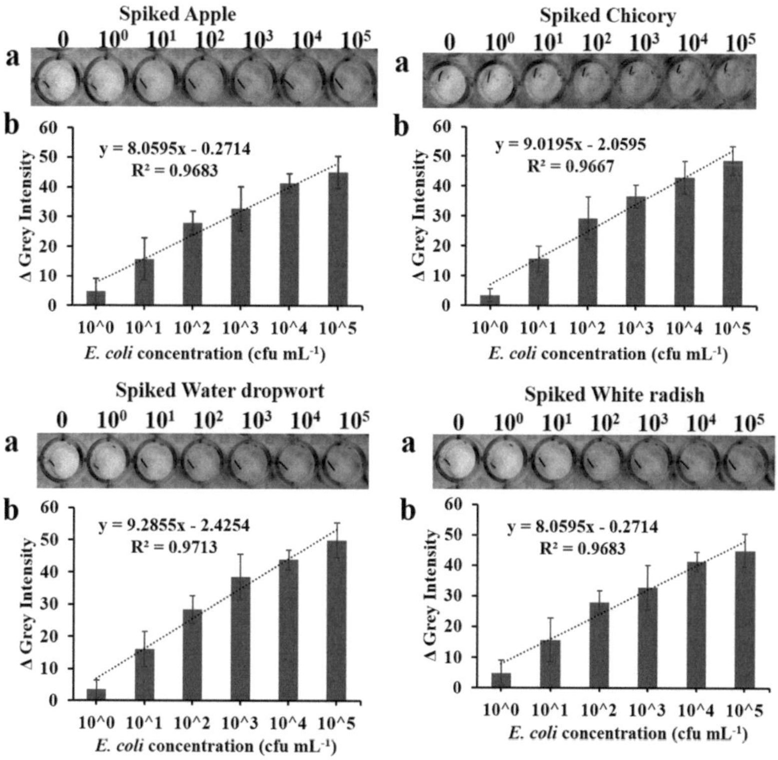

Figure 6. Linear relationship between Δ gray intensity and bacterial concentrations from 0 to 10^5 cfu mL^{-1} in spiked samples such as apple, chicory, water dropwort, and white radish. (a) Grayscale image. (b) Δ gray intensities of different concentrations, derived from ImageJ analysis.

4. Conclusions

In this study, we demonstrated the performance of the HRPzyme-integrated PCR-based colorimetric method for the simple, sensitive, and selective detection of 16S rRNA sequences from various food pathogens. The proposed strategy showed several advantages such as label-free, simple and easy procedure, ultrasensitive (detection limit up to single cfu mL^{-1}), highly selective, detection within 70 min, affordable at remote areas, easily integrated into smartphone-based image processor. PCR amplification is carried out with 16S rRNA-specific primers modified at the 5′-end with HRPzyme sequences. After PCR, in the presence of hemin, unamplified primers fold into a G-quadruplex structure, and a colorimetric signal is then generated in the presence of a chromogenic substrate. We successfully detected the presence of foodborne bacteria, including *E. coli* O157:H7, *B. cereus*, *L. monocytogenes*, and *V. parahaemolyticus* at levels as low as a single cfu mL^{-1} in buffer as well as in spiked fruit and vegetable samples. We believe that this method could be employed in the detection of pathogenic bacteria from biological samples by simply modifying existing primers with the HRPzyme sequence at the 5′ end. Further, this method could be integrated with a field-portable PCR instrument for the on-site detection of pathogens in resource-limited areas.

Acknowledgements

This research was supported by a grant from the World Institute of Kimchi, funded by the Ministry of Science, ICT and Future Planning (KE1701-5), Republic of Korea, and by the GIST (Gwangju Institute of Science and Technology), Korea, under the Practical Research and Development support program, supervised by the GTI (GIST Technology Institute), Republic of Korea.

Conflict of interest

The authors declare no financial or commercial conflict of interest.

Author details

Bhagwan S. Batule[1], Seong U. Kim[2], Hyoyoung Mun[1], Won-Bo Shim[3] and Min-Gon Kim[1,2]*

*Address all correspondence to: mkim@gist.ac.kr

1 Department of Chemistry, School of Physics and Chemistry, Gwangju Institute of Science and Technology, Gwangju, Republic of Korea

2 Advanced Photonics Research Institute, Gwangju Institute of Science and Technology, Gwangju, Republic of Korea

3 Department of Agricultural Chemistry and Food Science and Technology, Gyeongsang National University, Republic of Korea

References

[1] Priyanka B, Patil RK, Dwarakanath SA. Review on detection methods used for food-borne pathogens. The Indian Journal of Medical Research. 2016;**144**(3):327-338. DOI: 10.4103/0971-5916.198677

[2] Scallan E, Hoekstra RM, Angulo FJ, Tauxe RV, Widdowson M-A, Roy SL, et al. Foodborne illness acquired in the United States—Major pathogens. Emerging Infectious Diseases. 2011;**17**(1):7-15. DOI: 10.3201/eid1701.P11101

[3] Mandal P, Biswas A, Choi K, Pal U. Methods for rapid detection of foodborne pathogens: An overview. American Journal of Food Technology. 2011;**6**(2):87-102. DOI: 10.3923/ajft.2011.87.102

[4] Velusamy V, Arshak K, Korostynska O, Oliwa K, Adley C. An overview of food-borne pathogen detection: In the perspective of biosensors. Biotechnology Advances. 2010;**28**(2):232-254. DOI: 10.1016/j.biotechadv.2009.12.004

[5] Zhao X, Lin C-W, Wang J, Oh DH. Advances in rapid detection methods for food-borne pathogens. Journal of Microbiology and Biotechnology. 2014;**24**(3):297-312. DOI: 10.4014/jmb.1310.10013

[6] Jokerst JC, Adkins JA, Bisha B, Mentele MM, Goodridge LD, Henry CS. Development of a paper-based analytical device for colorimetric detection of select foodborne pathogens. Analytical Chemistry. 2012;**84**(6):2900-2907. DOI: 10.1021/ac203466y

[7] King W, Raposa S, Warshaw J, Johnson A, Halbert D, Klinger J. A new colorimetric nucleic acid hybridization assay for *Listeria* in foods. International Journal of Food Microbiology. 1989;**8**(3):225-232. DOI: 10.1016/0168-1605(89)90017-2

[8] Feng P. Impact of molecular biology on the detection of foodborne pathogens. Molecular Biotechnology. 1997;**7**(3):267-278. DOI: 10.1007/BF02740817

[9] Wang RF, Cao WW, Cerniglia C. A universal protocol for PCR detection of 13 species of foodborne pathogens in foods. Journal of Applied Microbiology. 1997;**83**(6):727-736. DOI: 10.1046/j.1365-2672.1997.00300.x

[10] Lampel KA, Orlandi PA, Kornegay L. Improved template preparation for PCR-based assays for detection of food-borne bacterial pathogens. Applied and Environmental Microbiology. 2000;**66**(10):4539-4542. DOI: 10.1128/AEM.66.10.4539-4542.2000

[11] O'sullivan N, Fallon R, Carroll C, Smith T, Maher M. Detection and differentiation of *Campylobacter jejuni* and *Campylobacter coli* in broiler chicken samples using a PCR/DNA probe membrane based colorimetric detection assay. Molecular and Cellular Probes. 2000;**14**(1):7-16. DOI: 10.1006/mcpr.1999.0274

[12] Naravaneni R, Jamil K. Rapid detection of food-borne pathogens by using molecular techniques. Journal of Medical Microbiology. 2005;**54**(1):51-54. DOI: 10.1099/jmm.0.45687-0

[13] Wei S, Zhao H, Xian Y, Hussain MA, Wu X. Multiplex PCR assays for the detection of *Vibrio alginolyticus, Vibrio parahaemolyticus, Vibrio vulnificus,* and *Vibrio cholerae* with an internal amplification control. Diagnostic Microbiology and Infectious Disease. 2014;**79**(2):115-118. DOI: 10.1016/j.diagmicrobio.2014.03.012

[14] Xu X, Qiao J, Li N, Qi L, Zhang S. Fluorescent probe for turn-on sensing of L-cysteine by ensemble of AuNCs and polymer protected AuNPs. Analytica Chimica Acta. 2015;**879**: 97-103. DOI: 10.1016/j.aca.2015.03.036

[15] Kim S, Ngoc HT, Kim J, Yoo SY, Chung H. Toehold-mediated DNA displacement-based surface-enhanced raman scattering DNA sensor utilizing an au–ag bimetallic nanodendrite substrate. Analytica Chimica Acta. 2015;**885**:132-139. DOI: 10.1016/j.aca.2015.04.037

[16] Mao K, Liu Y, Xiao H, Chen Y, Wu Z, Zhou X, et al. A novel platform for detection of protooncogene based on Au nanocluster enhanced fluorescence. Analytical Methods. 2015;**7**(1):40-44. DOI: 10.1039/C4AY02117G

[17] Raghunath P, Karunasagar I, Karunasagar I. Improved isolation and detection of pathogenic *Vibrio parahaemolyticus* from seafood using a new enrichment broth. International Journal of Food Microbiology. 2009;**129**(2):200-203. DOI: 10.1016/j.ijfoodmicro.2008.11.026

[18] Duan N, Wu S, Chen X, Huang Y, Wang Z. Selection and identification of a DNA aptamer targeted to *Vibrio parahemolyticus*. Journal of Agricultural and Food Chemistry. 2012;**60**(16):4034-4038. DOI: 10.1021/jf300395z

[19] Wu S, Duan N, Shi Z, Fang C, Wang Z. Simultaneous aptasensor for multiplex pathogenic bacteria detection based on multicolor upconversion nanoparticles labels. Analytical Chemistry. 2014;**86**(6):3100-3107. DOI: 10.1021/ac404205c

[20] Duan N, Wu S, Zhu C, Ma X, Wang Z, Yu Y, et al. Dual-color upconversion fluorescence and aptamer-functionalized magnetic nanoparticles-based bioassay for the simultaneous detection of *Salmonella* typhimurium and *Staphylococcus aureus*. Analytica Chimica Acta. 2012;**723**:1-6. DOI: 10.1016/j.aca.2012.02.011

[21] Travascio P, Witting PK, Mauk AG, Sen D. The peroxidase activity of a hemin–DNA oligonucleotide complex: Free radical damage to specific guanine bases of the DNA. Journal of the Americal Chemical Society. 2001;**123**(7):1337-1348. DOI: 10.1021/ja0023534

[22] Chinnapen DJ, Sen D. Hemin-stimulated docking of cytochrome c to a hemin–DNA aptamer complex. Biochemistry. 2002;**41**(16):5202-5212. DOI: 0.1021/bi015785f

[23] Pavlov V, Xiao Y, Gill R, Dishon A, Kotler M, Willner I. Amplified chemiluminescence surface detection of DNA and telomerase activity using catalytic nucleic acid labels. Analytical Chemistry. 2004;**76**(7):2152-2156. DOI: 10.1021/ac0352191

[24] Wang G, Zhu Y, He X, Chen L, Wang L, Zhang X. Colorimetric and visual determination of melamine by exploiting the conformational change of hemin G-quadruplex-DNAzyme. Microchimica Acta. 2014;**181**(3-4):411-418. DOI: 10.1007/s00604-013-1122-4

[25] Li T, Wang E, Dong S. G-quadruplex-based DNAzyme for facile colorimetric detection of thrombin. Chemical Communications. 2008:3654-3656. DOI: 10.1039/B805565C

[26] Ali MM, Li Y. Colorimetric sensing by using allosteric-DNAzyme-coupled rolling circle amplification and a peptide nucleic acid–organic dye probe. Angewandte Chemie. 2009;**121**(19):3564-3567. DOI: 10.1002/ange.200805966

[27] Yin BC, Ye BC, Tan W, Wang H, Xie CC. An allosteric dual-DNAzyme unimolecular probe for colorimetric detection of copper (II). Journal of the American Chemical Society. 2009;**131**(41):14624-14625. DOI: 10.1021/ja9062426

[28] Cheng K, Pan D, Teng J, Yao L, Ye Y, Xue F, et al. Colorimetric integrated pCR protocol for rapid detection of *Vibrio parahaemolyticus*. Sensors. 2016;**16**(10):1600. DOI: 10.3390/s16101600

[29] Bhadra S, Codrea V, Ellington AD. G-quadruplex-generating polymerase chain reaction for visual colorimetric detection of amplicons. Analytical Biochemistry. 2014;**445**:38-40. DOI: 10.1016/j.ab.2013.10.010

[30] Seok Y, Byun JY, Mun H, Kim MG. Colorimetric detection of PCR products of DNA from pathogenic bacterial targets based on a simultaneously amplified DNAzyme. Microchimica Acta. 2014;**181**(15-16):1965-1971. DOI: 10.1007/s00604-014-1297-3

[31] Cheglakov Z, Weizmann Y, Beissenhirtz MK, Willner I. Ultrasensitive detection of DNA by the PCR-induced generation of DNAzymes: The DNAzyme primer approach. Chemical Communications. 2006:3205-3207. DOI: 10.1039/B605205C

[32] Cheng X, Liu X, Bing T, Cao Z, Shangguan D. General peroxidase activity of G-quadruplex– hemin complexes and its application in ligand screening. Biochemistry. 2009;**48**(33):7817-7823. DOI: 10.1021/bi9006786

[33] Travascio P, Li Y, Sen D. DNA-enhanced peroxidase activity of a DNA aptamer-hemin complex. Chemistry & Biology. 1998;**5**(9):505-517. DOI: 10.1016/S1074-5521(98)90006-0

[34] Chakravorty S, Helb D, Burday M, Connell N, Alland D. A detailed analysis of 16S ribosomal RNA gene segments for the diagnosis of pathogenic bacteria. Journal of Microbiological Methods. 2007;**69**(2):330-339. DOI: 10.1016/j.mimet.2007.02.005

[35] Kim SU, Batule BS, Mun H, Shim W-B, Kim MG. Ultrasensitive colorimetric detection of *Salmonella enterica* typhimurium on lettuce leaves by HRPzyme-integrated polymerase chain reaction. Food Control. 2018;**84**:522-528. DOI: 10.1016/j.foodcont.2017.09.010

[36] Rajwa B, Mcnally HA, Varadharajan P, Sturgis J, Robinson JP. AFM/CLSM data visualization and comparison using an open-source toolkit. Microscopy Research and Technique. 2004;**64**(2):176-184. DOI: 10.1002/jemt.20067

[37] Busa LSA, Maeki M, Ishida A, Tani H, Tokeshi M. Simple and sensitive colorimetric assay system for horseradish peroxidase using microfluidic paper-based devices. Sensors and Actuators B: Chemical. 2016;**236**:433-441. DOI: 10.1016/j.snb.2016.06.013

[38] Busa LSA, Komatsu T, Mohammadi S, Maeki M, Ishida A, Tani H, et al. 3, 3′, 5, 5′-Tetramethylbenzidine oxidation on paper devices for horseradish peroxidase-based assays. Analytical Sciences. 2016;**32**(8):815-818. DOI: 10.2116/analsci.32.815

[39] Gautam S, Batule BS, Kim HY, Park KS, Park HG. Smartphone-based portable wireless optical system for the detection of target analytes. Biotechnology Journal. 2017;**12**(2):1-9. DOI: 10.1002/biot.201600581

[40] Yu J, Zhang Y, Li H, Yang H, Wei H. Sensitive and rapid detection of *Staphylococcus aureus* in milk via cell binding domain of lysin. Biosensors and Bioelectronics. 2016;**77**:366-371. DOI: 10.1016/j.bios.2015.09.058

[41] Rohde A, Hammerl JA, Boone I, Jansen W, Fohler S, Klein G, et al. Overview of validated alternative methods for the detection of foodborne bacterial pathogens. Trends in Food Science & Technology. 2017;**62**:113-118. DOI: 10.1016/j.tifs.2017.02.006

[42] Ma K, Deng Y, Bai Y, Xu D, Chen E, Wu H, et al. Rapid and simultaneous detection of *Salmonella, Shigella,* and *Staphylococcus aureus* in fresh pork using a multiplex real-time PCR assay based on immunomagnetic separation. Food Control. 2014;**42**:87-93. DOI: 10.1016/j.foodcont.2014.01.042

[43] Singh C, Agarwal GS, Rai GP, Singh L, Rao VK. Specific detection of *Salmonella Typhi* using renewable amperometric immunosensor. Electroanalysis. 2005;**17**(22):2062-2067. DOI: 10.1002/elan.200403334

[44] Wu W, Li J, Pan D, Li J, Song S, Rong M, et al. Gold nanoparticle-based enzyme-linked antibody-aptamer sandwich assay for detection of *Salmonella* typhimurium. ACS Applied Materials & Interfaces. 2014;**6**(19):16974-16981. DOI: 10.1021/am5045828

[45] Shim W-B, Song J-E, Mun H, Chung D-H, Kim M-G. Rapid colorimetric detection of *Salmonella* typhimurium using a selective filtration technique combined with antibody–magnetic nanoparticle nanocomposites. Analytical and Bioanalytical Chemistry. 2014;**406**(3):859-866. DOI: 10.1007/s00216-013-7497-6

[46] Ma X, Song L, Zhou N, Xia Y, Wang ZA. Novel aptasensor for the colorimetric detection of *S.* Typhimurium based on gold nanoparticles. International Journal of Food Microbiology. 2017;**245**:1-5. DOI: 10.1016/j.ijfoodmicro.2016.12.024

[47] Bakthavathsalam P, Rajendran VK, Saran U, Chatterjee S, Ali BMJ. Immunomagnetic nanoparticle based quantitative PCR for rapid detection of *Salmonella*. Microchimica Acta. 2013;**180**(13-14):1241-1248. DOI: 10.1007/s00604-013-1052-1

[48] Joo J, Yim C, Kwon D, Lee J, Shin HH, Cha HJ, et al. A facile and sensitive detection of pathogenic bacteria using magnetic nanoparticles and optical nanocrystal probes. The Analyst. 2012;**137**(16):3609-3612. DOI: 10.1039/C2AN35369E

[49] Park JY, Jeong HY, Kim MI, Park TJ. Colorimetric detection system for *Salmonella* typhimurium based on peroxidase-like activity of magnetic nanoparticles with DNA aptamers. Journal of Nanomaterials. 2015;**2015**:2. DOI: 10.1155/2015/527126

[50] Zhu C, Hong Y, Xiao Z, Zhou Y, Jiang Y, Huang M, et al. Colorimetric determination of *Salmonella* typhimurium based on aptamer recognition. Analytical Methods. 2016;**8**(35):6560-6565. DOI: 10.1039/C6AY01918H

[51] Denis N, Zhang H, Leroux A, Trudel R, Bietlot H. Prevalence and trends of bacterial contamination in fresh fruits and vegetables sold at retail in Canada. Food Control. 2016;**67**:225-234. DOI: 10.1016/j.foodcont.2016.02.047

[52] Schrader C, Schielke A, Ellerbroek L, Johne R. PCR inhibitors–occurrence, properties and removal. Journal of Applied Microbiology. 2012;**113**(5):1014-1026. DOI: 10.1111/j.1365-2672.2012.05384.x

FRET-Based Enzyme Activity Reporter: Practical Hints for Kinases as Indicators of Virulence

Corentin Spriet, Angelina Kasprowicz,
Dave Trinel and Jean-François Bodart

Additional information is available at the end of the chapter

http://dx.doi.org/10.5772/intechopen.72388

Abstract

Modulation of protein kinases activity is often requested for pathogenicity or virulence. This chapter provides several hints for one who might be interested in using FRET-based kinase activity reporters. The archetypes of these reporters, which are now within the arsenal of biosensors, were devoted to the detection and characterization of the activity of the cAMP-Protein kinase A pathway. Based on the principle of this biosensor, other FRET-based kinase activity reporters emerged. Here, the choice of the kinase to be monitored, the artifacts that might be met, and the flexibility and amenability of the FRET-based kinase activity reporters both for high-throughput analysis and dissection of protein kinase functions are discussed.

Keywords: genetically encoded biosensor, KAR, fret, MAPK, ERK

1. Introduction

Biological signatures of parasitic diseases may (1) involve the production and release of specific proteases, which are called to promote host invasion, to evade host defenses or to provide nutrients from the local environment [1] or (2) rely on the modulation of specific protein kinases activity such as mitogen-activated protein kinase (MAPK)/extracellular regulated kinase (Erk, *Toxoplasma gondii* [2], *Leishmania* spp. and *Trypanosoma cruzi* [3]). The abovementioned enzymes have been regarded from two angles, leading either to the development of inhibitory strategies or biosensors development [4].

Herein, we discuss several aspects related to use of biosensors in living cell contexts, which are of high interest in the perspective of biosensing in living organisms. Nevertheless, we restrain our talk to signaling pathways and focus on protein kinases. One shall note that biosensor is a generic term describing the various analytical devices incorporating a biological sensing element. Back in the 1980s, biosensors were mainly either sophisticated laboratory machines or amenable portable devices [5] based on electric currents [6] or conductivity [7]; optical properties [8] or other physico-chemical measurements. In the 1990s, emerged a plethora of new tools, conforming to the biosensor definition, and reporting enzymes activities. The latter were built and developed in different contexts (living cells, lysates), aiming at benefiting either from high sensitivity or selectivity. To these extents, devices like amperometric biosensors [9], bioluminescent-based sensors *in vivo* [10, 11] and functionalized nanoparticles were used [12, 13], exhibiting high sensitivity and selectivity, which are mandatory for diagnosis, especially in case of pathogens [14].

Among biosensors, genetically encoded Förster Resonance Energy Transfer (FRET) biosensors raised hope to focus on both enzymatic activities and ion concentration with high spatiotemporal resolution in both living cells and organisms. It relies on Förster Resonance Energy Transfer, or FRET, a radiationless coupling from a donor fluorophore to an acceptor molecule. Several conditions must be met for this transfer to occur (spectral overlap between fluorophore, dipole relative orientation or distance). The most useful property is that the donor and acceptor molecules must be in close vicinity (for commonly used fluorophore pairs, <10 nm) and that the FRET level depends on the sixth power of the distance between fluorophores. FRET biosensors are thus built to switch between two configurations where the distance between donor and acceptor are above and below this threshold distance (**Figure 1**). They are made of an adapted

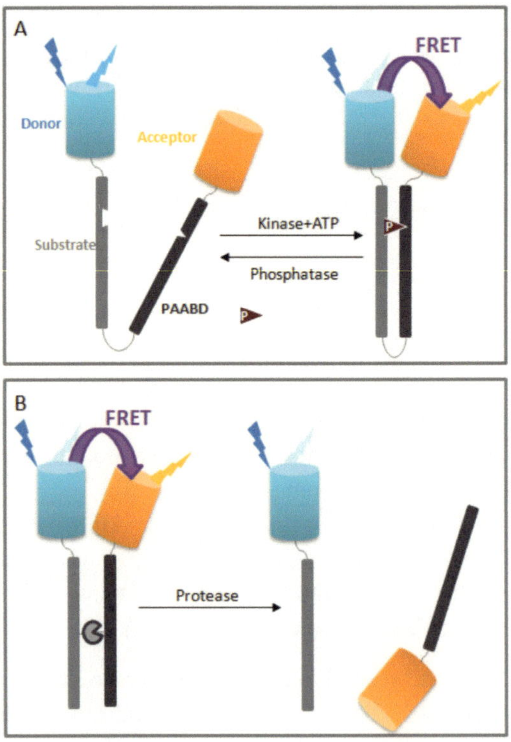

Figure 1. Scheme representing two categories of FRET-based biosensors. A, Kinase activity reporters reflect the balance between specific kinase and phosphatase; protease reporters (B) rely on an irreversible cleavage. Regarding interpretation, an increase in kinase activity will be reflected by an increase in FRET level, while the protease activation will induce a loss in the original FRET signal.

bioreceptor tagged on both end with a donor and acceptor. The biosensor configuration will be specifically altered by the presence of either a second messenger or the action of an enzyme, inducing either an increase or decrease in FRET efficiency. A FRET event will induce changes in most properties of light such as fluorophores excitation and emission or donor fluorescence polarization or lifetime. A variety of fluorescence-based methods are then derived from these changes to quantify biosensors' response with associated fluorescence microscopy benefits (selectivity, low toxicity, high temporal and spatial resolution, optical sectioning, etc.).

2. Kinase activity reporter archetypes

Being two FRET-based biosensors for protein kinase A activity, protein kinase A activity reporter (AKAR) and exchange proteins activated by cAMP (Epac) are considered as the archetypes for genetically encoded FRET reporters. Activity of protein kinase A (PKA) is controlled by cyclic adenosine monophosphate (cAMP) levels, which behaves as a second messenger for many cellular responses driven by external stimuli. The tandem cAMP-PKA is considered to play many essential functions within cellular life like cell cycle [15]. cAMP concentration is regulated by the activity of adenylyl cyclase, the latter being activated by G protein coupled receptor (GPCR), upon the specific interaction with its ligand. Under its inactive state, PKA is made up of regulatory subunit dimers associated with catalytic subunit dimers. The activation of PKA requests the fixation of four molecules of cAMP that are catalyzed on the regulatory subunit. Such fixation of the cAMP leads the catalytic dimer to dissociate (**Figure 2**). Counteracting the activity of adenylyl cyclase and phosphodiesterase downregulates PKA activity through cAMP degradation.

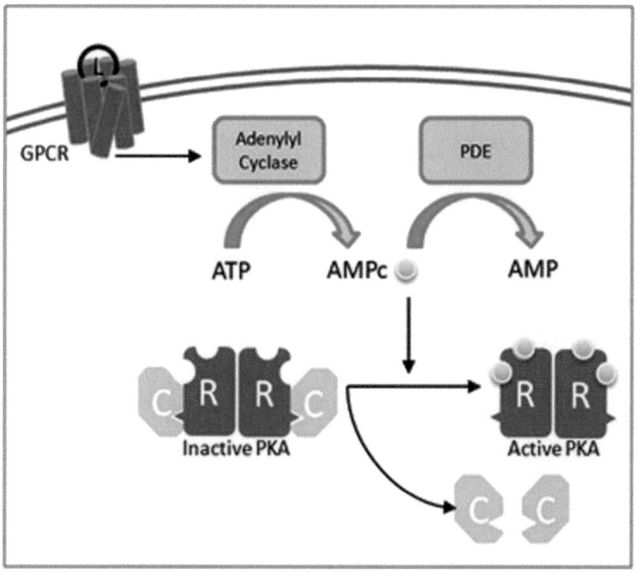

Figure 2. Focus on the PKA and cAMP signaling node. GPCR (G protein coupled receptor), R (regulatory subunit), C (catalytic subunit) of protein kinase A and PDE (PhosphoDiEsterase).

As mentioned earlier, two FRET-based biosensors have been developed and devoted to study the dynamics of c-AMP-PKA, mainly to overcome the shortcomings of the classical biochemical methodologies and to monitor individual cellular responses, which can either be sub-localized or transient. Both biosensors were based upon a similar structure: a specific phosphorylable peptide and a phosphoamino acid binding domain (PAABD), standing together between two fluorophores [16]. When phosphorylated, the peptide sequence interacts with PAABD, driving a conformational change bringing the fluorescent proteins in close vicinity. The latter enables the FRET to occur and provides measurable changes acknowledging for the activity of the considered enzyme, here PKA in case of AKAR. While AKAR mirrors the activities of kinase/phosphatases on a specific substrate of PKA [17], Epac proteins aimed at measuring the changes in

Specificity	Sensor name	References
Abl (Abelson murine leukemia viral oncogene homolog 1)	Crk indicator	*(Ting et al. 2001) [18]*
	EGFR indicator	*(Ting et al. 2001) [18]*
	PICCHU	*(Kurokawa et al. 2001) [19]*
Akt/PKB (Protein Kinase B)	AktAR	*(Gao and Zhang 2008) [20]*
	Aktus	*(Sato and Umezawa 2004) [21]*
	Akind	*(Yoshizaki et al. 2006) [22]*
	BKAR	*(Kunkel et al. 2005) [23]*
	GFP-PKB-RFP	*(Calleja et al. 2007) [24]*
	ReAktion	*(Ananthanarayanan et al. 2007) [25]*
AMPK (AMP-activated protein kinase)	AMPKAR	*(Tsou et al. 2011) [26]*
Aurora B kinase	Aurora B sensor	*(Chu et al. 2011) [27]*
ATM kinase	ATOMIC	*(Johnson, You, and Hunter 2007) [28]*
CyclineB1/cdk1	CyclineB1/cdk1 sensor	*(Gavet and Pines 2010) [29]*
EGFR (Epidermal Growth Factor Receptor)	EGFR-ECFP/PTV-EYFP	*(Offterdinger et al. 2004) [30]*
ERK (Extracellular signal-regulated kinase)	EKAR	*(Harvey et al. 2008) [31]*
	EAS	*(Green and Alberola 2005) [32]*
	Miu2	*(Fujioka et al. 2006) [33]*
FAK (Focal adhesion kinase)	FAK sensor	*(Seong et al. 2011) [34]*
Glucokinase	mCer-GCK-mVenus	*(Ding et al. 2011) [35]*
Histone H3 phosphorylation	H3 Reporter	*(Lin and Ting 2004) [36]*
Insulin receptor	Phocus	*(Sato and Umezawa 2004) [21]*
JNK	JNKAR	*(Fosbrink et al. 2010) [37]*
MK2 (MAP kinase activated protein kinase 2)	EGFP-MK2-EBFP	*(Neininger, Thielemann, and Gaestel 2001) [38]*
MARK (Microtubule affinity regulating kinase)	MARK sensor	*(Timm et al. 2011) [39]*
PLK1 (Polo like kinase 1)	Plk sensor	*(Macůrek et al. 2008) [40]*
PKA (Protein kinase A)	AKAR	*(Zhang et al. 2007) [41]*
	ART	*(Nagai et al. 2000) [42]*
PKC (Protein kinase C)	CKAR	*(Violin et al. 2003) [43]*
RSK (Ribosomal s6 kinase)	Eevee-RSK	*(Komatsu et al. 2011) [44]*
	Eevee-S6K	*(Komatsu et al. 2011) [44]*
Stress-activated protein kinase kinase kinase (SAP3K)	SAP3K activity reporter	*(Tomida et al. 2009) [45]*
Src (Proto-oncogene tyrosine-protein kinase)	Srcus	*(Sato and Umezawa 2004) [21]*
	Src indicator	*(Ting et al. 2001) [18]*

Table 1. Kinase activity reporters and associated references.

http://dx.doi.org/10.5772/intechopen.72388

concentration of cAMP. These biosensors unfold their structure upon the fixation of cAMP and break the vicinity of the donor and acceptor fluorescent proteins. Thus, while FRET increase is related to an increase in PKA activity in case of AKAR, a decrease in FRET activity is related to the increase of cAMP levels. The two biosensors provided complementary information regarding the levels of cAMP and PKA, being two angles of a same pathway.

From the initial development of kinase-specific biosensor for cAMP and kinases, several derivatives have been built as illustrated by the extracellular signal regulated kinase activity reporter (EKAR) variants (see **Table 1**) [18–45]. Indeed, kinase activity reporters (KAR) follow fluorophores' optimizations for FRET assay, thereby increasing their sensitivity and robustness. Furthermore, microscopy measurements allow sub-localization of kinase activity, which may be mandatory for the understanding of signaling nodes. KAR versions directed toward the different subcellular compartments were thus developed.

3. Choosing the right kinase activity to report: the needle in a haystack

Biological messages are mediated by intracellular signaling pathways, whose dynamics and interplays have not yet been fully deciphered. Biosensors are focused on specific elements of the networks conveying the information and interpretation shall be carried out accordingly. One has to carefully consider the complexity of pathways where protein kinases could be nodes within networks (**Figure 3**) [46]. Monitoring the phosphorylation of one particular sequence within the sensors will not necessarily reflect its involvement in all functions of the considered kinase.

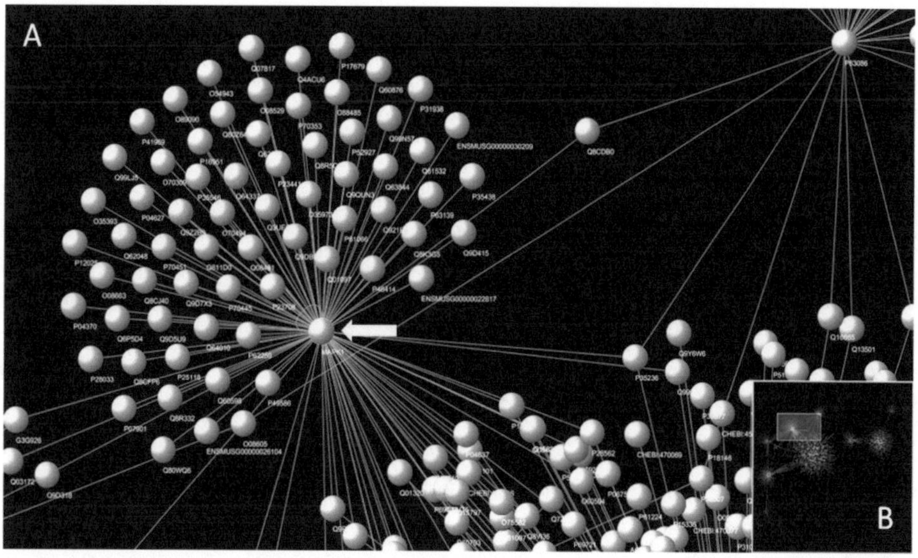

Figure 3. Scheme of MAPK1 interactom generated through Cytoscape. MAPK1 is highlighted by the white arrow, spheres correspond to interactors. A focus on MAPK1 node and B represent the overall network.

Modulation of protein kinase activities might be requested for pathogenicity or virulence [47]. Mitogen-activated protein kinase (MAPK)/extracellular regulated kinases (Erk) can be taken as a school case, since the latter activity is solicited in many different aspect of cellular life, that is, proliferation, migration and differentiation. On the one hand, MAPK are inhibited by several pathogens such as anthrax [48, 49], mycobacteria [50], *Vibrio parahaemolyticus* [51], herpes simplex virus 1 (HSV-1) [52] or *Yersinia* spp. [53]. Activation of MAPK/Erk can also be manipulated by diverse families of virus to favor their replication. For example, enteropathogenic coronavirus like the porcine epidemic diarrhea virus are infecting cells, due to the activity of MAPK/Erk [54]. Impairing the activation of MAPK drives the suppression of viral progeny production. As well, MAPK activity might be enrolled in human immunodeficiency virus of type 1 (HIV-1) replication [55]. Increase in other protein kinase activities may be requested for life cycle of other pathogens. A recent meta-analysis of data from different ribonucleic acid interference (RNAi) screening revealed a potential role for the members of Polo-like kinase for *Influenza A* virus infections [56]. Therefore, the latter Polo-kinase (Plk), which was more known for its pivotal role in cell cycle regulation, appeared as a therapeutic target and was extracted likely as a needle out of a haystack. Nevertheless, the function of Plk in this context remains elusive, but Plk might be required for the *Influenza* viral infection through the creation of an optimal environment for viral replication by balancing the apoptotic and antiapoptotic signaling pathways [57].

In this context, after identifying the hijacked node, researcher needs to monitor the pathogenic modulation of the kinase/phosphatase balance. FRET-based biosensors are thus optimal tool for dissecting these subtle alterations, far from binary modifications.

4. Discarding artifacts: chemical inhibitors and dead reporters

Insights gained by genetically engineered enzyme reporters are solely validated through adequate controls. Any response gathered using biosensors shall be carefully considered and fully analyzed: what you might see may not be what you will get as a response at the end of the analysis procedure [58]. Among other parameters, consensus sequence of the phosphorylable peptide, expression levels, kinetics and dynamic ranges have, for example, to be taken in account.

The choice of the peptide substrate is crucial and has to be defined accordingly to the specificity of the kinase, if known. For example, there is a current failure to determine a consensus site for p38MAPK. The latter inability to determine a sequence consensus hinders the amenability to construct any KAR for this particular kinase. The process of the KAR design can be optimized through a screening strategy for the best phosphopeptide sequence [59] or the linkers between the different segments and/or the fluorophores [17].

One shall also take a particular care to discriminate a specific response from the noise within the crowded environment of the intracellular compartments. The cellular noise depends upon the biophysical properties of the chosen cell lines to work with, as well as results from cell autofluorescence, intracellular pH and biosensors expression levels. In case of KAR, morphological changes are likely not to alter the signals, as observed for monitoring cyclin-dependent kinase 1 (Cdk1) activity during cell rounding at the beginning of mitosis [60].

http://dx.doi.org/10.5772/intechopen.72388

To discriminate the noise, several options might be undertaken to determinate the specificity and dynamical range of response. First is the use of chemical inhibitors to separate the balance of kinase/phosphatase activity from the cellular noise (*i.e.,* Cdk1/2 inhibitor of RO3306 for Cdk1 KAR [60] or U0126 for EKAR [17]). Second is the use of a dead reporter. The latter must be mandatory for any FRET-based enzyme reporter. A dead-reporter can be built upon a mutation that replaces, for example, a phosphorylable residue by another one, which cannot be phosphorylated. Thereby, the conformational change of the biosensor is never achieved, and the FRET changes shall be minimal, due to intrinsic flexibility of the structure, either in relaxed form or in a conformation with the fluorophores in close neighborhood. In case of KAR, dead reporter can be built, where the phosphorylable threonine of the phosphorylable peptide is substituted by an alanine. Thus, a control "baseline" can be monitored in these conditions (PKA [15–17], Erk [17]).

Though time-consuming, these steps of artifacts controls and intrinsic properties characterization of sensors are mandatory for proper analysis of KAR spatiotemporal profiles (**Figure 4**).

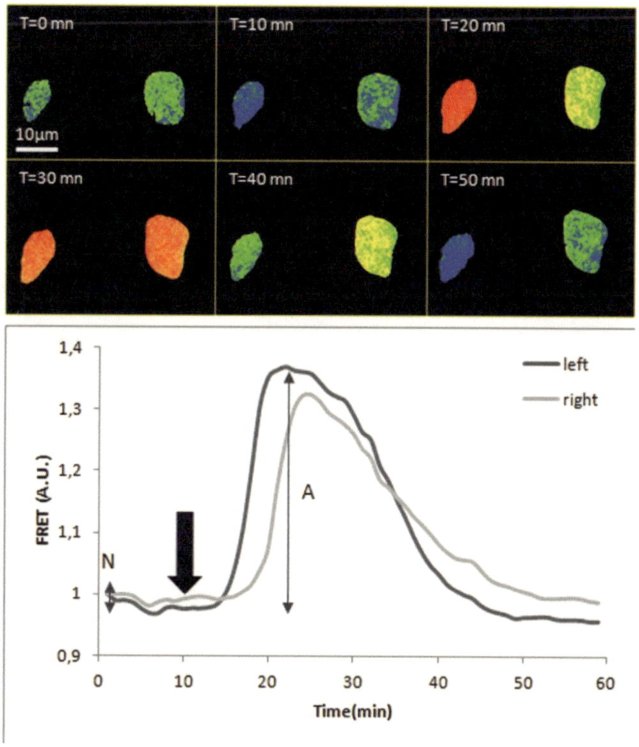

Figure 4. Time-lapse FRET measurement applied on MCF-7 cells expressing EKAR biosensor after EGF activation of the ERK pathway at 10 mn. The upper panel corresponds to FRET level color-coded from dark grey (low activity) to white (high activity). The bottom graph corresponds to the mean FRET measurement of both cells with N the biological "noise" and "A" the maximum amplitude achieved after induction. This state-of-the-art experiment illustrates the advantages of cell by cell analysis. Indeed, even two cells treated exactly in the same way can behave differently upon network activation. In this case, the maximum amplitude, the time needed to reach maximum activation and the duration before returning to the basal activity are different. Averaging these behaviors upon a large amount of cells can smooth or mask the individual response to stimuli and make it difficult to dissect regulatory networks.

5. A dynamic and flexible tool

Among the FRET-based biosensors, several categories exist and might have an impact on data interpretation. Especially, the change in FRET level can be due to either a configuration change or a cleavage of the sensor. In the first case, the sensor will be reversible as it is the case for most kinase activity reporters. Thus, the sensor will not monitor the kinase activity, but the balance between the kinase and its phosphatase counterpart. Cleavage-based reporters will have an irreversible response. In this case, the cumulative effect of the enzyme will be measured. Both behaviors are represented in **Figure 5**. In **Figure 5A**, a cyclic alternation of kinase and phosphatase

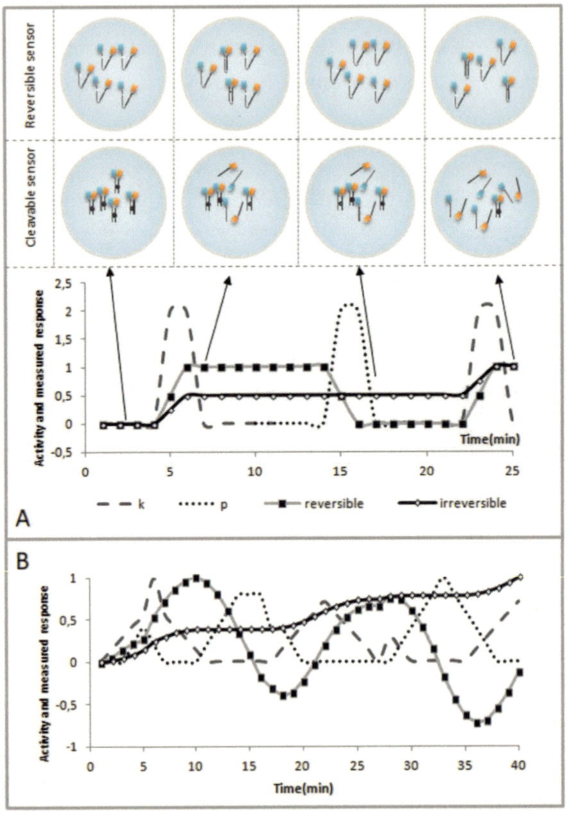

Figure 5. Illustration of sensor response to the balance between a kinase (k) and a phosphatase (p). (A) Sequential activation of a kinase and its phosphatase counterpart and associate response measured with either a reversible or an irreversible sensor. Upper panel: scheme representing both biosensors behavior after each activation step. Bottom panel: Associated activity and measured response. (B): Illustration of a more complex kinase/phosphatase oscillatory behavior with both sequential and simultaneous activation with different amplitudes and duration of activation. Irreversible sensors present a smooth response to kinase activity until cleavage of all available sensors. Reversible sensors are impacted by both kinase and phosphatase. While it offers a more realistic view of regulatory nodes, one shall keep in mind for interpretation that (i) the measure depends on the global state of the sensor. Kinase activation after a strong phosphatase period will take some time to change KAR conformation and thus to restore a positive response (T = 37 min). Thus, interpretation of time-lapse measurements is way easier than single acquisition. (ii) No difference can be made between no activity and a balance between kinase and phosphatase. Both will result in a constant behavior of the sensor (T = 18 min). (iii) An increase in the phosphatase activity can also result in activity measurements below the equilibrium value (T = 15 min).

action and associated biosensor response is depicted. While both behave in a similar manner upon the first kinase action, measurements diverge after the first phosphatase effect. Indeed, reversible sensors will then return to their basal level where the irreversible sensor will not be altered. Thus, while the second kinase activation will induce the same increase for both sensors, the final level will be different due to the cumulative effect observed for the irreversible version. More complex behavior is illustrated in **Figure 5B**.

From these simple schemes, it seems obvious that dissecting a node regulated by a kinase will be way easier with reversible sensors. Nevertheless, one should keep in mind that despite the name of sensors like KAR, reversibility mirrors the equilibrium of two enzymes. Thus, the measure corresponds to the kinase/phosphatase balance and biological interpretation should be made accordingly.

6. Amenability of FRET-based biosensors for high throughput

Perspectives are on different battleground for KAR use: (1) detection on environment or within living organisms and/or (2) untangling the host-pathogen interaction and the hijacking of host metabolism and signaling pathways (either to benefit from them or to mask host presence). Requested tools have therefore to be chosen accordingly to the purpose and to face the demand for high-throughput strategies or to face the complexity of molecular interactions within living organisms.

Energy transfer biosensors' sensitivity has been increased by the numerous multidisciplinary advances in the fields of photophysics, instrumentation and even nanomaterials. Above-mentioned advantages of KAR have thus made these tools amenable for high throughput [61] and led the kinase sensors to be cited as best biosensors in physiology [62].

Abbreviations

AKAR	Protein kinase A activity reporter
AktAR	Akt activity reporter
AMPK	AMP-activated protein kinase
AMPKAR	AMP-activated protein kinase activity reporter
ATM	Ataxia Telangiectasia mutated
ATOMIC	ATM observation method in cell
BKAR	B kinase activity reporter
cAMP	Cyclic adenosine monophosphate
Cdk1	Cyclin dependent kinase 1
EAS	ERK activity sensors

EGF	Epidermal growth factor
EGFR	Epidermal growth factor receptor
EKAR	Extracellular signal regulated kinase activity reporter
Epac	Exchange proteins activated by cAMP
Erk	Extracellular regulated kinase
FAK	Focal adhesion kinase
FRET	Förster Resonance Energy Transfer
GPCR	G protein coupled receptor
JNK	c-Jun N-terminal kinase
JNKAR	JNK activity reporter
KAR	Kinase activity reporters
MAPK	Mitogen activated protein kinase
MARK	Microtubule affinity regulating kinase
MK2	MAP kinase activated protein kinase 2
PAABD	Phosphoamino acid binding domain
PICCHU	Phosphorylation indicator of CrkII chimeric unit
PKA	Protein kinase A
PKB	Protein kinase B
PKC	Protein kinase C
Plk	Polo-kinase
RNAi	Ribonucleic acid interference
RSK	p90 Ribosomal S6 kinase
SAP3K	Stress-activated protein kinase

Author details

Corentin Spriet[1], Angelina Kasprowicz[1,2], Dave Trinel[1] and Jean-François Bodart[2*]

*Address all correspondence to: jean-francois.bodart@univ-lille1.fr

1 University Lille, TISBio, Lille, France

2 University Lille, Régulation des Signaux de Division Team, Lille, France

References

[1] McKerrow JH, Caffrey C, Kelly B, Loke P, Sajid M. Proteases in parasitic diseases. Annual Review of Pathology. 2006;**1**:497-536

[2] Robert-Gangneux F, Creuzet C, Dupouy-Camet J, Roisin MP. Mitogen activated protein kinases (MAPK) and *Toxoplasma gondii* host cell invasion. Annales Pharmaceutiques Françaises. 2001;**59**(5):297-304

[3] Soares-Silva M, Diniz FF, Gomes GN, Bahia D. The mitogen-activated protein kinase (MAPK) pathway: Role in immune evasion by Trypanosomatids. Frontiers in microbiology. 2016;**7**:183. DOI: 10.3389/fmicb.2016.00183

[4] Webb AJ, Kelwick R, Doenhoff MJ, Kylilis N, MacDonald JT, Wen KY, McKeown C, Baldwin G, Ellis T, Jensen K, Freemont PS. A protease-based biosensor for thedetection of schistosome cercariae. Scientific Reports. 2016;**6**:24725. DOI: 10.1038/srep24725

[5] Turner APF. Biosensors: Sense and sensibility. Chemical Society Reviews. 2013;**42**:3184

[6] Yoo EH, Lee SY. Glucose biosensors: An overview of use in clinical practice. Sensors (Basel). 2010;**10**(5):4558-4576. DOI: 10.3390/s100504558. Epub May 4, 2010. Review. PubMed PMID: 22399892; PubMed Central PMCID: PMC3292132

[7] Arshak K, Velusamy V, Korostynska O, Oliwa-Stasiak K, Adley C. Conducting polymers and their applications to biosensors: Emphasizing on foodborne pathogen detection. IEEE Sensors Journal. 2010;**9**(12):1942-1951

[8] Campbell K, Rawn DF, Niedzwiadek B, Elliott CT. Paralytic shellfish poisoning (PSP) toxin binders for optical biosensor technology: Problems and possibilities for the future: A review. Food Additives & Contaminants. Part A, Chemistry, Analysis, Control, Exposure & Risk Assessment. 2011;**28**(6):711-725. DOI: 10.1080/19440049.2010.531198

[9] Liu C, Li H, Jiang L, Luo X and Cai X. Electrochemical biosensors for the determination of glutamate pyravate transaminase and creatine kinase. International Journal of Nanoscience, 2006;**05**(06):865-870

[10] Herbst KJ, Allen MD, Zhang J. Luminescent kinase activity biosensors based on a versatile bimolecular switch. Journal of the American Chemical Society. 2011;**133**(15):5676-5679

[11] Van TN, Pellerano M, Lykaso S, Morris MC. Fluorescent protein biosensor for probing CDK/cyclin activity in vitro and in living cells. Chembiochem. 2014;**15**(15):2298-2305

[12] Yin H, Sun B, Dong L, Li B, Zhou Y, Ai S. A signal "on" photoelectrochemical biosensor for assay of protein kinase activity and its inhibitor based on graphite-like carbon nitride, Phos-tag and alkaline phosphatase. Biosensors & Bioelectronics. 2015;**64**:462-468

[13] Cui W, Parker LL. A time-resolved luminescence biosensor assay for anaplastic lymphoma kinase (ALK) activity. Chemical Communications. 2015;**51**(2):362-365

[14] Vidic J, Manzano M, Chang CM, Jaffrezic-Renault N. Advanced biosensors for detection of pathogens related to livestock and poultry. Veterinary Research. Feb 21, 2017;**48**(1):11. DOI: 10.1186/s13567-017-0418-5

[15] Vandame P, Spriet C, Trinel D, Gelaude A, Caillau K, Bompard C, Biondi E, Bodart JF. The spatio-temporal dynamics of PKA activity profile during mitosis and its correlation to chromosome segregation. Cell Cycle. 2014;**13**(20):3232-3240. DOI: 10.4161/15384101.2014.950907

[16] Vandame P, Sipieter F, Spriet C, Leray A, Vincent P, Trinel D, Bodart JF, Riquet FB, Héliot L. From FRET imaging to practical methodology for kinase activity sensing in living cells. Progress in Molecular Biology and Translational Science. 2013;**113**:145-216. DOI: 10.1016/B978-0-12-386932-6.00005-3

[17] Vandame P et al. Optimization of ERK activity biosensors for both ratiometric and lifetime FRET measurements. Sensors (Basel). 2013;**14**:1140-1115

[18] Ting AY, Kain KH, Klemke RL, Tsien RY. Genetically encoded fluorescent reporters of protein tyrosine kinase activities in living cells. Proceedings of the National Academy of Sciences of the United States of America. 2001;**98**(26):15003-15008

[19] Kurokawa K, Mochizuki N, Ohba Y, Mizuno H, Miyawaki A, Matsuda MA. Pair of fluorescent resonance energy transfer-based probes for tyrosine phosphorylation of the CrkII adaptor protein in vivo. The Journal of Biological Chemistry. 2001;**276**(33):31305-31310

[20] Gao X, Zhang J. Spatiotemporal analysis of differential Akt regulation in plasma membrane microdomains. Molecular Biology of the Cell. 2008;**19**(10):4366-4373. DOI: 10.1091/mbc.E08-05-0449

[21] Sato M, Umezawa Y. Imaging protein phosphorylation by fluorescence in single living cells. Methods. 2004;**32**(4):451-455

[22] Yoshizaki H, Aoki K, Nakamura T, Matsuda M. Regulation of RalA GTPase by phosphatidylinositol 3-kinase as visualized by FRET probes. Biochemical Society Transactions. 2006;**34**(Pt 5):851-854

[23] Kunkel MT, Ni Q, Tsien RY, Zhang J, Newton AC. Spatio-temporal dynamics of protein kinase B/Akt signaling revealed by a genetically encoded fluorescent reporter. The Journal of Biological Chemistry. 2005;**280**(7):5581-5587

[24] Calleja V, Alcor D, Laguerre M, Park J, Vojnovic B, Hemmings BA, Downward J, Parker PJ, Larijani B. Intramolecular and intermolecular interactions of protein kinase B define its activation in vivo. PLoS Biology. 2007;**5**(4):e95

[25] Ananthanarayanan B, Fosbrink M, Rahdar M, Zhang J. Live-cell molecular analysis of Akt activation reveals roles for activation loop phosphorylation. The Journal of Biological Chemistry. 2007;**282**(50):36634-36641

[26] Tsou P, Zheng B, Hsu CH, Sasaki AT, Cantley LC. A fluorescent reporter of AMPK activity and cellular energy stress. Cell Metabolism. 2011;**13**(4):476-486. DOI: 10.1016/j.cmet.2011.03.006

[27] Chu Y, Yao PY, Wang W, Wang D, Wang Z, Zhang L, Huang Y, Ke Y, Ding X, Yao X. Aurora B kinase activation requires survivin priming phosphorylation by PLK1. Journal of Molecular Cell Biology. 2011;**3**(4):260-267. DOI: 10.1093/jmcb/mjq037

[28] Johnson SA, You Z, Hunter T, Monitoring ATM. Kinase activity in living cells. DNA Repair (Amst). 2007;**6**(9):1277-1284

[29] Gavet O, Pines J. Activation of cyclin B1-Cdk1 synchronizes events in the nucleus and the cytoplasm at mitosis. The Journal of Cell Biology. 2010;**189**(2):247-259. DOI: 10.1083/jcb.200909144

[30] Offterdinger M, Georget V, Girod A, Bastiaens PI. Imaging phosphorylation dynamics of the epidermal growth factor receptor. The Journal of Biological Chemistry. 2004;**279**(35): 36972-36981

[31] Harvey CD, Ehrhardt AG, Cellurale C, Zhong H, Yasuda R, Davis RJ, Svoboda K. A genetically encoded fluorescent sensor of ERK activity. Proceedings of the National Academy of Sciences of the United States of America. 2008;**105**(49):19264-19269. DOI: 10.1073/pnas.0804598105

[32] Green HM, Alberola-Ila J. Development of ERK activity sensor, an in vitro, FRET-based sensor of extracellular regulated kinase activity. BMC Chemical Biology. 2005;**5**:1

[33] Fujioka A, Terai K, Itoh RE, Aoki K, Nakamura T, Kuroda S, Nishida E, Matsuda M. Dynamics of the Ras/ERK MAPK cascade as monitored by fluorescent probes. Journal of Biological Chemistry. 2006;**281**(13):8917-8926

[34] Seong J, Ouyang M, Kim T, Sun J, Wen PC, Lu S, Zhuo Y, Llewellyn NM, Schlaepfer DD, Guan JL, Chien S, Wang Y. Detection of focal adhesion kinase activation at membrane microdomains by fluorescence resonance energy transfer. Nature Communications. 2011;**2**:406. DOI: 10.1038/ncomms1414

[35] Ding SY, Nkobena A, Kraft CA, Markwardt ML, Rizzo MA. Glucagon-like peptide 1 stimulates post-translational activation of glucokinase in pancreatic beta cells. The Journal of Biological Chemistry. 2011;**286**(19):16768-16774. DOI: 10.1074/jbc.M110.192799

[36] Lin CW, Ting AY. A genetically encoded fluorescent reporter of histone phosphorylation in living cells. Angewandte Chemie International Edition (in English). 2004;**43**(22):2940-2943

[37] Fosbrink M, Aye-Han NN, Cheong R, Levchenko A, Zhang J. Visualization of JNK activity dynamics with a genetically encoded fluorescent biosensor. Proceedings of the National Academy of Sciences of the United States of America. Mar 23, 2010;**107**(12):5459-5464. DOI: 10.1073/pnas.0909671107

[38] Neininger A, Thielemann H, Gaestel M. FRET-based detection of different conformations of MK2. EMBO Reports. 2001;**2**(8):703-708

[39] Timm T, von Kries JP, Li X, Zempel H, Mandelkow E, Mandelkow EM. Microtubule affinity regulating kinase activity in living neurons was examined by a genetically encoded fluorescence resonance energy transfer/fluorescence lifetime imaging-based

biosensor: Inhibitors with therapeutic potential. The Journal of Biological Chemistry. 2011;**286**(48):41711-41722. DOI: 10.1074/jbc.M111.257865

[40] Macůrek L, Lindqvist A, Lim D, Lampson MA, Klompmaker R, Freire R, Clouin C, Taylor SS, Yaffe MB, Medema RH. Polo-like kinase-1 is activated by aurora a to promote checkpoint recovery. Nature. 2008;**455**(7209):119-123. DOI: 10.1038/nature07185

[41] Zhang L, Lee KC, Bhojani MS, Khan AP, Shilman A, Holland EC, Ross BD, Rehemtulla A. Molecular imaging of Akt kinase activity. Nature Medicine. 2007;**13**(9):1114-1119

[42] Nagai Y, Miyazaki M, Aoki R, Zama T, Inouye S, Hirose K, Iino M, Hagiwara MA. Fluorescent indicator for visualizing cAMP-induced phosphorylation in vivo. Nature Biotechnology. 2000;**18**(3):313-316

[43] Violin JD, Zhang J, Tsien RY, Newton ACA. Genetically encoded fluorescent reporter reveals oscillatory phosphorylation by protein kinase C. The Journal of Cell Biology. 2003;**161**(5):899-909

[44] Komatsu N, Aoki K, Yamada M, Yukinaga H, Fujita Y, Kamioka Y, Matsuda M. Development of an optimized backbone of FRET biosensors for kinases and GTPases. Molecular Biology of the Cell. 2011;**22**(23):4647-4656. DOI: 10.1091/mbc.E11-01-0072

[45] Tomida T, Takekawa M, O'Grady P, Saito H. Stimulus-specific distinctions in spatial and temporal dynamics of stress-activated protein kinase kinase kinases revealed by a fluorescence resonance energy transfer biosensor. Molecular and Cellular Biology. 2009;**29**(22): 6117-6127. DOI: 10.1128/MCB.00571-09

[46] Shannon P, Markiel A, Ozier O, Baliga NS, Wang JT, Ramage D, Amin N, Schwikowski B, Ideker T. Cytoscape: A software environment for integrated models of biomolecular interaction networks. Genome Research. 2003;**13**(11):2498-2504

[47] Krachler AM, Woolery AR, Orth K. Manipulation of kinase signaling by bacterial pathogens. Journal of Cell Biology. Dec 26, 2011;**195**(7):1083-1092. DOI: 10.1083/jcb.201107132

[48] Bodart JF, Chopra A, Liang X, Duesbery N, Anthrax MEK. cancer. Cell Cycle. 2002;**1**(1): 10-15

[49] Duesbery NS, Vande Woude GF. Anthrax lethal factor causes proteolytic inactivation of mitogen-activated protein kinase kinase. Journal of Applied Microbiology. 1999;**87**(2): 289-293

[50] Roach SK, Schorey JS. Differential regulation of the mitogen-activated protein kinases by pathogenic and nonpathogenic mycobacteria. Infection and Immunity. 2002;**70**(6):3040-3052

[51] Trosky JE, Li Y, Mukherjee S, Keitany G, Ball H, Orth K. VopA inhibits ATP binding by acetylating the catalytic loop of MAPK kinases. Journal of Biological Chemistry. 2007;**282**(47): 34299-34305

[52] Cthuluunbaatar U, Roller R, Mohr I. Suppression of extracellular signal-regulated kinase activity in herpes simplex virus 1-infected cells by the Us3 protein kinase. Journal of Virology. 2012;**86**(15):7771-7776. DOI: 10.1128/JVI.00622-12

[53] Mukherjee S, Keitany G, Li Y, Wang Y, Ball HL, Goldsmith EJ, Orth K. Yersinia YopJ acetylates and inhibits kinase activation by blocking phosphorylation. Science. May 26, 2006;**312**(5777):1211-1214

[54] Kim Y, Lee C. Extracellular signal-regulated kinase (ERK) activation is required for porcine epidemic diarrhea virus replication. Virology. 2015;**484**:181-193. DOI: 10.1016/j.virol.2015.06.007

[55] Yang X, Gabuzda D. Regulation of human immunodeficiency virus type 1 infectivity by the ERK mitogen-activated protein kinase signaling pathway. Journal of Virology. 1999;**73**(4):3460-3466

[56] Tripathi S, Pohl MO, Zhou Y, Rodriguez-Frandsen A, Wang G, Stein DA, Moulton HM, DeJesus P, Che J, Mulder LC, Yángüez E, Andenmatten D, Pache L, Manicassamy B, Albrecht RA, Gonzalez MG, Nguyen Q, Brass A, Elledge S, White M, Shapira S, Hacohen N, Karlas A, Meyer TF, Shales M, Gatorano A, Johnson JR, Jang G, Johnson T, Verschueren E, Sanders D, Krogan N, Shaw M, König R, Stertz S, García-Sastre A, Chanda SK. Meta- and orthogonal integration of influenza "OMICs" data defines a role for UBR4 in virus budding. Cell Host & Microbe. 2015;**18**(6):723-735. DOI: 10.1016/j.chom.2015.11.002

[57] Pohl MO, von Recum-Knepper J, Rodriguez-Frandsen A, Lanz C, Yángüez E, Soonthornvacharin S, Wolff T, Chanda SK, Stertz S. Identification of Polo-like kinases as potential novel drug targets for influenza A virus. Scientific Reports 2017;**7**(1):8629. DOI: 10.1038/s41598-017-08942-7

[58] Pouvreau S. Spatiotemporal mapping of PKA activity using biosensors. Cell Cycle. 2015;**14**(4):471. DOI: 10.1080/15384101.2015.1006555

[59] Kunkel MT, Newton AC. Spatiotemporal dynamics of kinase Signaling visualized by targeted reporters. Current Protocols in Chemical Biology. 2009;**1**(1):17-18

[60] Gavet O, Pines J. Progressive activation of CyclinB1-Cdk1 coordinates entry to mitosis. Developmental Cell. 2010;**18**(4):533-543. DOI: 10.1016/j.devcel.2010.02.013

[61] Rogers MS, Cryan LM, Habeshian KA, Bazinet L, Caldwell TP, Ackroyd PC, Christensen KA. A FRET-based high throughput screening assay to identify inhibitors of anthrax protective antigen binding to capillary morphogenesis gene 2 protein. PLoS One. 2012;**7**(6):e39911. DOI: 10.1371/journal.pone.0039911

[62] Oldach L, Zhang J. Genetically encoded fluorescent biosensors for live-cell visualization of protein phosphorylation. Chemistry & Biology. 2014;**21**:186-197. DOI: 10.1016/j.chembiol.2013.12.012